Psychopharmacology: Impact on Clinical Psychiatry

Donald W. Morgan, M.D., D.M.Sc.
Department of Neuropsychiatry and Behavioral Science
Professor and Vice Chairman
School of Medicine
University of South Carolina
Columbia, South Carolina

FIRST EDITION

Ishiyaku EuroAmerica, Inc.
St Louis • Tokyo • 1985

Ishiyaku EuroAmerica, Inc.

Book Edited By: Donald W. Morgan, M.D., D.M.Sc.

Index By: David Asher

Ishiyaku EuroAmerica, Inc.
11559 Rock Island Court, St. Louis, Missouri 63043

Library of Congress Catalogue Card Number 85-060909

Morgan, Donald W.
    Psychopharmacology: Impact on Clinical Psychiatry

ISBN 0-912791-06-3

Ishiyaku EuroAmerica, Inc.
St. Louis • Tokyo

Composition and design: Graphic World, Inc., St. Louis, Missouri
Printed in the United States of America

Contributors

LOWELL T. ANDERSON, Department of Psychiatry, New York University School of Medicine, New York, New York, U.S.A.

FRANK J. AYD, Jr., Baltimore, Maryland, U.S.A.

THOMAS A. BAN, Vanderbilt University and Tennessee Neuropsychiatric Institute, Nashville, Tennessee, U.S.A.

ROBERT H. BELMAKER, Jerusalem Mental Health Center—Ezrath Nashim, Jerusalem, Israel.

MAGDA CAMPBELL, Department of Psychiatry, New York University School of Medicine, New York, New York, U.S.A.

SHELLA CHAZAN, Jerusalem Mental Health Center—Ezrath Nashim, Jerusalem, Israel.

STEPHEN I. DEUTSCH, Department of Psychiatry, New York University School of Medicine, New York, New York, U.S.A.

DAVID DE WIED, Rudolf Magnus Institute of Pharmacology, Medical Faculty, University of Utrecht, Utrecht, The Netherlands.

EARL DICK, Psychiatry Service, St. Louis Veterans Administration Medical Center, St. Louis, Missouri, U.S.A.

JACQUES EISENBERG, Jerusalem Mental Health Center—Ezrath Nashim, Jerusalem, Israel.

RICHARD P. EBSTEIN, Jerusalem Mental Health Center—Ezrath Nashim, Jerusalem, Israel.

VACLAV FILIP, Department of Psychiatry, Medical Faculty, University of Utrecht, Utrecht, The Netherlands; and Department of Psychiatry, University of Prague, Prague, The Netherlands.

MARK S. GOLD, Fair Oaks Hospital, Summit, New Jersey, U.S.A.

SOLOMON C. GOLDBERG, Department of Psychiatry, Medical College of Virginia, Richmond, Virginia, U.S.A.

KENNETH E. GOOLSBY, William S. Hall Psychiatric Institute, Columbia, South Carolina, U.S.A.

WAYNE GREEN, Department of Psychiatry, New York University School of Medicine, New York, New York, U.S.A.

DAVID GREENBERG, Jerusalem Mental Health Center—Ezrath Nashim, Jerusalem, Israel.

LAWRENCE GREENBERG, Jerusalem Mental Health Center—Ezrath Nashim, Jerusalem, Israel.

WILLIAM GUY, Vanderbilt University and Tennessee Neuropsychiatric Institute, Nashville, Tennessee, U.S.A.

RAHEL HAMBURGER-BAR, Jerusalem Mental Health Center—Ezrath Nashim, Jerusalem, Israel.

EHUD KLEIN, Jerusalem Mental Health Center—Ezrath Nashim, Jerusalem, Israel.

HEINZ E. LEHMANN, Department of Psychiatry, McGill University, Montreal, Quebec, Canada.

BATSHEVA MANDEL, Jerusalem Mental Health Center—Ezrath Nashim, Jerusalem, Israel.

J. MENDLEWICZ, Department of Psychiatry, Erasme Hospital, University Clinics of Brussels, Free University of Brussels, Brussels, Belgium.

JOHN H. MONTI, Department of Psychiatry and The Neurosciences Program, University of Alabama, Birmingham, Alabama, U.S.A.

DONALD W. MORGAN, William S. Hall Psychiatric Institute and
Department of Neuropsychiatry and Behavioral Science,
University of South Carolina School of Medicine, Columbia, South
Carolina, U.S.A.

ROBERT J. PARY, William S. Hall Psychiatric Institute and
Department of Neuropsychiatry and Behavioral Science,
University of South Carolina School of Medicine, Columbia, South
Carolina, U.S.A.

ANGEL RODRIGUEZ, William S. Hall Psychiatric Institute, Columbia,
South Carolina, U.S.A.

YEHUDA SHAPIRA, Jerusalem Mental Health Center—Ezrath
Nashim, Jerusalem, Israel.

ELSA SHAPIRO, Jerusalem Mental Health Center—Ezrath Nashim,
Jerusalem, Israel.

JOHN R. SMYTHIES, Department of Psychiatry and The
Neurosciences Program, University of Alabama, Birmingham,
Alabama, U.S.A.

LELLAND C. TOLBERT, Department of Psychiatry and The
Neurosciences Program, University of Alabama, Birmingham,
Alabama, U.S.A.

DANIEL P. VAN KAMMEN, Western Psychiatric Institute and Clinic,
University of Pittsburgh, and Psychiatry Service, Veterans
Administration Medical Center, Pittsburgh, Pennsylvania, U.S.A.

WELMOET B. VAN KAMMEN, Western Psychiatric Institute and
Clinic, University of Pittsburgh, and Psychiatry Service, Veterans
Administration Medical Center, Pittsburgh, Pennsylvania, U.S.A.

JAN M. VAN REE, Rudolf Magnus Institute of Pharmacology,
University of Utrecht, Utrecht, The Netherlands.

KARL VEREBEY, State University of New York Downstate Medical
School, Brooklyn, New York.

FRANS H. M. VERHEY, Department of Psychiatry, Medical Faculty,
University of Maastricht, Maastricht, The Netherlands.

WIM M. A. VERHOEVEN, Department of Psychiatry, Medical Faculty, University of Utrecht, Utrecht, The Netherlands.

WILLIAM H. WILSON, Vanderbilt University and Tennessee Neuropsychiatric Institute, Nashville, Tennessee, U.S.A.

JOSEPH ZOHAR, Jerusalem Mental Health Center—Ezrath Nashim, Jerusalem, Israel.

Dedication

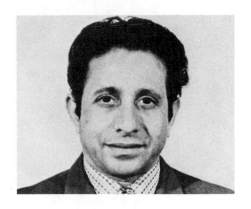

This book is dedicated to the memory of Nandkumar S. Shah, Ph.D. Doctor Shah died suddenly while working in his laboratory on May 23, 1983. The original outline of this book, as well as commitment from several contributors, had been completed at the time of his death. Doctor Shah was the driving force behind the symposium, "Advances in Psychopharmacology Research: Impact on Clinical Psychiatry," held at the William S. Hall Psychiatric Institute on October 25, 1982, which served as the core of this edition.

Doctor Shah was born in Nandurbar, India, in 1928. He received his B.S. and M.S. (biochemistry) from Poona University, India. In 1961, Doctor Shah came to the United States and continued his studies at the College of Medicine, University of Florida in Gainsville, Florida. After obtaining his Ph.D. in pharmacology at the University of Florida in 1965, he joined the staff at the Thudichum Psychiatric Research Laboratory, Galesburg, Illinois, and worked with Dr. Harold Himwich. His association with Doctor Himwich significantly influenced his reserach commitments in areas of neurochemical mechanisms in schizophrenia and in psychopharmacology.

From 1970 until the time of his death, Doctor Shah directed the Ensor Research Laboratory of the William S. Hall Psychiatric Institute. In 1978, he was appointed Research Professor, Department of Neuropsychiatry and Behavioral Science, University of South Carolina School of Medicine. In this position, he taught medical students, graduate students and psychiatry residents.

Doctor Shah was a dedicated teacher, researcher and colleague who is greatly missed.

Contents

Abbreviations

ABO—ABO blood types
Ach—acetylcholine
ACTH—adrenocorticotrophic hormone
ADD—attention deficit disorder
ADH—antidiuretic hormone
Adomet—5-adenosylmethionine
AER—average evoked response
AIRS—Amphetamine Interview Rating Scale
ATP—adenosine triphosphate
BE—or βE—beta endorphin
β-LPH—β-lipotropin
B.I.D.—twice daily
BPRS—Brief Psychiatric Rating Scale
BUN—blood urea nitrogen
COMT—catechol-o-methyltransferase
CBC—complete blood count
CCK—cholecystokinine
CGI—Clinical Global Impressions Rating Scale
CPRS—Children's Psychiatric Rating Scale
CPZ—chlorpromazine
CRF—corticotropin releasing factor
CSF—cerebral spinal fluid
CSF MHPG—cerebral spinal fluid methyoxy-hydroxy-phenyl-glycol
CT—computerized tomography
cyclic AMP or (c-AMP)—cyclic adenosine monophosphate
DA—dopamine
DA$_2$ receptor—dopamine A$_2$ receptors
DβH—dopamine-β-hydroxylase
DDAVP—1-desamino-8-D-arginine vasopressin
DEβE—des-enkephalin-β-endorphin
DGLA—dihomo-gamma-linolenic acid

DMI—desmethylimipramine
DMT—dimethyltryptamine
DNA—deoxyribonucleic acid
DTβE—des-tyr^1-β-endorphin
DQ—Gesell Language Developmental Quotients
DSM-III—Diagnostic and Statistical Manual, 3rd Edition
DST—dexamethasone suppression test
E—epinephrine
ECT or EST—electroconvulsive therapy
EEG—electroencephalogram
EKG or ECG—electrocardiogram
FAD—flavin adenine dinucleotide
FDA (F.D.A.)—Federal Drug Administration
5-HIAA—5-hydroxy indole acetic acid
5-HT—5-hydroxytryptamine (serotonin)
FB—free base
FMN—flavin mononucleotide
F.P.D.D.—familial pure depressive disease
FSH—follicle stimulating hormone
GABA—gamma-aminobutyric acid
G.C.—gas chromatography
GC/MS—gas chromatography/mass spectrometric
GH—growth hormone
GI—gastrointestinal
Ham-A—Hamilton Rating Scale for Anxiety
HAM-D—Hamilton Rating Scale for Depression
HLA—histocompatibility antigen
HPLC—high pressure liquid chromatography

HSCL—Hopkins Symptom Checklist
HVA—homvanillic acid
ICD-9—International Classification of Diseases, 9th Edition
INH—isonicotinic acid hydrozide
IRB—Institutional Review Boards
LH—luteinizing hormone
LRH—luteinizing-releasing hormone
LSD—D-lysergic acid diethylamide
LVP—lysine vasopressin
MAO—mono amine oxydase
MAOI—mono amine oxydase inhibitor
MAT—methionine adenosyltransferase
MBD—minimal brain dysfunction
MDD—major depressive disorder
MHPG—methoxy-hydroxy-phenyl-glycol
MSH—melano stimulating hormone
NAD—nicotinamide adenine dinucleotide
NADP—nicotinamide adenine dinucleotide
NA—sodium ion
NE—norepinephrine
NIMH—National Institute of Mental Health
NOSIE—Nurse's Observation Scale for Inpatient Evaluation
6-OCHS—6-hydroxycorticosteroids
11-OHCS—11-hydroxycorticosteroids
OMB—o-methylbufotenin
PC—phosphatidylcholine (lecithin)
PDR—Physician's Desk Reference
PE—phosphatidyl-ethanolamine
PG—prostaglandin
PGE—prostaglandin endoperoxide
Pl—phosphatidylinositol

PMT—phospholipid methyltransferase
POMC—pro-opiomelanocortin system
POMS—Profile of Mood Status
PS—phosphatdyl-serine
PSE—Present State Exam
PSSS—Patient Symptom Specific Scale
Q.I.D.—four times daily
RIA—radioimmunoassay
RBC—red blood cell
RDC—Research Diagnostic Criteria
REM—rapid eye movement
REM-latency—time to onset of first period of rapid eye movement sleep
REM sleep—rapid eye movement stage of sleep
RRA—radioreceptorassay
SADS—Schedule for Affective Disorders and Schizophrenia
SCL-56—Lipman-Rickels Symptom Checklist
SGOT—serum glutamate oxaloacetic transaminase
SGPT—serum glutamate pyruvate transaminase
SPH—sphingomyelin
SHMT—serine hydroxymethyltransferase
T.I.D.—three times daily
TPP—thiamine pyrophosphate
TRH—thyrotropin hormone-releasing hormone
U.S. DHEW—United States Department of Health, Education and Welfare
VMA—vanillylmandelic acid
WISC—Wechsler Intelligence Scale for Children

CHAPTER 1

Psychopharmacology: Past and Present

Donald W. Morgan, M.D., D.M.Sc.

This book describes the impact of psychopharmacology upon the treatment of the mentally ill and presents current theories supported by research data concerning the possible etiology of certain mental illnesses.

Historically, society's treatment of the seriously mentally ill has been shaped by fear, misunderstanding, and prejudice. Such individuals have been seen as evil or possessed by demons; therefore, worthy of punishment and contempt. Just as the lepers were seen as unclean and sinful to be banished from society because their illness was proof of God's displeasure, the mentally ill have been neglected and isolated from society. Families have been confused, frustrated, and overwhelmed in attempting to care for their mentally ill relatives. The overtones of guilt and shame interfered with the families' attempt to cope with mental disease. The chronic relapsing course of these illnesses depletes the families' financial and emotional resources. Those seriously mentally ill without family support were left to wander in the streets; and if their behaviors were extremely bizarre or "threatening", they were confined in jails or institutions. Exactly how much society's treatment of the chronically mentally ill differs today from times past is open to debate (Talbott, 1979). As we understand the basic physiology of the central nervous system and isolate the pathologic processes responsible for the various mental disorders, perhaps more effective treatments will evolve.

Like leprosy, perhaps mental illness will gradually become less mysterious, and its victims accepted as having legitimate medical illness rather than being ostracized by society. Modern psychopharmacology holds out great hope for advancing the understanding and treatment of

1

psychopathology. This chapter will briefly review the progress of somatic treatments in modern psychiatry so as to highlight the advances made since 1952 that are described in the remaining chapters. As Professor Lehmann cautions in the concluding chapter of this book, clinical psychiatry must continue to treat the total patient in society. We must not become so biologically oriented that we neglect the psychological and social facets of mental illness.

For the purposes of this review, let us define the beginning of modern psychiatric treatment with Phillippe Pinel's freeing of the insane from their chains at Bicetre in the last decade of the 1700's. Pinel clearly saw the mentally ill as suffering from a medical illness and described them in a medical model. About the same time in America, Benjamin Rush, a signer of the Declaration of Independence, studied the mentally ill at the Pennsylvania Hospital in Philadelphia. While the therapeutic efficacy of Doctor Rush's blood letting and circulating swing are seen as improbable today, these were attempts to apply the then current understanding of physiology and pathophysiology to the treatment of the mentally ill. The psychopharmacology and neurosciences of today will be seen by future generations as crude and even grossly incorrect. Nevertheless, it is the application of psychopharmacology in the clinical setting that holds the greatest promise for the severely mentally disturbed.

The early 1800's saw the beginning of humanistic treatment for the mentally ill. Dorothea Dix led the fight to secure government aid for the mentally ill. State legislatures enacted laws and created asylums in which patients would be given shelter, food, protection, and respect. Certainly, Dorothea Dix had no way of predicting that the asylums she helped create would fall into such disrupt (Goffman, 1961). She could not have anticipated that the demand for services would so far outstrip the resources provided.

By the end of the 1800's, mental illness became a legitimate area of study within medicine, and great advances in the field of psychiatry were made. Emiel Kraeplain contributed his descriptions of symptoms and course of illnesses. Sigmund Freud was introducing his "talking therapies" and theories concerning personality development. Julius von Waggner-Jauregg's clinical observation that fever was associated with remission of neurosyphillis (or general paralysis of the insane as it was then called) led him to the experiment of inoculating patients with tertian malaria. The dramatic response to the unorthodox treatment won him a Nobel prize (Stevenson, 1953). It is interesting to contrast Doctor Belmaker and his associates' views as they discuss, in the third chapter of this book, the current restrictions placed upon researchers. They cite the overrestriction of psychopharmacologic research by review boards and governments which they believe to be a disservice to patients. What grant review board would, today, approve the proposal of Doctor von Waggner-Jauregg? Yet, he is the only psychiatrist to win the Nobel prize. It is, of course, true that the real victory over syphillis did not appear until the discovery of the effectiveness of penicillin. This one pharmacologic agent prevented or cured mental illness in a group of patients who fifty years earlier would have been "incurable." Should clinical psychopharmacology wait until there is a drug such as penicillin to treat the other major mental illnesses; or, like von Waggner-Jauregg, should we match clinical observations with the methods of treatment currently available?

Another disease which often affected mental patients was pellagra. Marked by the triad of diarrhea, dermatitis, and dementia, this illness arose in patients in mental institutions and added new patients to the institutions. In the early 1900's, an infective process was postulated as the cause of this disorder. Joseph Goldberger had a highly unusual theory based upon his clinical observations that this disease was due to dietary deficiencies (Rapport and Wright, 1952). Years of experimentation and observation convinced Goldberger that the absence of fresh animal components—milk, eggs, butter, lean meat, and an overbalance of carbohydrates in the diet were associated with the illness. In 1916, Goldberger and his associates experimentally produced pellagra in a group of volunteer convicts by restricting their diets over a nine-month period. This well-documented work was met with great resistance from those of the medical community who were convinced that there was an infectious cause for pellagra. It took many years before nicotinic acid was isolated and shown to be effective in the treatment of pellagra. With our current enthusiasm for synthetic pharmacologic agents in the treatment of mental illness, are we as the infectionist who could not accept the findings of Doctor Goldberger, overlooking the role of nutrition as postulated by those who promote orthomolecular psychiatry (Autry, 1975)? Perhaps there are subgroups of mentally ill who would respond more effectively or maintain their remission for longer periods if their nutritional needs were adequately met.

The use of convulsive therapies in the treatment of mental illness during the 1930's was a significant advance. Cerletti and Bini introduced the method of generating seizures in patients by applying electrical current. Many refinements in these techniques have occurred over the succeeding years. The basic biological understanding of how the generalized seizure activity aids in treating mental disorders and particularly the depressive disorders presently escapes our full understanding. A controversy rages over the use of this technique (Ayd, 1975). Notwithstanding, the years of clinical experience and the findings of the American Psychiatric Association Task Force, social, political and other factors combine to cause a marked decline in the use of this proven effective treatment. Perhaps, when the neuroscientists unravel the mysteries of the mental disorders, they will also understand electroconvulsive therapy (ECT). In the future, I hope a less emotional and more rational discussion of this treatment modality will occur.

It is a fact that prior to the use of rapid tranquilization and the use of the major neuroleptics, patients who felt themselves losing control would ask to be placed in continuous tubs and cold wet packs. Other agitated patients were involuntarily treated by these methods. Even though these treatments appear barbaric by current standards, these techniques did calm patients and reduce assaultive behavior. The effectiveness of neuroleptics has completely erradicated these treatments from psychiatry. Perhaps those who advocate the seriously agitated mentally ill patient's right to refuse neuroleptic treatment would be less adamant in their views if they had assisted in trying to control patients by these continuous tubs and wet cold packs (Sadoff, 1982). Fortunately for the patients, court decisions are permitting the use of enforced treatment given appropriate safeguards (Appelbaum, 1983).

Prior to 1950, psychopharmacology was limited to bromides, paraldehyde, chloralhydrate, and barbiturates. These compounds did have sedative quieting effects upon patients, but they had little or no effect upon their psychotic thinking processes and bizarre behavior. In addition, the dangers of bromism and potential habituation to barbiturates caused these medicines to be reserved for the treatment of acutely-agitated, markedly-disturbed patients.

The age of modern psychopharmacology began with the introduction of reserpine, a rauwolfia alkaloid. This drug was a derivative of a naturally occurring substance that had been used in India for a number of years in the treatment of the mentally ill. Reserpine demonstrated a true antipsychotic effect. It also had a marked effect on blood pressure, causing in some patients orthostetic hypertension; and after prolonged use, some patients became depressed. Currently, reserpine is used primarily for its antihypertensive actions.

Shortly after the introduction of reserpine, chlorpromazine, developed in France, was introduced into American medicine (Lehmann, 1954). Thorazine has become the standard against which other neuroleptics can be measured. While it has many side effects, including hypertension, dermatological, hemotological, and neurological, (including the dyskinesias, dystonias, and pseudo-Parkinsonisms and akathisias), its clear effect on the psychotic symptoms of patients greatly outweighed the difficulties of its side effects. For the first time, the active symptoms of schizophrenia, i.e., hallucinations, delusions, agitation could be brought under control without excessive sedation. This ability to control psychotic features markedly enhanced the ability to provide an overall milieu treatment for patients. Consequently, the length of hospital stay shortened. General hospitals were far more accepting of psychiatric patients and created small wards for the treatment of patients who would have previously been destined for years of hospitalization. A number of patients were able to be discharged from hospital. These patients who had spent many years on locked wards in and out of restraints and seclusion could now be safely returned to the community. It became clear that the patients' ability to remain out of the hospital required that they be maintained on a continuous dose of neuroleptic medication. Further, it became apparent that these patients, while not having active symptoms, continued to suffer from many of the negative symptoms of their illness which made it impossible for them to be self-sufficient. Since 1952, more pharmaceutical companies began to invest in programs of research, looking for more effective neuroleptic medications. Many drugs have been introduced. For some patients, long-acting depo neuroleptics provided on biweekly injections have been helpful in controlling symptoms. The potential role of neuroleptic blood levels in clinical practice and patient compliance is described in Chapter 9. Much needs to be understood about the basic processes of the central nervous system. Presently, the psychiatric community eagerly awaits the development of more specific neuroleptics which will have fewer side effects. As the neurosciences continue to provide a better understanding of the biological basis and genetic control of these processes, we may someday understand why certain patients apparently respond exceedingly well to one neuroleptic, yet refuse to take or do not respond to another. Doctor Mendlewicz addresses some of the possible genetic factors in Chapter 4 of this book.

Another major medical problem impacted by psychopharmacology is depression. Unlike the schizophrenias, depression tends to be episodic and self-limiting. Electroconvulsive treatments mentioned above have been specific in effective treatment for depression. This treatment may still be the most effective, safest modality for major depression. The introduction of tricyclic antidepressants and monoamineoxidase inhibitors in the treatment of depression greatly expanded the opportunity for treating depressed patients as outpatients. The major drawback of these medications is the time period which is required prior to their having any antidepressant effect. Research continues to identify compounds which will be more rapid in onset of action and safer. Many primary care physicians prescribe tricyclic antidepressants for symptoms of depression which are related to acute situational disturbances or chronic personality disorders. Some investigators express considerable doubt as to whether any observed effectiveness goes beyond the mild sedative effect of these compounds. We must be alert to the danger of prescribing large numbers of the tricyclic antipressants since depressed patients tend to ingest medications in suicidal attempts. The number of successful suicides by individuals using these compounds argues for more thorough evaluation and careful monitoring. Nevertheless, the ability to treat major depressions and prevent relapse has been a significant advance in medicine.

Another significant psychopharmacological advance has been the introduction of the benzodiazepines. These compounds are highly effective and safe when compared to most other medications which are used for the treatment of situational anxiety and alcohol withdrawal. Doctor Ayd, in Chapter 14, reviews the history of these compounds and introduces a new compound which may, in fact, enhance our ability to treat chronic anxiety without the potential of habituation. These benzodiazepines are the most widely prescribed medication. General practitioners, family practitioners, internists, and surgeons use these compounds with relative safety. Benzodiazepines are currently a favorite preoperative drug to allay anxiety and assist in the induction of anesthesia. The usefulness of these drugs in chronic anxiety states needs study. However, the central nervous system effects of this increased tolerance cannot be compared to the devastating effects of chronic barbiturate use or dangers of barbiturate withdrawal. The American Psychiatric Association has taken a formal stand that these medications not be used in the chronic treatment of alcoholism; nevertheless, benzodiazepines' effectiveness in the short-term treatment of acute alcoholism is unsurpassed.

The introduction of lithium for the treatment of manic-depressive illness in the late 1960's brought about an almost miraculous control of this illness in a significant proportion of patients afflicted by it. Cade had suggested the value of lithium in treating mania in 1949. Because of the cardiotoxicity which occurred when lithium was used as a salt substitute, there was a marked delay in the availability of this drug in the United States. However, due to the favorable mass media publicity provided and the marked effectiveness in some patients, the general population is today well aware of the beneficial effects of lithium. In fact, this particular drug has done a great service to the general field of psychiatry by demonstrating that some individuals can return to a normal and productive life if properly diagnosed and treated. The number of patients with the diagnosis of manic-depressive illness has risen. This is, in part, due to the introduction of lithium as an effective treatment. Furthermore, the international studies which drew attention to the affective component of illnesses (Cooper et al, 1972) made the diagnosis more frequent. Whether or not the individuals suffering from cyclothymic disorder are on a true continuum with the manic-depressive illness is currently unknown. However, certain individuals who do not meet the criteria for manic-depressions, but do have cyclothymic disorder, have a great leveling of their mood swings with the institution of lithium. A complete review of the pharmacology and clinical usefulness of lithium will be found in Chapter 12.

For the practicing general psychiatrist, the explosion of information available in the neurosciences is overwhelming. New knowledge is being continuously accumulated about the numbers of neurotransmitters, their actions, and specific target sites within the central nervous system which has brought the practice of psychiatry to the molecular level. Clearly, we are only beginning to understand the enormous complexity and marvelous sophistication of the central nervous system. The interdependence of the brain to the endocrine system, interaction between the environment and the endocrine system, as well as the control of the major bodily functions has been explicated most recently. Some of these basic neuroscience hypotheses are presented in the following chapters.

The increasing knowledge in the neurosciences has been accomplished by a renewed interest in descriptive psychiatry. As Doctor Goldberg elaborates in the second chapter, the *Diagnostic and Statistical Manual III* (DSM-III), with explicit criteria for the disorders, has been a major benefit to psychiatry. As with all changes in the nomenclature, there are controversies (Klerman et al, 1984). From the view of a practicing psychiatrist, however, the ability to specifically communicate with other colleagues based upon observable criteria has to be the major advance provided by DSM-III. However, even with the manual's better delineation of the mental disorders, we still have a heterogeneous group within the schizophrenias and affective disorders. The charges leveled that a phenomenological approach omits the dynamic understanding of the patient and his social situation are weak. In fact, the multiaxial approach permits the emphasis on the person's personality traits and takes into account the psychosocial functioning and environmental stresses related to the episode of illness. It is difficult to practice a holistic approach to patients in any branch of medicine. Psychiatry is no exception; the *Diagnostic and Statistical Manual III* enhances classification and maintains a holistic perspective.

The ability to treat large numbers of psychiatric patients, who have formally been relegated to inpatient stay for their major mental disorders, on an outpatient basis presents a significant challenge to medicine. The pros and cons of deinstitutionalization have been debated in the psychiatric literature. In fact, we cannot expect that because we have effective medications to control symptoms that all patients will be compliant and that patients will have a proper support system which will permit them to function outside of the hospital. Those who have treated a significant number of individuals suffering with diabetes will understand the close analogy between the provision of effective treatment and the utilization of that treatment by patients. This is also true for chronic illnesses such as hypertension and cardiovascular disease. We must be conservative in selecting information concerning the treatment of these disorders in order to institute the most effective outpatient treatment for the chronically mentally ill. The current relegation of chronic mental illness to the domain of state mental health agencies has not led to the creation of an efficient care delivery system. The general involvement of medicine, particularly family practitioners, in the deinstitutionalization movement will be the critical factor in medicine's meeting its obligation to these severely disabled individuals.

This book has drawn together basic information and presented it in a way which the practicing psychiatrist, family practitioner, and general practitioner can use in the treatment of a wide spectrum of mental disorders in adults and children. The problems of classification, ethical issues related to research, review of the current theories, presentation of the recent data, and information concerning drugs which have not yet been released are discussed.

REFERENCES

Appelbaum, P.S.: Refusing treatment: the uncertainty continues. *Hosp. and Community Psychiatry* 34:11-12, 1983.

Autry, J.H.: Workshop on orthomolecular treatment of schizophrenia: a report. *Schizophr. Bull.* 12:94-103, 1975.

Ayd, F.J.: The contemporary attack on ECT. *International Drug Therapy Newsletter* 10(1):2-4, 1975.

Cade, J.F.: Lithium salts in the treatment of psychotic excitement. *Med. J. Aust.* 36:349, 1949.

Cerletti, M. and Bini, L.: L'Electroshock. *Arch. Gen. Neurol., Psichiatri, Psicoanal.* 19:266, 1938.

Cooper, J.E., Kendell, R.E., Gurland, B.J., Sharpe, L., Copeland, J.R.M. and Simon, R.: Psychiatric Diagnosis in New York and London, Oxford University Press, London, 1972.

Goffman, E.: Asylums, Aldine Publishing Company, Chicago, IL, 1961.

Klerman, G.L., Vaillant, G.E., Spitzer, R.L. and Michels, R.: A debate on DSM III. *Am. J. Psychiatry* 141:539-553, 1984.

Lehmann, H.E. and Hanrahan, G.E.: Chlorpromazine: New inhibiting agent for psychomotor excitement and manic states. *A.M.A. Arch. Neurol. Psychiat.* 71:227-237, 1954.

Rapport, S. and Wright, H.: Great Adventures in Medicine, The Dial Press, New York, 1952, pp. 586-605.

Sadoff, R.L.: Legal Issues in the Case of Psychiatric Patients, Springer Publishing Company, New York, pp. 36-53, 1982.

Stevenson, L.G.: Nobel Prize Winners in Medicine and Physiology, Henry Shuman Inc., New York, 1953, pp. 125-129.

Talbott, J.A.: Deinstitutionalization: avoiding disasters of the past. *Hosp. Community Psychiatry* 30:621-624, 1979.

Task Force on Electroconvulsive Therapy. Electroconvulsive Therapy. American Psychiatric Association. *Task Force Report No. 14,* September 1978.

CHAPTER 2

The Impact of Prediction of Drug Response on Psychiatric Diagnosis

Solomon C. Goldberg, Ph.D.

INTRODUCTION

Psychiatric diagnosis has undergone an evolution in conception and practice in the past century. It has had different meanings at differnet times. It has suffered from inadequate description resulting in poor communication of the operational process of making a diagnosis. The model that was emulated because of its great success was that of medical disease; i.e., every disease has a knowable and discoverable etiological agent whether that agent is an infection, a nutritional deficiency, a deranged metabolism, or a lesion.

DIAGNOSIS AS ETIOLOGY

The model of conceptualizing diseases as categorical processes is seductively simple for the practitioner. It is far more difficult to deal with patients on the basis of *all* the biological, psychological, and social dynamics that may obtain. It would be much simpler if disorders behaved in the same way as, for example, pregnancy, a non-disease process. The etiological act of impregnation eventually results in very lawful and predictable biological consequences. Anyone observing these biological consequences in a woman can easily "make the diagnosis" that she is pregnant. In this sense diagnosis refers to etiology. Some infectious and nutritional diseases behave in the same way. In following the medical disease model, some students of psychiatric manifestations accept as an article of faith the reality of psychiatric disorders as categorical process entities. Unfortunately in psychiatry, etiological agents are all but unknown, so how can the study of psychiatric diagnosis ever succeed in identifying disease entities? The difficulty in doing so has not deterred

9

theoreticians from making inferences about etiological agents from an analysis of syndrome patterns. The simplest inference is made when comparing a group of mental patients with a normal control group with regard to mental and behavioral manifestations. The inference is made that the patients are afflicted by some as yet undefined etiologies. Although one may never know what these etiologies are, it seems safe to say that the patient group but not the controls has them. There might then be some speculation on the possible nature of the etiology. There might be further differentiation of the patient group into relatively homogeneous syndromes with the further inference of different etiologies for different syndromes. Something of this kind was done by Kraepelin when he broadly distinguished dementia praecox from depression. Without knowing the etiological agents for each, researchers and practitioners began to regard these as real diagnostic entities and that if we look long and hard enough, we will discover the etiological agents.

SYNDROMAL DIAGNOSIS

We have now used the term diagnosis in two ways. The first is as an etiological agent which gives rise to a series of manifestations including the phenomenological syndrome that is observed in the clinic or the laboratory. The second use of diagnosis is as a syndromal classification, and this is the primary method available to psychiatry. Although the inference is made that a syndrome is associated with a specific etiology, there may never be the opportunity to test the inference.

A syndrome may be defined as a relatively frequently occurring (more than chance) pattern of mental, physical, and behavioral abnormalities. If the pattern occurs more frequently than chance, it follows that the elements of the pattern hang together and are correlated with each other. Thus, in schizophrenia delusional patients are also more likely to hallucinate and in depression, patients with psychomotor retardation are more likely to show sleep disturbance. It is interesting that there are some combinations of symptoms which occur less frequently than by chance alone. The mentally ill seem not to be a random combination of symptoms. Some symptoms hang together as syndromes and seem to imply some kind of functional unity as yet undefined.

In Table 1 is a hypothetical illustration of two uncorrelated symptoms each of which is dichotomously scored as present-absent. The table shows four symptom combinations but under our definition, no combination qualifies as a syndrome because none is more frequently occurring than chance.

Suppose, however, that the two symptoms were modestly correlated as in Table 2.

Now we see that the symptom combination of hallucinations and

TABLE 1. Cross tabulation of two dichotomously scored and uncorrelated symptoms

	Delusions	
	Present	Absent
Depression		
Present	25	25
Absent	25	25

TABLE 2. Cross tabulation of two dichotomously scored correlated symptoms

	Delusions	
	Present	Absent
Hallucinations		
Present	40	10
Absent	10	40

TABLE 3. Cross tabulation of two scaled correlated symptoms

	Delusions		
	High	Medium	Low
Hallucinations			
High	18	11	5
Medium	10	11	10
Low	5	11	18

delusions is one which occurs at a greater frequency than chance. If symptoms are scaled rather than scored dichotomously, the cross tabulation appears a bit more complicated as in Table 3.

A recent paper by Spitzer and Williams (1982) tests Klein's concept of hysteroid-dysphoria on whether it satisfies the requirements of a syndrome; they find very low correlations between the symptom elements presumably entering this syndrome-diagnosis and conclude it is not a bonafide syndrome. Without the requirement for correlation among elements, there would be an infinite number of syndromes.

In earlier years, Kraepelin would not have plotted cross tabulations to arrive at syndromes. Instead, he would simply be impressed in his run of patients that a frequently occurring symptom combination was hallucinations and delusions. It would be natural to regard this subgroup as some kind of categorical entity. However, in doing so there would be difficulty in classifying patients with high delusions and medium hallucinations or high hallucinations and medium delusions or medium on both symptoms. Are these low grade schizophrenics or nothing in particular?

It should become apparent from the last illustration that subgrouping according to extremes of distributions creates the false impression that these extreme groups are qualitatively different categorical types instead of combinations of quantitative symptoms.

Given the establishment of different syndromes, it is tempting to believe that they have different underlying etiologies. However, it is quite possible that the syndromes represent different stages of the same illness or are variant expressions of the same illness. For instance, hebephrenic silliness and blunted affect have been shown by Brill and Glass (1965) in longitudinal studies to be later stages of schizophrenia while some kinds of alcoholism have been shown by Winokur et al. (1969) to be a variant expression of depression in family studies; i.e., the females tend to be depressed and the males alcoholic.

VALIDATION OF SYNDROMES AGAINST ETIOLOGY

Ideally, to "validate" a syndrome, one needs to establish an association between it and an etiological variable. This has been done only rarely in the study of mental disorders, as, for instance, with phenylketonuria in some forms of mental retardation, in toxic psychoses, the new rare mental abberations of some nutritional deficiencies, and central nervous system syphillis. In all of these, knowledge of the etiology suggests an addition to a better understanding of the disorder.

Following the Danish adoption studies (Goodwin, et al., 1973; Kety, et al., 1971) there are now a number of psychiatric syndrome disorders for which genetic transmission has been implicated: schizophrenia, bipolar affective disorder, endogenous depression, alcoholism, and antisocial personality. There are probably more. The model of the adoption studies is to compare the adopted out newborns of ill parents with adopted out newborns whose biological parents are not ill. All these studies show a greater ultimate breakdown in the adoptees whose biological parents were ill. Although genetic transmission is implicated, the studies can say nothing about the nature of the genetic transmission and they can suggest nothing as an intervention except perhaps genetic counseling on the likelihood of having an ill child. Moreover, despite the fact of genetic transmission in schizophrenia, most schizophrenia syndrome patients (80-90%) according to Walker and Shaye (1982) do not have a family history of schizophrenia. Do they have a non-genetic etiology? It seems possible for a particular syndrome to have more than one etiology; and as a corollary, it is possible for a particular etiology to produce more than one syndrome as in the example of variant expressions.

Even though genetic schizophrenia is a relatively small proportion of all the schizophrenias, it may very well be a more homogeneous subgroup. There are now findings by Orzack and Kornetsky (1971), Walker and Shaye (1982), and Rutchmann et al. (1981), implicating deficits in the continuous performance task in genetic schizophrenia.

VALIDATION AGAINST CLINICAL COURSE

Aside from validating against etiology, what other evidence might validate a particular syndrome? One method employed by Kraepelin was naturalistic prognosis: he observed that the syndrome of dementia praecox tended toward deterioration while the syndrome of depression tended toward recovery.

VALIDATION AGAINST PREMORBID HISTORY

Another form of validation is in relation to social and developmental history. The level of premorbid competence has been shown by Goldstein et al. (1968) to be related to the presenting schizophrenic syndrome. Their results in the Table 4 show non-paranoids are mainly poor premorbid but paranoids mainly good.

VALIDATION AGAINST TREATMENT RESPONSE

The most recent validating process is in relation to treatment response. As was indicated earlier, one possible advantage of knowing etiology is that it might suggest a treatment and it is this that makes the diagnostic process a very utilitarian consideration. Until about 50 years ago, there were no firmly established treatments in psychiatry so there was not much selection of treatment to be done. By "firmly established" is meant studies in which there was random assignment to treatment under double-blind placebo controlled conditions. Today one can point to any number of firmly established psychiatric treatments in the form of neu-

TABLE 4. Paranoid status vs. premorbid competence in schizophrenia

	Premorbid competence		
	Good	Poor	Total
Paranoid	22	4	26
Non paranoid	28	44	72
Total	50	48	98

Goldstein, M.D., Held, J.M., and Cromwell, R.L.: Premorbid adjustment and paranoid-non paranoid status in schizophrenia.

roleptics for schizophrenia, antidepressants for depression, lithium for manics, anxiolytics for anxiety states, ECT for severe depressions, desensitization for simple phobias, and certain forms of family therapy for schizophrenia.

As soon as a treatment can be shown to be generally effective, we may begin to ask "what is the syndrome of those who respond most to treatment A vs. the syndrome of those who respond most to treatment B." If there is syndrome specificity for different treatments those syndromes may have different etiologies, or they may be different severities or variants of the same etiological process. Although we may never know, the practical utility is self evident. We are not implying that those who respond similarly to a treatment have the same diagnosis; rather those who respond differently to a treatment may be diagnostically different.

In the earlier days of clinical psychopharmacology research even when diagnostic specification was much looser than it is now, Donald Klein (1967) randomly assigned patients without regard to diagnosis to receiving chlorpromazine, imipramine, or placebo. One of his major findings as shown in Table 5 was that the responders to chlorpromazine tended to be diagnosed schizophrenic while the responders to the antidepressants tended to be diagnosed as depressed. These results would surprise no one today; yet they constitute broad evidence for there being *some* validity for the diagnostic concepts of schizophrenia and depression, loose as those diagnostic concepts were. This is not to say that these diagnostic concepts could not be made more valid and for that matter the current diagnostic procedures in the DSM-III for endogenous depression and schizophrenia are probably better predictors of response to antidepressants and to neuroleptics than were the diagnostic procedures at the time of Klein's study.

Another example of how psychopharmacology has had impact on diagnosis is in the discovery that lithium is effective in the treatment of mania. Up until that time mania was considered a disruptive but rare disorder. Since the advent of lithium there has been the experience of there being a greater number of manics than anyone thought existed, possibly because clinicians began to discover some patients that they

TABLE 5. Mean outcome ratins for schizophrenic and depressed patients in each drug group

Diagnoses	N	Placebo	Imipramine	CPZ + Procyclidine
Schizophrenics	142	0.9	1.4	3.5
Retarded depressions	17	3.8	6.9	4.3

From Klein, D.F., 1967.

ordinarily would not label as manic but who did respond to lithium. Thereafter they were more comfortable in trying lithium on some patients who in prior years they would have considered doubtful as manics. Since lithium was introduced some studies have shown manics to have many of the same symptom characteristics that are usually considered hallmarks of schizophrenia, such as delusions, hallucinations, and bizarre associations (Andreasen, 1979; Andreasen and Powers, 1974; Harrow and Quinlan, 1977). The DSM-III definition of mania arbitrarily holds that a diagnosis of schizophrenia must be ruled out before considering a diagnosis of mania. This arbitrariness in the distinction has been unsatisfactory to many clinicians and researchers such as Pope and Lipinski (1979). The use of lithium and a neuroleptic as pharmacological probes to distinguish mania from schizophrenia would be difficult because prior to lithium, neuroleptics had been used for the treatment of mania with modest success in symptom reduction. Nonetheless, in recent years practicing clinicians have discovered that there are a number of patients whom they would not have considered manic by an older diagnostic definition who now do respond to lithium. Some of these patients may have carried a diagnosis of excited schizophrenia and may have been treated with neuroleptics with modest but not great success. There are now a number of hospitals maintaining many patients on neuroleptics who are routinely giving each patient a trial on lithium, in the hope of discovering some lithium responders without necessarily knowing why they are responding. In time systematic research will characterize those patients who can and who cannot respond to lithium and by this means the diagnostic concept of mania will become more refined. The results on this line of research are not in yet but we await them eagerly.

RELATIVE VALIDITY

In the area of major depressive disorders, we have witnessed a variety of syndromal classifications such as endogeno-morphic, reactive, neurotic, primary versus secondary, psychotic, characterological, melancholia, atypical, and dysthymic reaction. Without going into the relative merits of any of those syndromal classifications some of them have been shown to be related to response to effective treatment such as tricyclic antidepressants or to electroshock therapy. To this extent those particular syndromal classifications have been shown to have some validity in predicting response to treatment. In this sense of validity it is possible for one syndromal classification to be relatively *more* valid than another even though both have *some* validity. In turn if a new system of classification could be shown to have greater validity for treatment response, it is this new system that would be preferred. An illustration of this example is in the review by Bielski and Friedel (1976) of prediction of response studies to antidepressants. Available diagnostic syndrome categories at the time of the review seemed to be less predictive of treatment response than did another list of symptoms, such as sleep disturbance, psychomotor disturbance, anorexia and weight loss, etc., all of which are similar but not identical to what many diagnosticians have called endogenous depression or melancholia. Since the DSM-III does contain a syndromal diagnosis called major depressive disorder with melancholia, an interesting study might compare the utility of DSM-III melancholia with that of the symptom list presented by Bielski and Friedel and if the latter showed greater utility in the sense of predictive efficiency for treatment response, it should be more useful for clinicians than the diagnosis of melancholia. It is through utility that diagnosis is refined.

BIOLOGICAL MARKERS AS SYNDROMES

Suppose further that if instead of clinical symptoms as predictors of treatment response and possibly etiology. The syndromal characterizaratory determined biological measures such as the dexamethasone suppression test or REM latency were able to predict treatment response *better* than the clinical measures, one would begin to have syndromal classifications in terms of an objective laboratory battery rather than subjective clinical observations. There is already a body of supporting evidence for this approach. When that day arrives in the future, patients suffering from dysphoria who present themselves for treatment would be evaluated by means of a battery of objective biological and behavioral tests to determine their likelihood of response to particular treatments.

DIFFERENT DIAGNOSES FOR DIFFERENT PURPOSES

All of this would be done without any regard necessarily for the question of the etiological agent. Diagnosis in this case has come to mean a characterization of the patient for the purpose of estimating response to treatment and perhaps long-term follow-up outcome. This is along the lines suggested by Fleck (1983). It is quite possible that the battery of predictors for short-term treatment response are somewhat different from the battery of predictors that would be associated with long-term outcome. In this case a patient would be characterized in both ways and it would be quite possible, for example, to state in the chart that the estimate of the patient's response to a particular treatment is high but that the estimate of his long-term outcome is modest at best. No longer does the term "diagnosis" imply that there is some categorical entity "out there" waiting to be discovered, into which a patient must be fit. Instead, diagnosis has come to mean working up and characterizing a patient in a way that allows predictive statements about his disposition and treatment. The ancient maxim still holds, "first diagnose and then treat." Originally, this meant that once one knew the cause, one would find the treatment flowing from that knowledge. Now the emphasis is no longer on cause but the maxim still holds.

SUMMARY

In the past, the study of psychiatric diagnosis has emulated the model of diagnosis in medical disease in assuming that any psychiatric disorder had a knowable etiology from which implications for treatment would flow. Since etiological agents are all but unknown in psychiatry, inferences concerning etiologies were made from the observations of differences in syndromes; individuals with different syndromes must have different etiologies. A syndrome is defined as a more frequently than chance occuring pattern of mental, physical, and behavioral abnormalities. Symptom characteristics which are uncorrelated with each other therefore cannot constitute a syndrome. The relevance of syndromes may be validated with regard to an etiological variable, clinical course, premorbid history, and finally against response to a known effective treatment. The relative validity of competing syndromes needs to be assessed so that the more valid one can be used. There has been some progress in the utilization of objective laboratory measures in constituting a syndrome which may be more valid (with regard to etiology, clinical course, premorbid history and treatment response) than syndromes based on clinical judgment. Diagnosis in clinical psychiatry has come to have a more complex meaning than the simplistic model that there are disease categories waiting to be discovered into which one can fit most patients. Instead, diagnosis has come to mean the characterization of a patient in ways that are relevant to premorbid history, clinical course, treatment response and possibly etiology. The syndromal characterization which best estimates premorbid history may be somewhat different from that which best estimates his response to treatment. Each characterization is valid for its own purposes. There is no *single* most valid way to characterize any patient. As the basic understanding of the central nervous system metabolism and function increases, we can look forward to more precise diagnostic categories. The discovery of psychopharmacological agents which are more specific and effective will continue to play an important role in our understanding of mental disorders.

REFERENCES

Andreasen, N.C.: Thought, language, and communication disorders. II. Diagnostic significance, *Arch. Gen. Psychiatr.* 36:1325-1330, 1979.

Andreasen, N.J.C. and Powers, P.S.: Overinclusive thinking in mania and schizophrenia, *Brit. J. Psychiatr.* 125:452-456, 1974.

Bielski, R.J. and Friedel, R.O.: Prediction of tricyclic antidepressant responses: A critical review, *Arch. Gen. Psychiatr.* 33:1479-1489, 1976.

Brill, Norman Q. and Glass, J.F.: Hebephrenic schizophrenic reactions, *Arch. Gen. Psychiatr.* 12:545-551, 1965.

Fleck, S.: A holistic approach to family typology and the axis of DSM-III, *Arch. Gen. Psychiatr.* 40:901-906, 1983.

Goldstein, M.J., Held, J.N. and Cromwell, R.L.: Premorbid adjustment and paranoid-nonparanoid status in schizophrenia, prepublication report, 1968.

Goodwin, D.W., Schulsinger, F., Hermansen, L., Guze, S.B. and Winokur, G.: Alcohol problems in adoptees raised apart from alcoholic biological parents, *Arch. Gen. Psychiatr.* 28:238-242, 1973.

Harrow, N. and Quinlan, D.: Is disordered thinking unique to schizophrenia? *Arch. Gen. Psychiatr.* 34:15-21, 1977.

Kety, S.S., Rosenthal, D., Wender, P.H., and Schulsinger, F.: Mental illness in the biological and adoptive families of adopted schizophrenics, *Am. J. Psychiatr.* 128:302-306, 1971.

Klein, D.F.: Importance of psychiatric diagnosis in prediction of clinical drug effects, *Arch. Gen. Psychiatr.* 16:118-126, 1967.

Orzack, M.H. and Kornetsky, C.: Environmental and familial predictors of atten-

tion behavior in chronic schizophrenics, *J. Psychiatr. Research* 9:21-29, 1971.

Pope, H.G., Jr., and Lipinski, J.F., Jr.: Diagnosis in Schizophrenia and manic-depressive illness: A reassessment of the specificity of 'schizophrenic symptoms' in the light of current research, *Arch. Gen. Psychiatr.* 35:811-828, 1978.

Rutschmann, J., Cornblatt, B. and Erlenmeyer-Kimling, L.: Sustained attention in children at risk for schizophrenia: Report on a continuous performance test, *Arch. Gen. Psychiatr.* 34:571-575, 1977.

Spitzer, R.L. and Williams, Janet B.W.: Hysteroid dysphoria: An unsuccessful attempt to demonstrate its syndromal validity, *Am. J. Psychiatr.* 139:1286-1291, 1982.

Walker, E. and Shaye, J.: Familial schizophrenia, *Arch. Gen. Psychiatr.* 39:1153-1156, 1982.

Winokur, George, Clayton, Paula J. and Reich, Theodore: *Manic Depressive Illness*, The C.V. Mosby Company, St. Louis, Missouri, 1969.

CHAPTER 3

Ethics and Psychopharmacologic Research

R.H. Belmaker
Ehud Klein
Earl Dick

INNOVATIVE TREATMENT AS EXPERIMENTATION

The Helsinki declaration notes that "in the treatment of the sick person, the doctor must be free to use a new therapeutic measure, if in his judgment it offers hope of saving life, reestablishing health, or alleviating suffering" (Levine, 1981). In this passage, the trial-and-error basis of much of medical practice is recognized. In psychiatry, for example, an endogenous depression can be effectively treated with an antidepressant drug such as imipramine. However, "effective treatment" means that drug treatment is significantly better than placebo. Our best estimates are that one-third of depressed patients will not respond to accepted, standard, effective pharmocologic treatment (Belmaker, et al., 1982). Evidence and clinical practice suggest that a considerable percentage of imipramine nonresponders will respond to a course of electroconvulsive therapy (ECT). However, some patients will refuse consent for ECT, others will have physical contraindications to ECT, and still other patients will fail to improve even after ECT. A clinical psychiatrist with such a patient will usually read about and consider numerous unproven treatments: He could try vitamins; estrogen therapy; stimulants such as amphetamines; an anticonvulsant such as carbamazepine, recently reported to have antidepressant properties; or many other possibilities. A clinical psychiatrist who decides on one of these unproven treatments with a depressed patient resistant to standard therapy should, of course, discuss the new treatment with his patient. Legally, in the United States or Israel, the clinical psychiatrist in this position may incur medicolegal risks and be required to obtain certain bureaucratic permissions. Ethically, however, the author submits that the clinical psychiatrist is in a no different position with one of the new, unproven drugs than he is with imipramine, the standard antidepressant therapy. The clinical psychiatrist weighs risks against benefits and advises his patient on treatment when the risk-benefit ratio is sufficiently favorable. The unproven treatments have greater risks, but the patient resistant to standard treatment is usually in greater need. Consent for such unproven treatment should include informing the patient that the treatment is not standard or proven. However, the consent procedure should not be in principle different from that required for imipramine. Requiring that the consent be formally written or a disclosure of every possible side effect is to prejudice the patient against treatment and increase his anxiety. Depressed patients are often hopeless and pessimistic. It is relatively easy to obtain consent for no treatment or referral to custodial institutions. It is much harder to obtain consent for new therapies that grate on the patient's sense of hopelessness. Moreover, the pessimism of depression often leads to overestimation of the seriousness and danger of side effects. Patients may demand to be "sent away to an institution" rather than risk side effects that they feel may create a burden on their families. Feeling worthless, they imagine that they do not deserve the time from their families and friends that a new treatment or its side effects may require.

A clear line cannot be drawn between an incompetent depressive whose guardian must give consent and a depressed patient able to consent for himself. In situations where the risk-benefit ratio is highly favorable for an unproven drug in a particular patient, it is, in our view, the doctor's duty to persuade as well as inform. Not to act is to act. No treatment is, in many ways, a treatment. It is accepted that it is the ultimate right of a competent patient to refuse treatment, even if the result is death (or in the case of depression, suicide). But this does not mean that the doctor must be neutral. He must be free to describe the new treatment orally to the patient in a manner designed to achieve a reasonable decision. A written informational document can be distorting and inappropriate for many patients. A patient whose father died of cancer, for instance, may not be properly able to evaluate a statement to the effect that "extremely rare cases of cancer have been reported" with a particular new drug.

Recently, studies of Institutional Review Boards (IRB) have sometimes used as a criterion for ethical research that a significant number of patients have exercised the right to refuse to participate. This would seem a very poor argument for ethical acceptability, since many patients might refuse beneficial, proven treatments if a frightening informational document is supplied. We know that a high percentage of patients voluntarily stop penicillin treatment of streptococcus pharyngitis, despite universal medical acceptance of the value of this treatment.

In summary, we have used the example of depression to illustrate that clinical medical practice may be "experimental" in the sense that it is not based on firm knowledge but on theoretical or empirical trial and error. We are in favor of informing patients of as much of the details of their treatment as possible, with the goal of enhancing autonomy and self-respect. Along with Beecher (1966), we feel that for most patients this is not an ethical requirement but a psychosocial secondary goal. Ethical consent to treatment is implied in the patient's coming to the physician and in the patient's taking of medication prescribed by the physician. A standard of the ethical acceptability of a trial of a new treatment would be, in our view, a statement by an independent review board that no better treatment of the condition is known other than the one administered.

The ethical boundaries of such a concept must be clear. If it is ethical to give carbamazepine, a new unproven drug, to depressed patients who did not respond to the standard imipramine, then it is by the same reasoning *unethical* to give carbamazepine to newly depressed patients who would be better treated with imipramine. Informed consent is in our view irrelevant here. A trial of carbamazepine in patients who could well be imipramine responders is to deny effective treatment. Patient consent might be obtained because of patient pessimism or hopelessness about all treatment, but that would not make the trial ethical. Only the highest standards of informed consent, with the patient clearly volunteering against his best interests, could possibly justify use of a new drug in a situation with known effective treatment. Withholding of treatment in a situation where there is a known effective treatment is as unethical as an unproven drug. It would seem strange indeed that the F.D.A. demands placebo-controlled data as evidence before it will register a new antidepressant, that a large number of depressed patients must receive placebo in order to prove the efficacy of a new potentially antidepressant compound. We would hesitate to participate in such a study; the review board at our hospital would probably not pass such a study; we would hesitate to refer a patient to such a study. Yet the standards of written informed consent for such a study are not different in some investigators' views from the standards required for adding carbamazepine to the treatment of a depressed patient refractory to imipramine. The fallacy, in our view, derives from the excessive reliance on informed consent as the criteria for ethical acceptability. A criterion of "what would a reasonable person do under these circumstances?" would lead to a less absurd result. The data needed by science for testing of efficacy of new drugs should be obtained in subgroups of patients who have physical contraindications to standard therapy (such as depressed patients with cardiac disease who might have a high risk for imipramine and who could possibly benefit from participation in a trial of a non-anticholinergic new antidepressant).

RANDOMIZED CONTROLLED TRIALS

Popular opinion tends to assume that physicians know the best treatment for disease, and that randomized controlled trials are done merely to accumulate "scientific" evidence to support their professional need for data. The truth, of course, is that many treatments are of unknown value; or more frequently, two treatments are available and knowledge is not available as to which treatment is better (Eisenberg, 1977). One may appear to work more quickly but have more side effects; the other may offer advantages in different clinical parameters. It should be noted that hypotheses of this type develop during the trial and error practice described above. Thus the impressions can be misleading because the early, clinical experience with a new drug tends to be in subgroups of patients with poor response to standard therapy.

When two clinical treatments are available and the clinician cannot choose which is optimal, a randomized controlled clinical trial is ethical. Patients are randomly assigned to one or the other treatment. If a treatment is not known to be better than placebo the clinician may randomize drug versus placebo. This procedure is ethically no different than giving the best available treatment, if the two treatments are indeed not known to be different. It is peculiar when consent forms for patients to participate in randomized clinical trials are written as if the patient can refuse research treatment and receive standard treatment: standard treatment in such cases would involve a flip of the coin choice between the same two procedures that are options in the randomized trial! Consider a recent clinical trial of neuroleptic only versus neuroleptic plus carbamazepine in excited schizoaffective patients (Klein, et al., 1984). Carbamazepine had been previously suggested to be a useful treatment in such conditions, although much stronger evidence supports the use of lithium in such cases (Biederman, et al., 1979). A trial was, therefore, designed in which patients with poor past lithium response or physical contraindications to lithium were randomized to neuroleptic plus carbamazepine versus neuroleptic plus placebo. Consent in such a trial, in our view, should not needlessly emphasize "research" or risks specific to the protocol. Consent should be given and obtained *as for optimal psychopharmacologic treatment*, which is what both options in this trial are. Presenting patients or their families with the details of the protocol would, in our view, not increase their likelihood of an intelligent choice. The issues are far too complex. To call such consent under such conditions "free choice" would be like attributing the random flipping of a coin to "heads" as its "free choice." A far more effective guarantor of patient rights would be a statement by a review board that no better treatments of the condition are known, and no compelling advantages of either treatment are known for the condition under study.

Random clinical trials can experience "ethical slippage" if they are extended to related conditions where better treatments *are* known. For instance, if *all* new excited schizoaffective patients came to be admitted to the neuroleptic plus carbamazepine study, effective known treatment with lithium would thereby be withheld in an unethical manner. Informed consent is a poor guarantor against such ethical slippage. Many manic and schizophrenic patients are dissatisfied with standard psychopharmacologic treatments, both realistically because of side effects and unrealistically because of poor insight into their ill behavior and need for treatment. Many are unreasonably willing to try new drugs and will sign consent forms with the openly-stated hope that the new drug will be "less strong" (i.e. less effective) than lithium or chlorpromazine. Only proper delineation of the study population by the review board, and not patient informed consent, can guarantee ethical standards in such clinical trials.

It is sometimes argued that patients receive less than optimal treatment in a random trial because the physician declines to use information that could predict in a specific patient a better response to one of the randomized treatments in the study. Clearly, this issue should be studied; the treatment outcomes in clinical research trials can be compared with those in non-research clinical practice. In principle, however, good science as well as ethics will dictate that only those patients enter the clinical trial about whose treatment a true open question exists. A trial of phlebotomy versus penicillin in pneumonia is of no scientific value: a study of carbamazepine in lithium-responsive, lithium-tolerant excited schizoaffective patients is similarly indefensible. If clinical data allows us to predict rapid lithium response in a subgroup of excited schizoaffectives, then such patients should be excluded from the population of the study. In the future, if data accumulates suggesting that carbamazepine is as effective and safe as lithium, it may become ethical to do a randomized clinical trial of the two compounds even in lithium-responsive patients.

NONTHERAPEUTIC RESEARCH

The above discussion concerned innovative therapy in a clinical context and therapeutic research in randomized controlled design. Such therapeutic research ideally advances treatment methods and helps the individual patient without conflict between the two goals. Sometimes, however, research aimed at understanding the etiology of mental illness holds little promise of help for the individual patient. Such nontherapeutic research usually requires much higher standards of informed consent than therapeutic research. For instance, research involving injections of small doses of epinephrine and measurement of the subsequent rise in plasma cyclic AMP in order to evaluate the -adrenergic receptor effects of lithium were done only in outpatient, euthymic, remitted manic-depressive patients who could give informed consent and not in acutely manic or depressed patients (Ebstein, et al., 1976). The rule of using only willing, competent volunteers is a safeguard that is necessary in the case of nontherapeutic research. In the case of therapeutic research a review board can ask whether the proposed treatments are the ones that a reasonable patient would want. However, in nontherapeutic research it is impossible to evaluate the reasons why another individual might or might not volunteer. The individual patient must volunteer after informed of relevant risks and benefits, although the review board must retain an important role in preventing experiments with excessive risk or little potential benefit from being proposed to possible patient volunteers (Katz, 1972).

The model of an autonomous patient volunteering for research that will benefit not him but others in the future has been the central model in discussions of ethical aspects of research (Humber and Almeder 1979). In the author's research experience, however, only a minority of research projects are nontherapeutic. In psychiatry, especially, we have many effective treatments and relatively few leads to the etiology of the psychoses. The model of voluntariness and nontherapeutic research has perhaps distorted the discussion of clinical research in general, has overemphasized the risks, deemphasized the benefits to the patient himself, and exaggerated the role of signed, formal informed consent (Annas, et al, 1977). The situation has occasionally reached reductio ad absurdum where patients had to sign long consent forms for a small drawing of blood; where epidemiologists wishing to survey patient records in hospital were asked to secure consent from thousands of scattered former patients; or where consent had to be obtained to use, for research purposes, the excess of an already drawn, clinically-necessary sample of spinal fluid. These excesses of informed consent doctrine have led to unnecessary antagonism between researchers and ethnicists and to some ridicule at the concept of informed consent itself. In order to remain an effective concept, informed consent should not be trivialized. New regulations from the US DHEW have indeed given institutional review boards new discretion to eliminate written informed consent for blood drawing and other procedures of minimal risk (Code of Federal Regulations, 1981). However, these regulations are worded so indirectly that researchers can justly assume that the regulation writers hesitate to come right out and exempt blood drawing from informed consent regulations. Indeed, many institutional review boards in the USA have not exercised their option to waive written informed consent for research involving blood drawing.

The authors feel that a concept of implied consent is required for nontherapeutic research involving minimal risk, such as blood-drawing; low-dose, diagnostic x-rays; psychological testing; and family interviews. Implied consent as a concept has been used in several settings: public figures lose, to some degree, their right to privacy or to sue for libel as their role in the public sphere implies consent to newspaper articles and photos of them. Motorists in some states are assumed to have given implied consent to alcohol breath testing if they use the public roads. In our view, a hospital patient assumes that his doctor may perform minor tests for the interests of science if the risk is minimal. Such has been the tradition of medicine and is widely known through public literature. Patients who object to such testing cannot be coerced, and a patient who asks the purpose of every blood test or x-ray and refuses if inadequate explanation is forthcoming cannot be deceived. However, patients who willingly put forth their arms for blood drawing or accept their doctor's requests for a special x-ray need not, in our view, be warned formally of their right to refuse as if the Miranda decision and the adversary concept of policeman and accused applied to medicine.

Sometimes, nontherapeutic and therapeutic research may interact in complex ways. For example, neurologists in many settings have often advised psychiatrists to do lumbar puncture for analysis of spinal fluid on newly-admitted patients with severe mental illness. The purpose is to rule out neurological disorders such as brain tumor, cerebrovascular hemorrhage or encephalitis, all of which can cause a clinical picture resembling psychosis. On many neurological services, including the one affiliated to our psychiatric hospital, lumbar punctures are considered a risk-free procedure akin to venipuncture and are routinely performed without written informed consent in the evaluation of disorders such as headache. Psychiatrists have usually not done spinal taps on newly-admitted psychotic patients, but more for reasons of training and clinical habit than reasoned judgment. Several years ago a group of physicians was interested in levels of a new biochemical variable, cyclic AMP, in the spinal fluid of schizophrenic patients (Biederman, et al., 1977). It was essential that the patients studied be free of drug treatment and in the acute phase of their illness. It was possible to accomplish the study by providing the "service" of a diagnostic spinal tap to the admitting psychiatrist of new psychotic patients. Those patients were usually not able to give informed consent because of the acute phase of their illness; delay to contact relatives was not possible because the patients required pharmacological treatment. The spinal taps were performed on admission by a physician, not a member of the regular staff, who was skilled at lumbar puncture and who arranged for clinical examination of the fluid for white cells, red cells, glucose and protein. Remaining fluid was used for the research test of interest, cyclic AMP.

Thinking about the ethics of the above study brings one to think about the motives of the researchers. Did they really feel that spinal taps were a worthwhile clinical addition to the admission diagnostic workup of psychosis or did they merely use this excuse for research? For comparison, however, let us consider the researcher who wishes to study lipoproteins in heart disease. Would it not be ethical, even without fully-informed consent, to draw blood for cholesterol and lipoproteins on newly-admitted patients with myocardial infarction? Or consider the researcher who wishes to study rennin in hypertension and arranges a complete reno-vascular workup for new hypertensive patients in a general clinic where they would otherwise probably be assumed to have hypertension and be treated accordingly. Is the provision of an additional service, albeit not entirely risk free, unethical if done for research motives? Clearly, there are financial and bureaucratic issues here as well, as the patient should not have to pay for procedures whose primary motive is research. Clearly, also, the patient should be informed as much as possible of the nature of the procedures that are proposed for him. However, to demand that the consent form emphasize research entirely is to distort the situation. Moreover, many "research" procedures, as described above, are routinely used in some expensive, private care setting. Does an expensive new procedure become ethical if it is done out of desire to maintain a prestigious private clinic, or desire to satisfy demanding patients who want only the best, or desire to profit from the insurance margin, but unethical if one of the motives is research? Mixed motives are present in every human endeavor. The unearthing of a research motive should not immediately require that a particular clinical practice be subject to the strictest considerations of nontherapeutic research protocols. A spinal tap, while not in the category of venipuncture for which we advocate implied consent, can be clinically justified for newly-admitted psychotic patients. A second spinal tap on the same patient later in treatment, however, should require informed consent as nontherapeutic research.

THE RISKS OF RESTRICTION

Leon Eisenberg (Eisenberg, 1977), has eloquently described the importance of medical research and the impotence of medicine based on clinical experience alone. We would like to add here one additional danger of excessive reliance on clinical experience, and that is physician hubris and paternalism. Advocates of detailed disclosure in all clinical and research settings have often decried physician paternalism and demand full patient partnership in clinical decision making. Yet, without hard data, even the most intelligent layman can do little but accept his physician's clinical impressions. We know how many clinical practices and impressions are based on mythology. Involvement in clinical research can subjugate the physician's decision-making process to empirical data and contribute toward preventing feds or arbitrary treatment. In schizophrenia treatment at the moment, for instance, it would be clearly beneficial if acute schizophrenic patients were randomized for high-dose, rapid neuroleptization treatment or standard dose treatment. Rapid, high-dose treatment of schizophrenia "is sweeping the world like an epidemic" in the words of one psychiatric clinician; its advocates rely on clinical impressions and uncontrolled data (Belmaker, et al., 1980). One controlled study (Lerner, et al., 1979) suggests no advantage for such high-dose, rapid treatment over standard neuroleptic treatment of acute schizophrenia. Formal informed consent demands would make a randomized, controlled trial of this treatment in schizophrenia impossible. Few acute schizophrenic patients are truly competent, and many relatives are unavailable early in the illness or too frightened to give consent. Formal legal guardians are sometimes not as concerned with the patient's medical welfare as they are with keeping the paperwork clean so that disability payments will continue to flow unimpeded. Ethically, we submit that our knowledge is so scant that patients could be randomized to the two dose schedules after consent to hospitalization and neuroleptic treatment. Such research randomization would be better for the patient than a randomization that depended on the clinical beliefs of the physician he happened to be treated by. Scientific demands for a controlled trial are the best defense against medical fadism; charges that "controlled trials are unethical" may be a smoke screen for an inefficacious practice. Paternalistic clinicians have often been afraid of controlled studies of their practices and medical ethics should not serve as a buttress of nonscientific medicine.

The argument of this paper that consent should be more flexible for some types of research does not derive from a lazy desire to protect the researcher's time or effort (Barber, 1976). Rather, consent must be flexible to allow large numbers of physicians and patients to take part in research and, thereby, to maintain continual scientific control of clinical practice. Medical research in isolated research institutes with normal volunteers and significant risks is only one model of medical research, albeit a popular stereotype. Multicenter, multiphysician clinical trials is another, at least as important, model. Nothing is as valuable for a physician, and his patients, as finding that his favorite treatment approach is inferior in controlled clinical trial.

THE PSYCHIATRIC PATIENT

Stanley and colleagues (Stanley and Stanley, 1981) have instituted a series of empirical research of informed consent in studies of psychiatric patients. In general, they find psychiatric patients as able to understand risks and judge risks as general medical patients. These findings of

Stanley et al (Stanley and Stanley, in press) are important in allowing competent psychiatric patients to volunteer for nontherapeutic research with risks when such research is required (Stanley, et al., 1981). However, we do not believe that these findings invalidate comments above about the tendencies of acute depressives, acute manics or acute schizophrenics regarding consent. Moreover, the possibility of obtaining detailed informed consent from psychiatric patients does not make it always ethically necessary for therapeutic research or minimal risk nontherapeutic research, as described above.

SUMMARY

Ethical considerations in research should place the patient first and foremost as follows:

1. The purpose of ethical standards in research is to prevent abuse of patients against their own interests, not to enhance an absolute concept of individual autonony;

2. When innovative therapy or randomized trials of the best available treatments present the patient with optimal therapy, consent is implied in the patient's choice of physician and cooperation with him;

3. When nontherapeutic research in patients presents minimal risk or discomfort such as blood drawing, consent can be seen as implied if the patient does not object to the procedure;

4. The existence of research motivation does not impose stricter standards on programs or procedures that are clinically justifiable and beneficial; and

5. Strict standards of informed consent after disclosure and voluntariness are necessary for nontherapeutic research involving significant risks but such research is probably a minority of human research and does not represent the central paradigm for discussion and regulation.

REFERENCES

Annas, G.J., Glantz, L.H. and Katz, B.F.: Informed Consent to Human Experimentation: The Subject's Dilemma. Ballinger Publishing Company, Cambridge, Massachusetts.

Barber, B.: The ethics of experimentation with human subjects. *Scientific American*, 234:25-31, 1976.

Beecher, H.K.: Ethics and clinical research. *New England Journal of Medicine*, 274:1354-1360, 1966.

Belmaker, R.H., Lerner, Y. and Ebstein, R.P.: Rapid neuroleptization reconsidered. *Amer. J. Psychiatry*, 137:129, 1980.

Belmaker, R.H., Lerer, B. and Zohar, J.: Salbutamol treatment of depression. In: Typical and Atypical Antidepressants, (E. Costa and G. Racagni, eds.) Raven Press, New York, pp. 181-193, 1982.

Biederman, J., Lerner, Y. and Belmaker, R.H.: Combination of lithium plus haloperidol in schizoaffective disorder: A controlled study. *Arch. Gen. Psychiatry*, 36:327-333, 1979.

Biederman, J., Rimon, R., Ebstein, R.P., Belmaker, R.H. and Davidson, J.T.: Cyclic AMP in the CSF of patients with schizophrenia. *Brit. J. Psychiatry*, 130:64-67, 1977.

Code of Federal Regulations.: Protection of human subjects. U.S. Public Health Service Department of Health and Human Services, 1981.

Ebstein, R.P., Belmaker, R.H., Grunhaus, L. and Rimon, R.: Lithium inhibition of adrenaline-sensitive adenylate cyclase in humans. *Nature*, 259:411-413, 1976.

Eisenberg, L.: The social imperatives of medical research. *Science*, 198:1105-1110, 1977.

Humber, J.M. and Almeder, R.F.: Biomedical Ethics and the Law. Plenum Press, New York and London.

Katz, J.: Experimentation With Human Beings. Russell Sage Foundation, New York, 1972.

Klein, E., Bental, E., Lerer, B. and Belmaker, R.H.: Carbamazepine and haloperidol versus placebo and haloperidol in excited psychoses. *Arch. Gen. Psychiatr.*, 41:165-170, 1984.

Lerner, Y., Lwow, E., Levitin, A. and Belmaker, R.H.: Acute high-dose parenteral haloperidol treatment of psychosis: A controlled study. *Amer. J. Psychiatry*, 136:1061-1064, 1979.

Levine, R.J.: Ethics and Regulation of Clinical Research. Urban and Schwarzenberg, Baltimore-Munich, 1981.

Stanley, B. and Stanley, M.: Testing competency in psychiatric patients: What is it, how is it assessed and is it necessary? IRB, in press.

Stanley, B., Stanley, M., Lautin, A., Kane, J. and Schwartz, N.: Preliminary findings on psychiatric patients as research participants: A population at risk? *Amer. J. Psychiatry*, 138:669-671, 1981.

Stanley, B.H. and Stanley, M.: Psychiatric patients in research: Protecting their autonomy. *Comp. Psychiatry*, 22:420-427, 1981.

CHAPTER 4

Genetic Aspects of Psychopharmacology

J. Mendlewicz

INTRODUCTION

Genetic factors play an important role in drug metabolism and drug response. These factors interact with environmental factors in determining therapeutic response and side effects, and are of primary importance in studying the action of psychotropic drugs in major psychiatric disorders, which are known to be partially genetically determined.

Various kinetic processes are involved in the fate of a drug from its absorption to its binding to plasma proteins or to various tissues, its biotransformation and interaction with receptor sites, and finally to its excretion. These five major processes take place simultaneously, and genetically transmitted variations can occur through DNA mutations inducing structural alterations in the specific proteins directly involved in these five processes. In a given person, more than one pharmacologically significant mutation can arise and such mutations may not be so rare, as illustrated by phenomena responsible for genetic polymorphisms such as the ABO or the HLA, the pseudocholinesterase and the INH-acetyl-transferase polymorphisms. Various distribution curves for a given dose of a drug may indicate the relationship between plasma drug level and drug response or side effects. The unimodal gaussian curve indicates genetic homogeneity or polygenic control, while the bimodal (mendelian autosomal dominant trait) or polymodal curve (autosomal recessive) are suggestive of a mechanism controlled by genes at a single locus.

The genetic and environmental factors involved in drug metabolism and drug response can be studied by various methods. The twin method, comparing identical and fraternal twins, makes it possible to evaluate to what extent variations in drug metabolism are genetically influenced. Differences in drug rates between one-egg and two-egg twins can provide an estimate of the "heritability", a theoretical concept expressing the genotypic variance as a proportion of the phenotypic variance. Family studies may also permit differentiation of environmental and genetic sources of variation in drug response by establishing regression of offspring values to averaged parent values and comparing spouse values.

GENETIC ASPECTS OF ANTIDEPRESSANT TREATMENTS

The inactivation of isoniazid is a classical example of a pharmacogenetic phenomenon which has relevance to psychopharmacology. This drug is inactivated in the liver by acetylation. Patients with rapid inactivation seem to respond less favorably than slow acetylators who have, however, more toxic side effects (Price Evans, 1960). Rapid acetylation is determined as an autosomal dominant trait while slow acetylation is transmitted as an autosomal recessive trait. Slow inactivators have a liver acetyl transferase which has a lower activity than the enzyme found in rapid inactivators. The acetyl transferase polymorphism is of great importance in psychopharmacogenetics since monoamine oxidase inhibitors (MAOI) are derivatives similar to isoniazid and are thus subject to liver acetylation. It is, therefore, conceivable that treatment response to MAOI may be related to acetylation status. This hypothesis has been tested with phenelzine, a compound similar to isoniazid, having a monosubstituted hydrazine side chain.

Evans et al. (1965), examined the response to phenelzine in an uncontrolled study of forty-seven depressive patients and found no significant correlation between improvement and acetylator status. Johnstone and Marsh (1973) performed a controlled study in seventy-two neurotic depressive patients and found phenelzine to be more effective in the slow acetylator group. It has also been suggested that depressed patients treated with imipramine respond to the same type of drugs in future relapses and that their affected blood relatives are also more likely to respond to the same compounds.

Pare and Mack (1971) have confirmed this hypothesis and suggest that drug response depends on the nature of the biochemical abnormality in depression. They hypothesized that there are at least two genetically different types of depression, one responding to the MAOI and another to the tricyclics. The recent discovery of multiple forms of MAO has brought a revival of interest not only in the enzyme but also in the synthesis of selective MAO inhibitors as antidepressants (Mendlewicz and Youdim, 1978).

Alexanderson et al. (1969) showed that large interindividual differences (sometimes forty-fold) exist in the steady-state plasma levels of nortriptyline hydrochloride, a phenomenon also seen with imipramine and desmethylimipramine, the active metabolite of imipramine. This suggests that the oral dose commonly used is not a satisfactory way to make sure that a patient is receiving adequate tricyclic treatment and that individual plasma level may be a better way of monitoring antidepressant treatment.

Alexanderson et al. (1969) also studied the contribution of genetic factors to plasma levels of tricyclic antidepressant drugs by using the twin method. Nineteen monozygotic and twenty dizygotic twins were given nortriptyline orally in doses of 0.2 mg/kg body weight, three times daily for eight days. The intrapair difference in steady-state plasma levels was not significant in identical twins, but was in fraternal twins. Most of the variations in steady-state plasma concentrations between unrelated persons appear to be controlled by a polygenic type of inheritance (Asberg et al., 1971). These genetic studies are of importance since toxic side effects and the therapeutic response to tricyclic drugs may well be correlated with the plasma concentration of the drug rather than the dose administered, although these results still need further confirmation.

Clinico-genetic studies of imipramine in depressive patients, where plasma levels have been monitored, provide further evidence. Therapeutic response to imipramine appears to be influenced by the genetic background of depressed patients. Comparing antidepressant responders and nonresponders, the first have significantly more familial unipolar illness and less familial schizophrenia than the latter (Perel et al., 1976).

Environmental factors also play a role in the kinetics of tricyclic antidepressant drugs, although to a lesser extent than hereditary factors. Methylphenidate (Ritalin) raises the steady-state plasma level of imipramine by liver microsomal enzyme inhibition mainly through the cytochrome P-450 reductase system (Wharton et al., 1971). This potentiation of imipramine by amphetamines is also said to cause clinical improvement in previously drug-resistant patients. Similarly 1-triiodothyronine has also been found to increase the effectiveness of tricyclic antidepressant in female depressed patients. This phenomenon is probably due to triiodothyronine decreasing action on plasma binding of imipramine.

Conversely, barbiturates and ethanol produce enzyme induction and decrease the steady-state level of tricyclics; thus, they are potentially able to diminish the clinical effectiveness of tricyclic antidepressants. Therefore, combinations of tricyclic drugs with barbiturates for therapeutic use should be avoided in the treatment of depression. Nonbarbiturate hypnotics should then be used. The same phenomenon is present if one would combine some neuroleptics like haloperidol and tricyclic drugs (Gram et al., 1974). Cigarette smoking is also an important variable influencing the rate of metabolism of imipramine. The mean steady-state level of imipramine in heavy smokers was found to be significantly lower when compared to nonsmokers, thus indicating the negative influence of tobacco on plasma levels of imipramine (Perel, personal communication).

A better knowledge of genetic-environmental interaction in the metabolism of antidepressant drugs will no doubt result in a more rational approach to the pharmacological treatment of depression. Genetic factors have been studied quite extensively in the schizophrenias and affective disorders, but the possible relationship between hereditary factors and the outcome of pharmacological treatment is still an open field. Our present knowledge of the genetics of the major psychoses would indicate that familial data could predict response to treatment. For example, a positive family history of schizophrenia in the relatives of a patient presenting an unclear psychotic clinical picture, including depressive symptoms, is an indication that this patient's illness may be genetically related to schizophrenia and would probably not benefit from antidepressant therapy alone.

GENETIC FACTORS AND DRUG-INDUCED SYNDROMES

Another area of great interest in psychopharmacogenetics is the role played by hereditary predisposition in the production of drug-induced syndromes. This question has been examined in a study of Parkinson patients experiencing affective syndromes (depression or mania) while treated with L-Dopa (Mendlewicz et al., 1976).

Thirty such probands were matched with thirty controls (i.e. Parkinson patients with no psychiatric reaction while on L-Dopa), and family studies were conducted blind on both groups. The risks for affective illness in the first-degree relatives of the probands were significantly greater than in the relatives on the controls. The probands also had more affective episodes in their past than did the controls. These results suggest that Parkinson patients presenting affective syndromes on L-Dopa may be genetically predisposed to affective illness. Several enzymes involved in the metabolism of biogenic amines are being extensively studied in animals and man. Monoamine oxidase (MAO), catechol-o-methyltransferase (COMT) and dopamine-β-hydroxylase (DBH) in particular, are the subject of investigations in normal and psychiatric subjects because of the apparent involvement of biogenic amine anomalies in the major psychiatric disorders.

Clinical and epidemiological studies have shown that the incidence of depressive disorders tends to increase with age and among female patients. Platelet and plasma MAO activities were also found to be higher in older subjects and in females as compared to males, and there is evidence from twin studies that plasma and platelet MAO activity in man is genetically determined. This genetic influence seems to be present for both the mitochondrial MAO activity to platelets and soluble MAO activity of plasma regardless of the substrate used to measure MAO activity. Furthermore, lower platelet MAO activity has been proposed as a genetic marker for the predisposition to schizophrenia, since there was no significant difference between platelet MAO activity in monozygotic twins discordant for schizophrenia (Wyatt et al., 1975).

Murphy and Weiss (1972) showed a decrease in platelet MAO activity in bipolar depression and an increase in MAO activity in unipolar depression. This study should be related to an interesting report by Robinson et al., (1975), indicating that female depressed patients with a lower MAO activity responded better to phenelzine (MAOI) than depressed females with high MAO activity. It is not yet known whether MAO activity will eventually be used as a genetic marker of depression or schizophrenia, since these results are still controversial, but the finding that MAO activity can predict response to MAOI treatment in depression is of evident interest in pharmacogenetic studies.

Erythrocyte catechol-O-methyltransferase (COMT) has also been studied in affective disorders with conflicting results but most investigators agree that hereditary factors play a role in the control of the red blood cell activity of this enzyme (Weinshilboum et al., 1974). The data on Dopamine-β-hydroxylase (DBH) are also difficult to interpret. It is clear that the plasma activity of this enzyme is determined to a large extent by genetic factors, as evidenced by family and twin studies (Mendlewicz et al., 1974).

The heritability estimate for serum DBH activity in these twin studies were found to be close to one, a value indicating a strong genetic influence. However, plasma DBH activity measured through one sampling procedure has not been shown to vary consistently in psychiatric disorders as compared to normal controls, but the significance of these results is unclear. These enzyme studies will probably contribute to a better understanding of pharmacogenetic factors in psychiatric illnesses.

Our knowledge of the contribution of genetic and environmental influences in drug metabolism and drug response is an essential research area that will hopefully lead to the establishment of predicting factors in drug treatment response. There is an increasing number of genetic systems which could be investigated in psychopharmacological research as exemplified by the recent report of Smeraldi et al. (1976), suggesting a relationship between positive response to chlorpromazine in some subtypes of schizophrenia and a determined immunogenetic phenotype expressed by the histocompatibility antigen A1 (HLA-A1).

GENETIC ASPECTS OF LITHIUM RESPONSE

Since lithium treatment is often considered as a prophylactic therapy, thus advocated for months and years, the early recognition of objective criteria for predicting long-term lithium response is a fundamental clinical issue in psychiatry today. There are, however, important clinical questions on lithium prophylaxis which remained unsolved. Among them are: is lithium response or nonresponse a permanent feature of the illness; do acute studies give us any clue as to the prophylactic benefit of lithium therapy; and do social and personality variables significantly influence the outcome of long-term lithium treatment?

Similar questions should be raised for the biological parameters investigated in those studies attempting to differentiate lithium responders from nonresponders. Are the observed biological criteria state-dependant, or can they be considered as biological markers of an underlying vulnerability to mental disorders? Because of these limitations, one should be cautious and critical in interpreting results on biological and clinical predictors of lithium response.

Nevertheless, the predictive approach is obviously of considerable importance in the field of lithium therapy. Recent promising prediction studies are reviewed here, and some of our contributions are described. In analyzing the current literature, one should first differentiate between acute and long-term studies in reference to depression and mania. That adequate plasma lithium levels are used in the studies is assumed.

Serry (1969) and Serry and Andrews (1969) in Australia were among the first investigators to propose a pharmacokinetic test for predicting lithium response to mania: the so-called lithium excretion test. Serry reported that 70 percent of manic patients responding to lithium were "retainers", i.e. demonstrated slow urinary lithium excretion. Lithium nonresponders were found to be rapid excretors.

Although it has been shown that patients during mania tend to retain more lithium, the predictive value of the lithium excretion test has been disputed in subsequent reports (Epstein et al., 1965; Geisler et al., 1971; Almy and Taylor, 1973).

So far, EEG neurophysiological studies have not been effective in predicting lithium response to mania. Most studies show that the lithium-induced EEG changes in contingent negative variation have no predictive value, (Platman and Fieve, 1969; Johnson et al., 1970; Small et al., 1971; Bowers and Heninger, 1977). However, Kupfer et al (1974) studying the sleep EEG have shown lithium responders to present a reduction in REM sleep and an increase in delta sleep. This was also observed by Chernik et al. (1974), who questioned the predictive value of this sleep EEG effect, considering it to be drug-induced. Most investigation on central amine metabolism based on CSF studies of 5-HIAA, HVA, or urinary MHPG in relation to lithium response in mania have been inconclusive as of today.

One report, Sullivan et al. (1977), indicates that low platelet MAO activity may be associated with poor response to lithium treatment during mania, but this observation has not yet been confirmed.

ACUTE STUDIES IN DEPRESSION

The question of biological predictors of lithium response in depression is much complicated by the heterogeneous nature of the depressive syndromes and by the rarity of well-designed controlled studies in depression.

Friedel (1976) has claimed that higher plasma lithium levels (>1.mEq/L) are needed to achieve an antidepressant effect in comparison to the antimanic effect. This pharmacokinetic parameter (a therapeutic level) does not have the same significance in the depressive as compared to the manic phase. Platelet MAO, electrolytes and EEG variables have been investigated in lithium-treated depression with disappointing results (Carroll, 1979).

One study, Beckmann et al., (1975), has reported low uninary MHPG (noradrenaline-deficient) patients showing a better antidepressant response to lithium. It is not clear, however, whether low uninary MHPG levels in patients are primarily related to mood state, physical activity or antidepressant response.

Conversely, Goodwin et al. (1973) have reported a low probenecid-induced increment in CSF 5-HIAA to predict good antidepressant response to lithium, but this has not been confirmed by Bowers and Heninger (1977). A recent study shows that patients experiencing strong mood elevation after a single dose of d-amphetamine tend to respond better to lithium, but this one study needs replication.

Electrophysiological parameters have also been implicated. The augmenting average evoked response (AER) pattern is more often seen in lithium responders while nonresponders tend to have reducing AER patterns (Buchsbaum et al., 1971). Again, this characteristic has been linked to bipolar illness and may, thus, not be indicative of lithium response alone.

Finally, good lithium response has also been associated with high baseline calcium/magnesium ratios and elevation of serum magnesium during successful lithium treatment, while the opposite was seen in nonresponders, (Carman et al., 1974).

The question raised by long-term lithium studies has to consider separately, mood stabilization, depression and mania prophylaxis. It may be more fruitful to investigate overall mood stabilization after a reasonable study period (± 12 months). The decision as to whether a patient will turn out to be a lithium responder or lithium failure is not so obvious and may differ from one study to the other. Despite these limitations, several studies have proposed some biological predictors of long-term lithium response. Genetic factors have been associated with various patterns of lithium prophylaxis. Bipolar patients with a positive family history of bipolar illness seem to have a better long-term lithium response than patients without family history (Mendlewicz et al., 1973; Stallone et al., 1973). These results have now been confirmed by several groups, (Zvolsky et al., 1974; Prien et al., 1974; Taylor and Abrams, 1975; Kupfer et al., 1975; Mendlewicz et al., 1978; Ananth et al., 1979; Cazullo and Smeraldi, in press), although one study (Misra and Burns, 1977) reported nonresponders to lithium prophylaxis to have more relatives with affective illness than lithium responders. This association was not observed, however, for the presence of unipolar illness in relatives of bipolar patients, (Mendlewicz et al., 1973; Stallone et al., 1973). These genetic results indicate that there may be several distinct genetic subgroups of bipolar illness showing different treatment response to lithium.

The genetic heterogeneity of long-term lithium response in bipolar illness is further evidenced by twin studies. A higher concordance rate for affective illness is found in both monozygotic and dizygotic twin pairs when the proband had experienced good long-term response to lithium (Mendlewicz, 1979; Mendlewicz et al., 1978).

In those twin pairs where the proband was considered as a lithium nonresponder, the concordance rate for affective illness was much lower. Furthermore, concordant twin pairs, with better lithium prophylaxis in the index case, had higher morbidity risks for affective illness than discordant pairs. The above family and twin studies indicate that genetic factors are to be considered as useful biologic predictors of long-term lithium prophylaxis. These genetic data also underline the importance of the concept of genetic heterogeneity of bipolar illness in relation to long-term lithium prophylaxis.

The histocompatibility antigenic system has also been studied in an attempt to find immunogenetic markers of lithium prophylaxis, (Perris et al., 1978). The HLA-A3 antigen was more frequently found in bipolar patients who were long-term lithium failures, while long-term lithium responders showed reduction in the HLA-B18 antigen (Perris et al., 1978). This is certainly an interesting observation relevant to the membrane hypothesis of affective illness, since some of the antigens in the HLA system may be implicated in membrane transport mechanisms, but this study needs further replication. The membrane hypothesis of affective illness has recently stimulated considerable research into the physiological mechanisms of lithium transport across the red blood cell (RBC). Claims were made that the lithium RBC/plasma ratio may serve as a pharmacokinetic indicator of short- and long-term lithium response in the affective illness, (Mendels and Frazer, 1973; Mendels et al., 1976; Frazer et al., 1978). Although these claims have been disproved, (Mendlewicz et al., 1978; Carroll, 1979; Mendlewicz, 1979) very important knowledge has been gained in the physiology of the transport of the lithium ion across the red cell membrane (Greil et al., 1979). It is also now clear that genetic factors do play an important role in the membrane lithium transport (Schless et al., 1975; Dorus et al., 1975; Mendlewicz et al., 1978; Mendlewicz, 1979).

The lithium RBC/plasma ratios have also been shown to have heterogeneous distribution (two separate subgroups) in patients who are nonresponders to lithium prophylaxis. Patients responding well to lithium prophylaxis clearly showed an homogeneous pattern of lithium RBC/plasma ratio distribution (Mendlewicz, 1978; Mendlewicz, 1979). More recently, Dorus et al., 1979, have reported higher in vitro lithium RBC/plasma ratios in some relatives (secondary cases) of bipolar patients, suggesting that higher lithium RBC/plasma ratios may be biological indicators of a membrane vulnerability to bipolar illness. Similar results are found by us (higher lithium/RBC/plasma ratios) in monozygotic and dizygotic twins concordant for affective illness when compared to discordant twins.

One investigation (Bert et al., 1977) has reported an increase in Stages 3-4 slow-wave sleep in long-term lithium responders, a promising electrophysiological predictor of lithium response if confirmed in later studies.

CONCLUSION

After many years of the clinical use of lithium in psychiatry, although its therapeutic efficacy has now been demonstrated both for acute stages of affective illness as well as for affective prophylaxis, the question of long-term therapeutic outcome and prediction still remains poorly defined. A multidisciplinary approach combining genetic, pharmacokinetic, neurophysiological, neuroendocrine and neurochemical parameters along with well-designed, long-term clinical outcome studies will be needed to shed more light on one of the key issues in lithium treatment, that is, the need for specific biological and clinical predictors of lithium preventive treatment in affective illness.

SUMMARY

In this review, methods of establishing new data attesting to genetic influences upon the pharmacotherapy of psychiatric illness have been presented briefly. The by-now classical approaches used in animal pharmacogenetics such as the "animal inbred strain" method and the "recombinant" method which are aimed at studying inbred strains of animals with various behavioral and biochemical characteristics have not been discussed. We have attempted, instead, to illustrate the importance of the genetic approach as applied to human psychopharmacological research. It is clear that the nature-nurture dichotomy is a fallacy, for what better examples can there be of gene-environment interaction than those provided by pharmacogenetics.

REFERENCES

Alexanderson, B., Evans, D.A. and Sjovist, F.: Steady-state plasma levels of nortriptyline in twins: Influence of genetic factors and drug therapy, Br. Med. J. 4:764-768, 1969.

Almy, G.L. and Taylor, M.A.: Lithium retention in mania, Arch. Gen. Psych. 29: 232-234, 1973.

Ananth, J., Engelsmann, F., Kiriakos, R. and Kolivakis, T.: Prediction of lithium response, Acta Psych. Scand. 60:279-286, 1979.

Asberg, M., Evans, D.A. and Sjoquist, F.: Genetic control of nortriptyline kinetics in man: A study of relatives of propositi with high plasma concentrations, J. Med. Genet. 8:129-135, 1971.

Beckmann, H., St-Laurent J. and Goodwin, F.K.: The effect of lithium on urinary MHPG in unipolar and bipolar depressed patients, Psychopharmacologia 42:277-282, 1975.

Bert, J., Saier, J., Dufour, H., Scotto, J.C., Julien, R. and Sutter, J.M.: Modification du sommeil provoquees par le lithium en administration aigue et an administration chronique, Electroenceph. and Clinical Neurophys. 43:745-748, 1977.

Bowers, M.B., Jr. and Heninger, G.R.: Lithium: Clinical effects and cerebrospinal fluid acid monoamine metabolites, Commun. Psychopharmacol. 1:135-145, 1977.

Buchsbaum, M., Goodwin, F., Murphy, D. and Borge, G.: AER in affective disorders, Am. J. Psychiatry 128:19-25, 1971.

Carman, J.S., Post, R.M., Teplitz, T.A. and Goodwin, F.K.: Divalent cations in predicting antidepressant response to lithium, Lancet 2:1454, 1974.

Chernik, D.A., Cochrane, C. and Mendels, J.: Effects of lithium carbonate on sleep, J. Psych. Res. 10:133-146, 1974.

Carroll, B.J.: Prediction of treatment outcome with lithium, Arch. Gen. Psychiatry 36:870-878, 1979.

Cazullo, C.L. and Smeraldi, E.: HLA system in psychiatry and psychopharmacology, Progress in Neuropsychopharmacology, in press.

Dorus, E., Pandey, G.N. and Davis, J.M.: Genetic determinant of lithium ion distribution. An in vitro and in vivo monozygotic-dizygotic twin study, Arch. Gen. Psych. 32:1097-1100, 1973.

Dorus, E., Pandey, G.N., Shaughnessy, R., Gaviria, M., Val, E., Ericksen, S. and Davis, J.M.: Lithium transport across red cell membrane: A cell membrane abnormality in manic-depressive illness, Science 205:932-934, 1979.

Epstein, R., Grant, L., Herjanic, M. and Winokur, G.: Urinary excretion of lithium in mania, J.A.M.A. 192:409, 1965.

Evans, D.A., Davison, K. and Pratt, R.T.: The influence of acetylator phenotype on the effects of treating depression with phenelzine, Clin. Pharmacol. Ther. 6:430-435, 1965.

Frazer, A., Mendels, J., Brunswick, D., London, J., Pring, M., Ramsey, T.A. and Rybakowski, J.: Erythrocyte concentrations of the lithium ion: Clinical correlates and mechanisms of action, Am. J. Psychiatry 135:1065-1069, 1978.

Friedel, R.O.: Lithium and depression, Am. J. Psychiatry 133:976, 1976.

Geisler, A., Schou, M. and Thomsen, K.: Renal lithium elimination in manic-depressive patients: Initial excretion and clearance, Pharmacopsychiatry 10:149-155, 1971.

Goodwin, F.K., Post, R.M., Dunner, D.L. and Gordon, E.K.: Cerebrospinal fluid amine metabolites in affective illness: The probenecid technique, Am. J. Psychiatry 130:73-79, 1973.

Gram, L.F., Over, K.F. and Kirk, L.: Influence of neuroleptics and benzodiazepines on metabolism of tricyclic antidepressants in man, Am. J. Psychiatry 131:863-869, 1974.

Greil, W., Becker, B.F. and Duhm, J.: On

the relevance of the red blood cell/plasma lithium ratio. In: Lithium Controversies and Unresolved Issues (T.B. Cooper, S. Gershon and N.S. Kline, eds.), pp. 209-217, *Excerpta Medica*, Amsterdam, 1979.

Johnson, G., Maccario, M., Gershon, S. and Korein, J.: The effects of lithium on electroencephalogram, behavior and serum electrolytes, *J. Nerv. Ment. Dis.* 151:273-289, 1970.

Johnstone, E.C. and Marsh, W.: Acetylator status and response to phenelzine in depressed patients, *Lancet* i:567-570, 1973.

Kupfer, D.J., Reynolds, C.F., Weiss, B.L. and Foster, G.: Lithium carbonate and sleep in affective disorders: Further considerations, *Arch. Gen. Psychiatry* 30:79-84, 1974.

Kupfer, D.J., Pickar, D., Himmelhoch, J.M. and Detre, T.P.: Are there two types of unipolar depression?, *Arch. Gen. Psychiatry* 32:866-871, 1975.

Mendels, J. and Frazer, A.: Intracellular lithium concentration and clinical response: Towards a membrane theory of depression, *J. Psych. Res.* 10:9-18, 1973.

Mendels, J., Frazer, A., Baron, J., Kukopulos, S., Reginald, D., Tondo, L. and Caliari, B.: Intra-erythrocyte lithium ion concentration and long-term maintenance treatment, *Lancet* i:966, 1976.

Mendelwicz, J., Fieve, R.R. and Stallone, F.: Relationship between the effectiveness of lithium therapy and family history, *Am. J. Psychiatry* 130:1011-1013, 1973.

Mendlewicz, J., Levitt, M. and Fleiss, J.L.: A genetic study of plasma dopamine-beta-hydroxylase activity in man, *Acta. Gent. Med. Gemellolog.* 24:105-110, 1975.

Mendelwicz, J., Yahr, F. and Yahr, M.D.: Psychiatric disorders in Parkinson's disease treated with L-dopa: A genetic study. In: Advances in Parkinsonism (W. Birkmayer and O. Hornykiewicz, eds.), pp. 103-107, Editions Roche, 1976.

Mendelwicz, J., Verbanck, P., Linkowski, P. and Wilmotte, J.: Lithium accumulation in erythrocytes of manic-depressive patients: An in vivo twin study, *Brit. J. Psychiatry* 133:436-444, 1978.

Mendlewicz, J. and Youdim, M.B.: Anti-

depressant potentiation of 5-hydroxytryptophan by L-deprenyl, an MAO "Type B" inhibitor, *J. of Neural Transmission* 43:279-286, 1978.

Mendelwicz, J.: Prediction of treatment outcome: Family and twin studies in lithium prophylaxis and the question of lithium red blood cell/plasma ratios. In: Lithium: Controversies and Unresolved Issues (T.B. Cooper, S. Gershon and N.S. Kline, eds.) pp.●●-●● *Excerpta Medica*, Amsterdam, 1979.

Misra, P.C. and Burns, B.H.: Lithium nonresponders in a lithium clinic, *Acta Psychiat. Scand.* 55:32-40, 1977.

Murphy, D.L. and Weiss, R.: Reduced monoamine oxidase activity in blood platelets from bipolar depressed patients, *Am. J. Psychiatry* 128:1351-1357, 1972.

Pare, C.M. and Mack, J.W.: Differentiation of two genetically specific types of depression by the response to antidepressant drugs, *J. Med. Genet.* 8:306-309, 1971.

Perel, J.M., Mendlewicz, J., Shostak, M., Kantor, S.J. and Glassman, A.H.: Plasma levels of imipramine in depression. Environmental and genetic factors, *Neuropsychobiology* 2:193-202, 1976.

Perris, C., Stransman, E., and Wahlby, L.: HLA antigens and the response to prophylactic lithium, 11th C.I.N.P. Congress Vienna, 9-14, 1978, in press.

Platman, S.R. and Fieve, R.R.: The effect of lithium carbonate on the electroencephalogram of patients with affective disorders, *Brit. J. Psychiatry* 115:1185-1188, 1969.

Price Evans, D.A.: Genetic variations in the acetylation of isoniazid and other drugs, *Ann. N.Y. Acad. Sci.* 151:723-733, 1960.

Prien, R.F., Caffey, E.M., Jr. and Klett, C.J.: Factors associated with treatment success in lithium carbonate prophylaxis: Report of the Veteran's Administration and National Institute of Mental Health Collaborative Study Group, *Arch. Gen. Psychiatry* 31:189-192, 1974.

Robinson, D.S., Nies, A., Lamborn, K.R., Ravaris, C.L. and Ives, J.O.: Patterns of monoamine oxidase activity in man. In: Neuropsychopharmacology (J.R. Boissier, H. Hippius and P. Pichot, eds.) pp. 989-994, Elsevier, Amsterdam, 1975.

Schless, A.P., Frazer, A., Mendels, J., Pandey, G.N. and Theodorides, V.J.: Genetic determinant of lithium ion metabolism: II. An in vivo study of lithium ion distribution across erythrocyte membranes, *Arch. Gen. Psychiatry* 32:337-390, 1975.

Serry, M.: The lithium excretion test: I. Clinical application and interpretation, *Aust. N.Z. J. Psych.* 3:390-394, 1969.

Serry, M. and Andrews, S.: The lithium excretion test: II. Practical and biochemical aspects, *Aust. N.Z. J. Psych.* 3:395-397, 1969.

Small, J.G., Small, I.F. and Perez, H.C.: EEG evoked potential, and contingent negative variations with lithium in manic depressive disease, *Biol. Psychiatry* 3:47-58, 1971.

Smeraldi, E., Bellodi, L., Sacchetti, E. and Cazzullo, C.L.: The HLA system and the clinical response to treatment with chlorpromazine, *Br. J. Psychiat.* 129:486-489, 1976.

Stallone, F., Shelley, E., Mendlewicz, J. and Fieve, R.R.: The use of lithium in affective disorders. III: A double-blind study of prophylaxis in bipolar illness, *Am. J. Psychiat.* 130:1006-1010, 1973.

Sullivan, J.L., Cavenar, J.O., Jr., Maltbie, A. and Stanfield, C.: Platelet-monoamine-oxidase activity predicts response to lithium in manic-depressive illness, *Lancet* ii:1325-1327, 1977.

Taylor, M.A. and Abrams, R.: Acute mania: Clinical and genetic study of responders and nonresponders to treatments, *Arch. Gen. Psychiatry* 32:863-865, 1975.

Weinshilboum, R.M., Raymond, F.A., and Elveback, L.R.: Correlation of erythrocyte catechol-O-methyltransferase activity between siblings, *Nature* 252:490-491, 1974.

Wharton, R.N., Perel, J.M., Dayton, P.G. and Malitz, S.: A potential clinical use for methylphenidate with tricyclic antidepressants, *Am. J. Psychiat.* 127:1619-1625, 1971.

Wyatt, R.J., Belmaker, R. and Murphy, D.L.: Low platelet monoamine oxidase and vulnerability to schizophrenia. In: Genetics and Psychopharmacology (J. Mendlewicz, ed.), Vol. 10, (Th. A. Ban, F.A. Freyhan, P. Pichot and W. Poldinger, series eds.), pp. 38-56, 1975.

Zvolsky, P., Vinarova, E. and Dostal, T.: Family history of manic-depressive and endogenous depressive patients and clinical effect of treatment with lithium, *Act. Nerv. Sup.* (Praha) 16:194-195, 1974.

CHAPTER 5

Amphetamine Response in Schizophrenia: An Episode Marker

Daniel P. van Kammen, M.D. Ph.D.
Welmoet B. van Kammen, Ph.D

INTRODUCTION

One way to test the dopamine hypothesis of schizophrenia is to study the behavioral response to dopamine agonists. Studies of dopamine agonists have focused upon the increase in psychosis observed with doses that do not induce psychosis in non-schizophrenic subjects (Angrist et al., 1974, 1981; Janowsky and Davis, 1976). The dopamine agonist challenge test was developed as a consequence of the dopamine hypothesis of schizophrenia (Meltzer and Stahl, 1976; Snyder, 1976; van Kammen, 1979). However, not all schizophrenic patients respond with an increase in psychosis to the challenge test, particularly when they are in remission or when they are in a stabilized psychotic state (Janowsky and Davis, 1976; van Kammen et al., 1982a). Furthermore, improvement has been noted following dopamine agonists in schizophrenic patients as well (Belart, 1942; Bischoff, 1951; Inanaga et al., 1975; Gerlach and Luhdorf, 1975; Tamminga et al., 1978). This heterogeneous response raises the question whether the amphetamine induced increase in psychosis is a trait marker for schizophrenia or whether this response reflects changes associated with change in clinical state (i.e., a state or episode marker).

According to Zubin (1980) schizophrenia is an episodic illness. This episodic nature and the uncertainty how long an episode lasts after symptoms have decreased with antipsychotic drugs makes it difficult for the clinician to decide whether or not the patient should be withdrawn from neuroleptic drugs (Davis et al., 1980). If a patient is withdrawn prior to the end of his psychotic episode, he will relapse rapidly; whereas the patient whose episode has passed completely may remain symptom-free for a longer period of time. Among others, Zubin (1980) has stressed the importance of being able to define the beginning and the end of a psychotic episode. Because psychotic decompensation is a dynamic process that develops in stages over time (Docherty et al., 1978; Szymansky et al., 1983) we may be able to identify biological markers of the pre-psychotic condition. The amphetamine challenge test could become one of such markers.

In this chapter, I review our studies of repeated d-amphetamine infusions under different clinical and treatment conditions (van Kammen et al., 1980, 1982 abcd, 1984). The results of these studies indicate that the effect of amphetamine on psychosis is a state dependent trait marker. Amphetamine as a pharmacological stressor will be considered, and finally, I will address the possibility of using the stimulant challenge test as a clinical tool to assess the need for continued neuroleptic drug treatment and to aid in the choice of pharmacological treatment.

METHODS

Forty-five schizophrenic patients (20 women and 25 men, age range 18-55 years, mean 23 years) who were voluntarily admitted to an inpatient clinical research unit at the National Institute of Health participated in this study. They were physically healthy and adhered to a controlled monoamine, low caffeine and alcohol-free diet. They were diagnosed as having schizophrenia (n = 39) or schizoaffective disorder (mainly schizophrenic) (n = 6) using 1978 Research Diagnostic Criteria (RDC). In addition, to be included in the study, the patients had to show four or more (mean $\pm$ SE = 6.8 $\pm$ .2) of the 12 differentiating symptoms of the flexible system of the International Pilot Study of Schizophrenia, thus providing a high probability for the diagnosis of schizophrenia. They also were evaluated for the presence of Schneiderian first rank symptoms, duration of illness and age of onset. Patients signed informed consent forms and informed consent was evaluated on an on-going basis. When it was indicated, a relative signed the consent forms as well.

Study I

Twenty mg d-amphetamine and a saline placebo were administered to all 45 patients over 30 seconds in a running IV of .9% saline solution 3-5 days apart in a double-blind randomized design. Patients were drug-free for a mean of 34 days, (range 21-54 days) before the study. The first amphetamine infusion is referred to as the index infusion compared to subsequent infusions. The infusions took place 1 to 1½ hours after the patient had been awakened. Vital signs were monitored every five minutes by a nurse familiar to the patient. During a semi-structured interview, patients' acute behavioral responses to d-amphetamine were rated before and after the infusion by means of the Brief Psychiatric Rating Scale (BPRS) and the Amphetamine Interview Rating Scale (AIRS) as designed by us (van Kammen et al., 1982a). The AIRS includes the following items: psychosis (a 1-7 modification of the Bunney-Hamburg Global Psychosis item), delusions, increased speech, elation, and dysphoria. All of these items were rated on a scale from one (not present) to seven (most severe). A score of two points indicated some residual psychotic symptoms. The changes in scores in BPRS and AIRS items were calculated by subtracting the pre-infusion rating from those obtained 30 to 45 minutes following the infusion. The raters were instructed that the change of one point in the seven point psychosis item (AIRS) had to indicate a clearly observable, clinically meaningful change in psychotic symptoms. The patients with a decrease in psychosis of one point or more were designated "improved"; those with an increase in psychosis of one point or more were designated "worsened" and those with no ratable change were designated "not changed." A second independent rater observed the patients' behavior during the interview from behind a one/way mirror and provided ratings for determining the interrater reliability of the global psychosis score (interclass correlation = .913). The patients were well known to the raters. Change in psychosis ratings correlated significantly with the change in the composite scores for psychosis on the BPRS, i.e., the thinking disturbance cluster which consists of unusual thought content, hallucinatory behavior, and conceptual disorganization (r = .81, p < .0001) and 9 items of the schizophrenia cluster (r = .79, p < .0001).

Study II

Seventeen patients received a repeat 20 mg d-amphetamine infusion during a second drug-free condition up to four months following the first infusion. Almost all had received one or more amphetamine infusions between Study I and II, as described in studies IV, V, and VI or during lithium treatment.

Study III

A repeat infusion occurred during pimozide treatment (n = 30) after 37 ± 2 days of pimozide pre-treatment (range 15-54 days) with the daily dose of pimozide ranging from 1-20 mg with a mean of 8 ± mg pimozide per day. Pimozide is an investigational neuroleptic of the diphenylbutlypiperdine type designed for use in chronic schizophrenia (McNeil-Orap).

Study IV

Twelve patients participated in an amphetamine infusion and this infusion which took place 7 days after pimozide was discontinued. This study included 6 patients who responded with an increase in psychosis and 6 who remained unchanged during Study I.

Study V

Fifteen patients from Study III were followed after pimozide discontinuation for up to three months while being treated with placebo. Six patients who showed an increase in psychosis with the amphetamine infusion and seven who did not respond were included in this study. The remaining two patients who showed a decrease in psychosis are excluded from direct analysis as they did not meet the criteria of staying the same or relapsing following pimozide withdrawal (i.e. relapse prediction).

RESULTS

Study I   Placebo controlled amphetamine response in patients off medication

Of the 45 patients receiving randomized placebo controlled index infusions of 20 mg d-amphetamine; thirteen patients improved one point or more on the psychosis item of the AIRS and 18 worsened. After the placebo infusion, six patients improved and six worsened (Fig. 1). Over 69% of the patients changed one point or more in psychosis in either direction after the d-amphetamine infusion while only 27% changed after placebo infusion, indicating that d-amphetamine significantly more frequently induced a change in psychosis than placebo (Fig. 2). Paired t-tests revealed that psychosis ratings were not significantly affected by d-amphetamine (2.9 ± .35 vs. 3.2 ± .32) or placebo (2.9 ± .25 vs. 2.8 ± .22) but the variance in the absolute changes following d-amphetamine and placebo infusion was significantly different (p<.01).

Pre-infusion Conditions and Changes in Psychosis

Pre-infusion global psychosis ratings were significantly different among patients who improved, did not change and worsened (4.3 ± .4 vs. 1.7 ± .2 vs. 2.7 ± .4, p < .0001) even though there was considerable overlap in ratings among these three groups. Similarly, the pre-infusion profile of the BPRS and AIRS items of the three groups showed a significant and fairly consistent difference in level (p < .002) (Fig. 3), but there was not a significant interaction effect with repeated measures of ANOVA. The pre-infusion difference in symptom level indicates that the intensity of symptoms (clinical state) rather than the type (i.e., individual symptoms) was related to the direction of change in psychosis following d-amphetamine (i.e., state dependency). The type of response

AMPHETAMINE EFFECTS ON
PSYCHOSIS IN SCHIZOPHRENIA

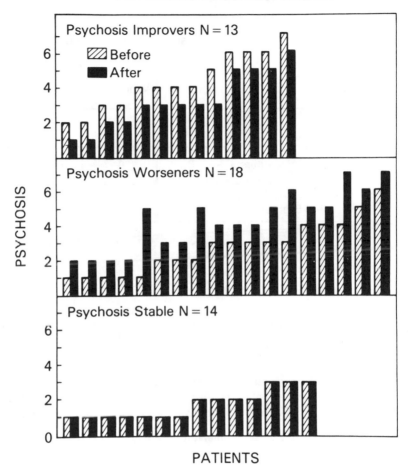

FIG. 5-1. Bunney-Hamburg psychosis rating before and after d-amphetamine infusion. Patients in solid remissions did not change in psychosis ratings after d-amphetamine.

was determined by the patient's clinical state. However, the height of intensity of the psychosis during an episode was not the same for each patient. Traditional clinical and demographic variables failed to differentiate the patients who improved from those who worsened or those who did not change in psychosis. No significant differences were observed among the three types of response groups for any of the following: diagnostic subgroups, twelve differential symptoms, number of

COMPARISON OF THE D-AMPHETAMINE AND PLACEBO EFFECTS UPON PSYCHOSIS

		Response to d-Amphetamine Infusion			
		Improvers	Worseners	Phychosis Stable	
Response to Placebo Infusion	Improvers	**1**	5	0	6
	Worseners	2	**1**	3	6
	Psychosis Stable	10	12	**11**	33
	Total	13	18	14	

Stuart-Maxwell X^2 = 14.5, df = 2, p < .001

Kappa = −.046, p = NS

FIG. 5-2. The distribution of the responses following infusions of placebo and d-amphetamine in the same people. This suggests strongly that the responses were not identical to the two infusions.

Schneiderian symptoms, prognostic indicators, premorbid functioning, age, gender, age of onset, duration of illness, months of hospitalization, and number of hospitalizations.

Study II   Repeat amphetamine infusions in drug-free condition

During a similar drug-free condition and four months after the index infusion, we retested 17 patients with 20 mg of d-amphetamine. All had one or more amphetamine infusions between Study I and II, as described in Study III, IV and V or during lithium treatment.

The patients who received the repeat infusion during the second drug-free period under similar conditions as during the index infusion (Study I) showed considerably less response (Fig. 4). Negative symptoms improved significantly. However, most patients had changed in the manifest intensity of their illness; many had gone into remission and two had relapsed compared to their index infusion. Of the eight who worsened following the index infusion, only three did so again. Two of the three who had improved initially were still psychotic or had become psychotic again when retested, and improved once again acutely during

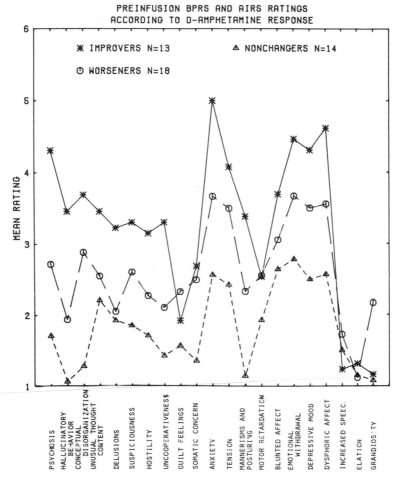

FIG. 5-3. The pre-infusion symptom profile according to the three responses following d-amphetamine.

this infusion (Fig. 5). The third improving patient was not psychotic at the time of the repeat infusion and did not show a change in psychosis. Another patient who relapsed during the interim period improved briefly during the repeat infusion (with a preinfusion psychosis score of 4). This man had not shown a change following the index infusion when he was non-psychotic (psychosis score of 1).

Study III   Pimozide pretreatment interaction with response to amphetamine

Of the 30 patients who received a repeat amphetamine infusion during pimozide treatment, eight had improved during the index infusion, 12

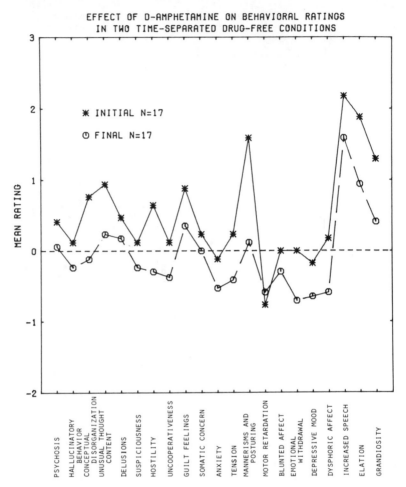

FIG. 5-4. Behavioral response profile of the amphetamine infusions during the two drug-free conditions. The final d-amphetamine infusion induced significantly less of a behavioral response than the first infusion. The decrease in activation and stimulation response in particular is intriguing as this response is genetically controlled.

had worsened, and 10 did not change. During pimozide three improved, 10 worsened and 17 did not change (Fig. 6). The type of response during pimozide was not significantly different from the type of response during the drug-free condition. The patients who worsened, improved or did not change in psychosis with the index/amphetamine infusion did not receive significantly different doses of pimozide. The dose of pimozide did not correlate significantly with the amphetamine effect on psychosis

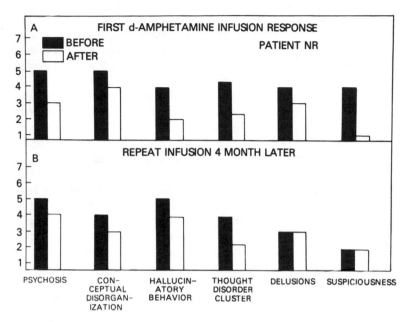

FIG. 5-5. An example of a patient who responded twice with improvement with amphetamine. Baseline state had remained the same.

D-AMPHETAMINE EFFECT ON PSYCHOSIS BEFORE AND AFTER PIMOZIDE

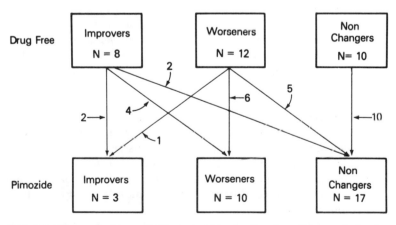

FIG. 5-6. This graph shows what happened during the pimozide d-amphetamine infusions compared to during the index infusions. Half of the patients who worsened, worsened again.

during the pimozide treatment infusion either (r_s = .06). The number of days of pimozide treatment also was not significantly different in the three groups (worsened in psychosis 35 ± 3 days; improved in psychosis 39 ± 3 days; stable 37 ± 2 days, p = NS). Figure 5 shows the effect of amphetamine infusion during pimozide treatment in the 12 patients who worsened during the index infusion. The psychosis related changes in behavior were significantly less in these patients compared to the whole group while the activating responses i.g., increased speech, elation and grandiosity were not affected. Of the ten pimozide treated patients who worsened in response to d-amphetamine, seven apparently showed a reversal of the antipsychotic effect of pimozide. These 7 patients had become less psychotic with pimozide (decreases between 1.5 and 5.3 points of the Bunney-Hamburg Psychosis Scale). In an additional patient psychosis ratings lessened one point with pimozide. Two patients did not change in psychosis with d-amphetamine: one patient was already nonpsychotic and one had become more psychotic since his index infusion. Three patients did not change their response to d-amphetamine following pimozide treatment (decrease of 3.4, 6.6, and 7.4 points on the Psychosis Scale). Of the other four patients who did not change in psychosis with the infusion, three had been non-psychotic prior to pimozide (psychosis ratings less than 4).

Study IV   Amphetamine response during pimozide withdrawal

When 12 patients were retested during the period of hypothetical dopamine receptor supersensitivity, 7 days after pimozide withdrawal, three patients worsened, one improved, and eight did not change. Of the three worseners, one had previously not changed with the index infusion, and four of the patients who had previously worsened did not change at this time, suggesting that neuroleptic drugs had induced a stabilization in the majority of patients. However, one patient improved with d-amphetamine at this particular time (Fig. 7).

Study V   Relapse Prediction

Six patients experienced an increase in psychosis and seven patients showed no change after the pimozide amphetamine infusion. The 6 worseners after the d-amphetamine infusion relapse following pimozide withdrawal within 4 to 20 days (mean 10.5 days); only one of the seven patients who showed a lack of change after the pimozide amphetamine infusion relapsed 31 days following pimozide withdrawal (Fisher Exact Test p < .005).

The two additional patients who improved acutally with amphetamine during this infusion and on whom sufficient follow-up data were available showed further improvement following discontinuation of pimozide.

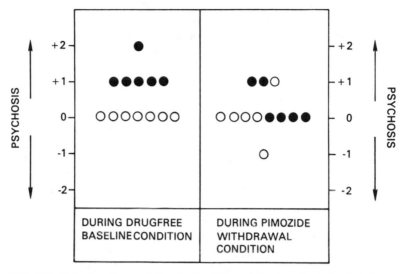

FIG. 5-7. Only 2 patients of the 6 who did so following the index infusion, worsened in response to d-amphetamine following the d-amphetamine infusion during the pimozide withdrawal (dopamine receptor supersensitivity phase). Of the 6 who did not change, one worsened and one improved. We could demonstrate an increased response to d-amphetamine post-pimozide in one patient only. 0 = no change in psychosis during the index infusion.

DISCUSSION

The most striking observation of our studies is the state dependency of the effect of the amphetamine challenge test on psychosis. During a stable psychotic or a stable non-psychotic period patients do not respond to d-amphetamine with a change in psychosis. However, during the height of decompensation or after patients have shown some improvement with neuroleptic treatment but have not yet entered a stable state, acute improvement or worsening (reversal of neuroleptic induced improvement) with amphetamine may be observed. In other words, when schizophrenics are in an unstable condition they are likely to show a response to the amphetamine challenge test. Because schizophrenia is an episodic illness, the periods of instability may come and go over time. The amphetamine challenge test may help us to delineate the unstable states of the illness preceding and following psychotic decompensation. To find the cause of this instability is probably fundamental to our understanding of schizophrenia.

Our data show an association between the response to amphetamine during neuroleptic treatment and prediction of relapse after neuroleptic withdrawal. Patients who did not respond to the amphetamine challenge test and therefore seemed to be in stable clinical state as a consequence of their neuroleptic treatment were still in the same stable clinical state three months after neuroleptic withdrawal. The patients who responded to the challenge test with an increase in psychosis, did relapse when taken off medication. The two patients who responded with an acute improvement, showed this improvement following neuroleptic drug withdrawal as described by Marder et al. (1979). Angrist et al. (1982) and Lieberman et al. (1983) showed similar results using the same paradigm with amphetamine and methylphenidate. To date approximately 50 patients have been studied this way. It is therefore fair to conclude that the challenge test as a predictor of relapse after neuroleptic withdrawal shows promise for clinical application. Studies are underway to find other biological markers to assess the continuation of neuroleptic treatment.

Amphetamine is considered to be a pharmacological stressor in man because it increases plasma cortisol, growth hormone, prolactin, beta-endorphin and norepinephrine levels (Schulz et al, 1981; van Kammen et al., 1984a). Amphetamine as a stressor in animals has recently been reviewed by Antelman and Chiodo (1983). The heterogeneous stress response to the challenge test in schizophrenia has a parallel in the response to environmental stressors. Schizophrenic episodes can be provoked by such stressors as going to college, death of a pet, military draft, etc. On the other hand severe stress (hospital fire, evacuation because of war acts) can decrease temporarily psychotic symptoms in some patients. We therefore propose that schizophrenia is an illness with abnormal behavioral responses to stress that vary over time and depend on the clinical state of the patient. Neuroleptics protect schizophrenics partially against environmental stresses (Vaughn and Leff, 1976). The psychotogenic effect of the challenge test during pimozide treatment reveals that the underlying stress sensitivity or responsiveness has not gone away.

In Study II (repeat drug-free infusion) we noticed a general decrease in response to amphetamine compared to the index infusion (Fig. 4). The decrease in response was not only observed in behavior, but also in blood pressure and pulse rate. This decrease was not observed with infusions during lithium and pimozide treatment. According to Antelman and Chiodo (1983), the intermittent use of amphetamine leads to decreased stress sensitivity in rats. This concept may explain the decreased response following intermittent amphetamine administration and provide direction for further studies in schizophrenia. For instance, intermittent amphetamine administration several weeks apart may lead to protection against stress induced decompensation and a decrease in psychotic episodes, in contrast to continuous amphetamine administration which is frequently associated with paranoid psychosis.

Improvement with amphetamine in schizophrenia may be due to relative pre and post synaptic dopamine receptor stimulation. We found CSF MHPG to predict amphetamine induced improvement (Fig. 8) which advocates a role for NE in schizophrenia as well. We reviewed elsewhere the NE system in schizophrenia (van Kammen and Antelman,

CSF MHPG ON PROBENCID vs PSYCHOSIS CHANGE AFTER D-AMPHETAMINE

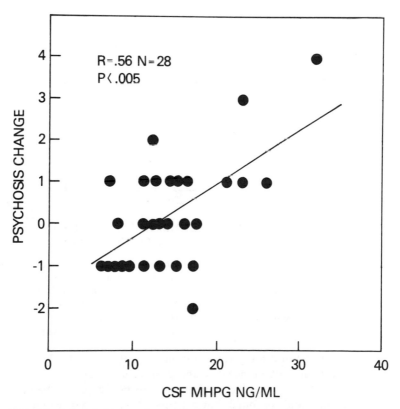

FIG. 5-8. Spinal fluid 3 methoxy-4 hydroxy-phenylglycol (MHPG) levels prior to the d-amphetamine infusion correlated significantly with the response to d-amphetamine. This MHPG level also predicted the d-amphetamine response during pimozide response in these who underwent Study III.

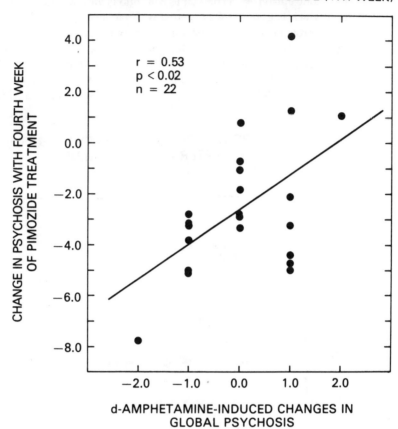

FIG. 5-9. The psychosis change during the 4th week of double-blind pimozide treatment correlated significantly with the response to d-amphetamine. Those who improved with d-amphetamine improved the most with pimozide. Those who worsened, improved with pimozide frequently also, but less so than those who showed acute improvement with amphetamine.

in press) and are presently examining the role of NE agonist in the treatment of both negative and positive symptoms.

We evaluated the amphetamine response versus the pimozide response and we found that patients who improved with amphetamine the most, also improved the most with pimozide (van Kammen et al, 1982c) (Fig. 9) (Boronow and van Kammen, 1982). Lithium has been shown to have antipsychotic effects in schizophrenia (Alexander et al,

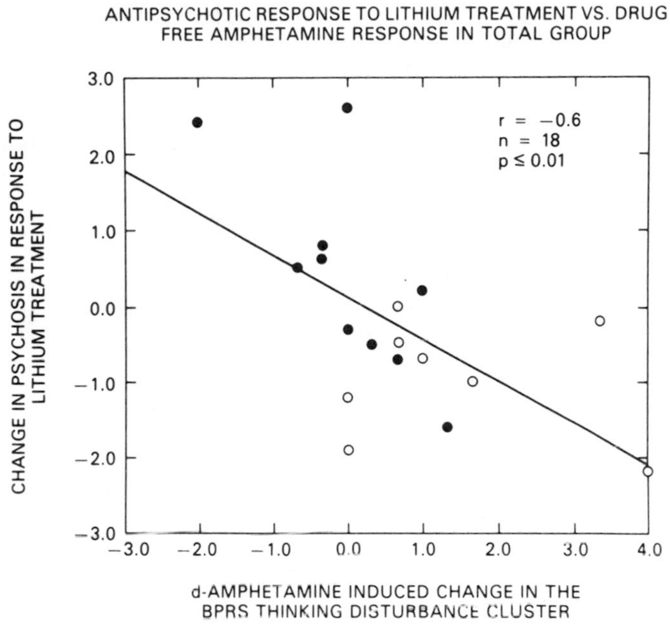

ANTIPSYCHOTIC RESPONSE TO LITHIUM TREATMENT VS. DRUG
FREE AMPHETAMINE RESPONSE IN TOTAL GROUP

FIG. 5-10. The relationship between the change in psychosis with amphetamine and the (modest) anti-psychotic response to lithium is more strongly present in the males (●) then in the female patients (○). There were no female improvers to d-amphetamine in this sub-group.

1979; Braden et al, 1982). In contrast to the pimozide response prediction study, amphetamine induced *worsening* predicted consistently a therapeutic effect of lithium (van Kammen et al, 1981) (Fig. 10). Since treatment responses to lithium and pimozide are state dependent, it is no surprise that we found amphetamine response which is also state dependent to predict treatment response to these two different drugs. Further studies are needed to establish the role of the amphetamine challenge test as an aid in the choice of pharmacological treatment.

Conceptually it seems promising to approach schizophrenia as a chronic stress susceptible disorder. This stress susceptibility leads to episodes of stress sensitivity and desensitivity. The duration of each state depends on neuroleptic treatment, spacing of environmental stressors interacting with the biochemical substrate and other unknown variables. The underlying hypothesized biochemical disregulation involves the dopamine system with NE as the major regulator of dopamine mediated behavior.

REFERENCES

Alexander, P.E., van Kammen, D.P. and Bunney, W.E., Jr.: Antipsychotic effects of lithium in schizophrenia. *Am. J. Psychiatry* 136:283-287, 1979.

Angrist, B., Sathananthan, G., Wilk, S. and Gershon, S.: Amphetamine psychosis: behavioral and biochemical aspects, *J. Psychiatry Res.* 11:13-23, 1974.

Angrist, B., Rotrosen, J. and Gershon, S.: Responses to apomorphine, amphetamine, and neuroleptics in schizophrenic subjects, *Psychopharmacology* 67:31-38, 1980.

Angrist, B., Peselow, E., Rotrosen, J. and Gershon, S.: Relationship between responses to dopamine agonists, psychopathology, neuroleptic treatment response, and need for neuroleptic maintenance in schizophrenic subjects. In: Recent Advances in Neuropsychopharmacology, Oxford, Pergamon Press, pp. 49-54, 1981.

Angrist, B., Peselow, E., Rubinstein, M., Corwin, J. and Rotrosen, J.: *Psychopharmacology* 78:128-30, 1982.

Antelman, S.M. and Chiodo, L.A.: Amphetamine as a stressor. In: Stimulants: Neurochemical, Behavioral and Clinical Perspectives, (I. Crease, ed.), Raven Press, New York, pp. 269-299, 1983.

Antelman, S.M., Eichler, A.J., Black, C.A. and Kocan, D.: Interchangeability of stress and amphetamine in sensitivation, *Science* 207:329-331, 1980.

Belart, W.: Pathogenetisches und therapeutisches aus pervitinversuchen bei schizophrenia, *Schweiz Med. Wochenschr* 2:41-42, 1942.

Bischoff, A.: Ueber eine therapeutische Verwendung der sogenannten 'Weckamine' in der Behandlung schizophrener Erregungszustande, *Monatssch. Pschyiatry Neurol.* 121:329-344, 1951.

Boronow, J.J. and van Kammen, D.P.: Scientific Proceedings, *American Psychiatric Association Meeting*, May 19, Toronto, New Research Abstract #61, 1982.

Braden, W., Fink, E.B., Qualls, C.B., Ho, C.K. and Samuels, W.O.: Lithium and chlorpromazine in psychotic inpatients, *Psychiatry Res.* 7:69-81, 1982.

Davis, J.M., Schaffer, C.B., Killian, G.A., Kinard, C. and Chan, C.: Important issues in the drug treatment of schizophrenia. *Schizophrenia Bull.* 6:70, 1980.

Docherty, J.P., van Kammen, D.P., Siris, S.G. and Marder, S.R.: Stages of onset of schizophrenic psychosis. *Am. J. Psychiatry* 135:420-426, 1978.

Gerlach, J. and Luhdorf, K.: The effect of L-DOPA on young patients with simple schizophrenia, treated with neuroleptic drugs: A double-blind crossover trial with madopar and placebo, *Psychopharmacologia* 44:105-110, 1975.

Inanaga, K., Nakazawa, Y. and Inoue, K.: Double-blind controlled study of L-DOPA Therapy in schizophrenia, *Folia Psychiatr Neurol J.* 29:123-143, 1975.

Janowsky, D.S. and Davis, J.M.: Methylphenidate, dextroamphetamine, and levamphetamine. Effects on schizophrenic symptoms, *Arch. Gen. Psychiatry* 33:304-308, 1976.

Lieberman, J.A., Kane, J.M., Gadaleta, D., Brenner, R., Lesse, M.S. and Kinon, B.: Scientific Proceedings, *American Psychiatric Assn. Meeting*, New Research Section, May 5, New York, New Research Abstract #119, 1983.

Marder, S.R., van Kammen, D.P. and Docherty, J.P.: Predicting drug-free improvement in schizophrenic psychosis, *Arch. Gen. Psychiatry* 36:1080-1085, 1979.

Meltzer, H.Y. and Stahl, S.M.: The dopamine hypothesis of schizophrenia: A review, *Schizophrenia Bull.* 2:19-76, 1976.

Schulz, S.C., van Kammen, D.P., Rogol, A.D., Ebert, M., Pickar, D., Cohen, M.R. and Naber, D.: Amphetamine increases prolactin but neither growth hormone nor beta-endorphin immunoreactivity in schizophrenic patients. *Psychopharmacology Bull.* 17:193-195, 1981.

Snyder, S.H.: The dopamine hypothesis of schizophrenia: Focus on the dopamine receptor, *Am. J. Psychiatry* 133:197-202, 1976.

Szymanski, H.V., Simon, J.C. and Gutterman, N.: Recovery from schizophrenic psychosis, *Psychiatry* 140:335-338, 1983.

Tamminga, C.A., Schaffer, M.H. and Smith, R.C.: Schizophrenic symptoms improve with apomorphine, *Science* 200:567-568, 1978.

van Kammen, D.P.: The Dopamine hypothesis in schiozophrenia revisited. *Psychoneuroendocrinology* 4:37-46, 1979.

van Kammen, D.P., Docherty, J.P. and Marder, S.R.: Lack of behavioral supersensitivity to d-amphetamine after pimozide withdrawal, *Arch. Gen. Psychiatry* 37:287-290, 1980.

van Kammen, D.P., Docherty, J.P., Marder, S.R. and Bunney, Jr., W.E.: Acute amphetamine response predicts antidepressant and antipsychotic responses to lithium carbonate in schizophrenic patients, *Psychiatry Res.* 4:313-325, 1981.

van Kammen, D.P., Bunney, Jr., W.E., Docherty, M.D., Marder, S.R., Ebert, M.H., Rosenblatt, J.E. and Rayner, J.N.: d-Amphetamine-induced heterogeneous changes in psychotic behavior in schizophrenia, *Am. J. Psychiatry* 139:991-997, 1982a.

van Kammen, D.P., Docherty, J.P. and Marder, S.R. et al.: Antipsychotic effects of pimozide in schizophrenia: treatment response prediction with acute dextroamphetamine response, *Arch. Gen. Psychiatry* 39:261-266, 1982b.

van Kammen, D.P., Docherty, J.P., Marder, S.R. and Bunney, Jr., W.E.: Long-term pimozide pretreatment differentially affects behavioral responses to dextroamphetamine in schizophrenia, *Arch. Gen. Psychiatry* 39:275-281, 1982c.

van Kammen, D.P., Docherty, J.P. and Bunney, Jr., W.E.: Prediction of early relapse after pimozide discontinuation by response to d-amphetamine during pimozide treatment. *Biol. Psychiatry* 17:233-242, 1982d.

van Kammen, D.P., Schulz, S.C. and Rogol, A.D.: Hormonal responses to d-amphetamine in schizophrenia, *Psychoneuroendocrine Dysfunc.* 549-567, 1984.

van Kammen, D.P. and van Kammen, W.B.: Amphetamine induced psychotogenic effect: A stressor. In: Catecholamines and Stress, (R. Kvetnansky and E. Usdin, eds.), 1984a. In Press.

Vaughn, C.E. and Leff, J.P.: The measurement of expressed emotion in the families of psychiatric patients. *Br. J. Soc. Clin. Psychol.* 15(2):157-165, 1976.

Zubin, J.: Chronic schizophrenia from the standpoint of vulnerability. In: Perspectives in Schizophrenia Research, (C.F. Baxter and T. Melnechuk, eds.), New York, Raven Press, pp. 269-294, 1980.

CHAPTER 6

Psychopharmacology in the Understanding of the Schizophrenias

Thomas A. Ban, M.D.
William Guy, Ph.D.
William H. Wilson, Ph.D.

INTRODUCTION

Schizophrenic disorders occur in 0.86% of the general population. This implies that 86 out of 10,000 people randomly chosen from the general population will develop one or another schizophrenic disorder during their lifetime (Tsuang and Vandermay, 1980). Almost half of all patients diagnosed as schizophrenic will need long-term treatment; and it has been estimated that 30 to 60% of all new long-term patients suffer from these disorders (Mann and Cree, 1976). There is evidence that 15% of patients who are diagnosed today as suffering from a schizophrenic disorder will become chronically hospitalized at some time in the future. Consequently, it is estimated that 1/3 to 1/2 of all psychiatric beds, i.e., 1/6 to 1/4 of all hospital beds—since nearly 50% of all beds are psychiatric—are occupied by schizophrenic patients (Todd et al., 1977).

The problem is compounded by the early onset of these disorders (Woodruff, et al., 1974). The genetic risk for children if one parent suffers from a schizophrenic disorder is approximately 12.3%, and, if both parents are schizophrenic, the risk increases to 36.6% (Slater and Cowie, 1971). Although the genetic basis and/or hereditary pattern of schizo-

This study was supported in part by grant 1-R01-M435720 from the National Institute of Mental Health.

61

phrenia are far from being fully understood, these figures imply that the risk for children of schizophrenic parents is 15 to 40 times that of the general population.

ANTIPSYCHOTIC (NEUROLEPTIC) DRUGS

Considering the size of the schizophrenic population and the availability of treatment resources, the most efficient treatment approach is the pharmacologic one. The pharmacologic agents which are the most generally effective in the treatment of schizophrenic patients are antipsychotic drugs. They are not an etiological treatment and certainly not exclusive for these disorders. Nevertheless, neuroleptics can exert rapid control in psychiatric emergencies created by the disease, can shorten the manifestations of severe psychopathology seen during an acute episode or exacerbation, can maintain patients in remission and may even prevent relapse.

The first drug was chlorpromazine, a phenothiazine consisting of 2 benzol rings connected to each other by a sulfur and nitrogen atom. It was given for the first time to a psychiatric patient by Hamon, et al. (1952) at Val de Grace, the famed military hospital in Paris. From Val de Grace, chlorpromazine therapy in psychiatry raced through the mental hospitals of France within a single year (Delay and Deniker, 1952). Swiss psychiatrists introduced chlorpromazine in January of the next year (Staehelin and Kielholz, 1953), and, by the spring of 1953, the "psychopharmacologal revolution" was well underway throughout continental Europe. The first American publication (Lehmann and Hanrahan, 1954) appeared as early as February, 1954; and one year later, the first Australian (Webb, 1955) and Russian (Tarasov, 1955) publications were also in print (Ban, 1972).

Since the introduction of chlorpromazine, a great number of neuroleptics have been synthesized. Today there are at least 19 neuroleptics distributed among five different chemical classes available for clinical use in the United States. All of these drugs are secondary or tertiary amines containing at least one aromatic ring linked to the amine position by an intermediate chain. Most of these drugs are active inhibitors of apomorphine-induced vomiting in dogs, apomorphine or amphetamine-induced stereotypic chewing and non-stereotypic agitation, and norepinephrine or epinephrine-induced mortality in rats. They also inhibit intracranial self-stimulation and conditioned operant behavior in all laboratory animals. At somewhat higher doses, neuroleptics induce cataleptic immobility with a reduction of spontaneous motility and indifference towards the environment; and, at considerably higher doses, they induce ptosis, ataxia, prostration and other symptoms of CNS depression (Janssen, 1973).

NEUROLEPTICS: ACTION MECHANISMS

Neuroleptics share numerous common clinical biochemical actions. It is rather difficult to decide which of these actions are relevant to their therapeutic effects. By stabilizing cell membrane, neuroleptics interfere with the pathophysiological action of alpha 2-globulin—the plasma protein factor allegedly responsible for schizophrenic psychopathology; by inhibiting the action of the N-methyl-transferase enzyme system, they decrease the formation of epinephrine—the precursor of the allegedly psychotoxic adrenochrome; and, by decreasing adenosine/triphosphate utilization, they interfere with increased transmethylation—presumed responsible for the production of psychotoxic dimethylated indolamines and catecholamines (Ban and McEvoy, 1982).

Since the early 1960's, there has been considerable attention paid to the dopamine (DA) receptor blockage produced by neuroleptics. The original observation that neuroleptics increase the nialamide-induced accumulation of 3-O-methylated metabolities of DA and norepinephrine, i.e., 3-methoxytyramine and normetanephrine, was made by Carlsson and Lindquist as early as 1963. However, it was more than a decade later before it was possible to demonstrate with x-ray crystallography that DA receptor blockage actually takes place (Creese et al., 1975). Furthermore, by employing radioligand-binding techniques, it was revealed that clinical potencies of neuroleptics correlate well with the binding affinities at DA_2 receptors, i.e., receptors which can be selectively labeled with 3H-haloperidol and 3H-spiroperidol (Kebabian and Calne, 1979). In addition, there is some evidence that neuroleptics also have opiate receptor binding properties (Jacquet and Marks, 1976).

BIOCHEMICAL HYPOTHESES
Dopamine: Excess or Deficiency

The finding that clinical potencies, i.e., the mg/Kg potencies of neuroleptics, correlate well with binding affinities at DA_2 receptors prompted several laboratories to search for alterations in the levels of DA and/or DA receptors in post-mortem brains of schizophrenic patients. As a result, a significantly increased number of DA_2 receptors was found in schizophrenic brains (Owen et al., 1978) as well as a 50% increase in DA content (Bird et al., 1977). There were indications, however, that the increase in the number of DA_2 receptors may have been related to neuroleptic treatment.

Supporting the hypothesis that a DA excess is related to the psychopathology seen in schizophrenic patients are the findings that their psychopathology may be precipitated and/or aggravated by the administration of methylphenidate or ethanol (both releasers of DA) and that the therapeutic effects of neuroleptics may be potentiated by adding alphamethyl-paratyrosine—a specific tyrosine hydroxylase inhibitor, or alpha-methyldopa—a non-specific dopa decarboxylase inhibitor, i.e., substances which interfere with the formation of DA, to the treatment regime (Snyder, 1976).

Nevertheless, recent findings have created some doubt about the DA excess hypothesis (Fischman, 1983). The essential point in the argument against the hypothesis is based on the amphetamine model of schizophrenia. The timing of the onset of amphetamine psychosis coincides more closely with DA depletion than with increased availability (Alpert and Friedhoff, 1980). Furthermore, there are even data in favor of a DA deficiency hypothesis of schizophrenia. Fukuda and Mitsuda (1979) found that amphetamines may enhance the therapeutic effects of neuroleptics; and Van Kammen et al. (1982) showed that amphetamines may reduce psychotic symptoms in some schizophrenics.

Prostaglandin: Deficiency or Excess

The link between the DA excess hypothesis and the prostaglandin deficiency (PG) hypothesis of schizophrenia is prolactin, a potent stimulator of PG synthesis. Since the release of prolactin is controlled by DA, the neuroleptic-induced DA receptor blockage produces an excess of prolactin and consequently an increase in PG synthesis.

The hypothesis that schizophrenia is a PG deficiency disease has evolved from observations that schizophrenic patients are relatively resistant to pain and inflammation and are free of rheumatoid arthritis, i.e., conditions in which PG plays an important role; PG antagonists, e.g., chloroquine, quinine, quinacrine, may, in high doses, induce schizophrenic-like states; therapeutically effective neuroleptics stimulate the production of prolactin and drugs which precipitate or aggravate schizophrenia, e.g., levodopa, cortisol, suppress secretion and/or block prolactin effects (Horrobin, 1977). Further, the results of two pilot studies in which penicillin, a substance which mobilizes dihomo-gamma-linolenic acid (DGLA)—the rate limiting step in PGE_1 synthesis, has shown some therapeutic effects in chronic schizophrenics (Chouinard et al., 1978).

In opposition to the proposition that schizophrenia is a PG deficiency disease, it has been suggested that schizophrenia is a disease of PG excess, i.e., the result of an excessive release of PGE_1 into the hypopothalamus with an accompanying elevation of temperature (Feldberg, 1976). Although Falloon et al. (1978) found no evidence that paracetamol,—a substance which reduces PGE_1 levels—had any therapeutic effect in acute schizophrenic patients, Gjessing (1953) reported febrile episodes in two-thirds of his special group of catatonic patients.

Endorphins: Excess or Deficiency

Beta-endorphin has been shown to have the diametrically opposite effect to that of prolactin in PGE synthesis in that it blocks the mobilization of DGLA and the formation of PGE_1. Terenius et al. (1976) reported on elevated CSF beta-endorphin levels in schizophrenic patients. Since successful neuroleptic treatment decreased CSF beta-endorphin concentrations, the possibility of a positive relationship between CSF endorphin concentrations and the severity of schizophrenic psychopathology was raised. Further, since naloxone, by occupying endorphin receptors, reversed beta-endorphin induced catatonia in animals, it was hypothesized that naloxone might have a therapeutic effect in schizophrenia. However, the initial favorable therapeutic effects of intravenous naloxone administration could be replicated only in two out of eight subsequent clinical experiments (Volavka et al., 1977).

Conversely, it has also been suggested that decreased availability of beta-endorphin to the cerebral opiate receptor sites may have the same effect (Jacquet and Marks, 1976). Within this latter frame of reference, the catatonia induced by beta-endorphin in rats was conceived to be similar to that seen with neuroleptics. Schizophrenic psychopathological symptoms were believed to be the result of a deficiency in the production of an endogenous neuroleptic peptide which can be replaced by exogenous neuroleptic drugs. In favor of this hypothesis is the opiate receptor binding property of endorphins and neuroleptics; and the finding that, of all CNS regions, the striatum has the highest opiate-binding capacity. Also supportive of this position are the findings that, in at least three schizophrenic patients, intravenous beta-endorphin administration produced a reduction and/or disappearance of auditory hallucinations, paranoid ideation and pathological pressure of thought (Kline et al., 1977).

NEUROLEPTICS: LONG-TERM EFFECTS

The origin of the DA excess hypothesis lies in careful studies on the action mechanism of neuroleptics. However, while it is acceptable to make inferences on the nature of a disorder from the action mechanism of drugs with exclusive effectiveness in well-defined diseases, similar tactics in case of an ill-defined illness are questionable. It is difficult to understand how the DA excess hypothesis of schizophrenia actually evolved, because antipsychotic/neuroleptics are far from being exclusive treatment for schizophrenia; they are just as effective a treatment for mania and for some of organic psychoses. They certainly don't "cure" schizophrenia and are useful only in some schizophrenic patients in the prevention of relapse. Considering this, it should not be surprising that this artificially-created "neuroleptic responsive" singular disease eludes definition and creates a situation in which even the opposite hypothesis becomes defensible. Indeed, the DA deficiency, PGE_1 excess and beta-endorphin deficiency hypotheses of schizophrenia are even less defendable than the DA excess, PGE_1 deficiency and beta-endorphin excess hypotheses.

It is rather paradoxical that while some biochemists and pharmacologists want to "invent a disease," some sociologists, along with some psychiatrists, are trying to deny the existence of a group of disorders. Neuroleptics, together with the improvement of milieu in psychiatric hospitals, have considerably transformed the prevailing manifestations of schizophrenic disorders. Perhaps this has made it possible for Szasz (1961), a professor of psychiatry, to argue that mental illness is a myth and for Scheff (1970), a professor of sociology, to assert that mental illness is nothing but a label for a wide "residual" category of social offenders.

Another consequence of the transformation in the prevailing manifestations of schizophrenia is that a large proportion of patients who previously would have been hospitalized are now discharged from hospitals. As a result, there is an increase in the psychiatric population within the community with a comparable increase in fertile marriages among community-based schizophrenics (Erlenmeyer-Kimling et al., 1969). Implicit in these fertility gains relevant to the general population is a small, but important, shift in the structure of the population gene pool. This, of course, is not expected to lead to an abrupt rise in the incidence of schizophrenia. What can be forseen, however, is the gradual accumulation of alleles, the gradual dispersion of alleles throughout larger segments of the population and an eventual increase in the proportion of persons who may be affected.

Irrespective of the possible consequences on society, long-term treatment with neuroleptics may produce serious adverse effects in patients receiving them. While skin pigmentation occurs in less than 0.1% of all patients treated with phenothiazines for a period of two years or more (Lehmann and Ban, 1974), the estimated incidence of ocular changes is as high as 20 to 35% in patients receiving phenothiazines over an extended period. The prevalence of tardive dyskinesia, the most serious long-term complication, ranges from 0.5 to 40% (Ban, 1979).

To reduce the occurrence of these complications and eliminate at least those attributable to the indiscriminate use of neuroleptic drugs, it is of crucial importance to develop techniques which can identify those schizophrenic patients who require maintenance treatment from those who do not. While there is little, if any, evidence that patients with different types of schizophrenia, as classified by the DSM-III or ICD-9, would respond differentially to neuroleptics, there are indications for differential therapeutic responsiveness to neuroleptics in the different subtypes of schizophrenia described in Leonhard's classification.

LEONHARD'S CLASSIFICATION AND RESPONSE
TO NEUROLEPTICS

Leonhard's classification of the schizophrenias is divided into unsystematic schizophrenias and systematic schizophrenias. Leonhard believes these schizophrenias have essentially nothing to do with each other, and one rarely has any trouble differentiating between systematic and unsystematic schizophrenia because the symptom picture and course are different. The systematic schizophrenias display a creeping progressive course while the unsystematic may go into remission. Within the unsystematic schizophrenias are found (1) affect-laden paraphrenia—in which there is anxiety related to the ideas of reference and hallucinations; (2) cataphasia (schizophasia)—lively, confused, compulsive speech as if they were speaking in a foreign language; and (3) periodic catatonia involves both hyperkinetic and akinetic states, negativistic behavior, little motivation followed by sudden outbursts of exaggerated laughter, senseless movements, and sterotyped postures. Remission of symptoms regularly follow acute outbursts. The systematic schizophrenic pictures are found in the end state of the disease. Systematic forms of the disease generally have a creeping onset. Systematic schizophrenias are divided into catatonic forms—parakinetic affected, proskinetic, negativistic voluble, sluggish; hebephrenic forms—silly, eccentric, insipid, autistic; and paranoid forms—hypochondriacal, phonemic, incoherent, fantastic, confabulatory, expansive. These subgroups are defined by the prominent symptom picture.

In a clinical study involving 474 chronic schizophrenic patients, Fish (1964) found that 117 out of 123 nonsystematic schizophrenics (95%) showed a favorable therapeutic response to neuroleptics, while only 279 out of 351 systematic schizophrenics (69%) showed a favorable response. Further, among the nonsystematic schizophrenics, the favorable therapeutic response was rated marked to moderate in 79% of the treatment responsive patients, while among the systematic schizophrenics only 23% were so rated. Fish also noted that, despite the generally favorable neuroleptic response found among nonsystematic schizophrenic patients, patients suffering from periodic catatonia responded somewhat less favorably than patients with affect-laden paraphrenia or cataphasia. Further analyses of the FISH data revealed that, although 79% of the patients from the group of disorders under systematic schizophrenia showed a favorable therapeutic response, therapeutic responsiveness was not evenly distributed among the three major classes of illness within this group; i.e., paraphrenia hebephrenia and catatonia. Thus, while as many as 40% of the paraphrenics showed a moderate or marked therapeutic response to neuroleptics, only 23% of the hebephrenics and 0.9% of the systematic catatonics showed a similar response pattern. Paradoxically, catatonia is the only class among the systematic schizophrenias which has shown a significant decrease during the past years as reflected in the differences between a German (Leonhard, 1974) sample (21.7%) and a Norwegian (Astrup, 1979) sample (8.2%). It is important to note, however, that the decrease in the number of systematic catatonics appears to have begun prior to the neuroleptic era and with the introduction of milieu therapies in mental hospitals. Considering all this, treatment with DA receptor blocker neuroleptics may not have a major role in the therapy of catatonic disorders.

Supporting this contention are the observations of a 14-year old boy who was admitted to the hospital because of sudden onset of delusional thinking with catatonic manifestations; e.g., waxy flexibility, mutism and bizarre posturing. Associated with these symptoms during the first ten days were high temperature (101°F), tachycardia (130/min), hypertension (160/100 Hg mm), epistaxis, nausea and vomiting—and, apart from low (1.6 ng/ml) testosterone levels, no other abnormal laboratory findings, raising the diagnostic possibility of febrile catatonia. Febrile catatonia, according to Feldberg (1976), may be related to PG excess, since PGE_1, when injected in the third ventricle of cats, produces catalepsy along with fever. The patient was treated with haloperidol in gradually increasing dosages up to 200 mg/day—later supplemented with 400 mg of chlorpromazine daily. Since the patient failed to respond to this treatment regime after four weeks, chlorpromazine was discontinued and haloperidol tapered off to 30 mg/day. With the lowering of dose, the patient improved sufficiently to be allowed to go home on a trial visit. He returned to the hospital exhibiting a dramatic exacerbation of symptoms. During the efforts to identify factors responsible for the exacerbation, it was found that the patient's mother had withheld medication during his home visit and that the exacerbation closely followed our "re-initiation" of haloperidol treatment. Neuroleptics were then discontinued completely and delusional thinking and catatonic manifestations remitted within a couple of weeks. Three months later, on follow-up, the patient continued to remain symptom-free without medication. Since these catatonic manifestations were present prior to neuroleptic administration, the possibility that they were drug-induced can be excluded. The nature of the patient's thought disorder excluded a diagnosis of an affective episode. The findings that an increase in the dosage of neuroleptics was associated with exacerbation, a decrease in dosage with amelioration, and discontinuation of medication with remission of psychopathological symptoms suggest that neuroleptics may have played a role in sustaining psychopathology in this patient (Kelwala and Ban, 1981a).

Systematic Hebephrenias

In the aforementioned patient whose differential diagnosis within Leonhard's system of classification was between periodic catatonia (a nonsystematic subtype) and hyperkinetic-akinetic motility psychosis (a type of cycloid psychosis), neuroleptics seemed to have a negative therapeutic effect. In two shallow hebephrenic patients, the usefulness of maintaining neuroleptic treatment was questionable.

Insipid hebephrenia is one of the subtypes of the systematic schizophrenias and is characterized by extreme flatness of affect, meager symptomatology and episodic outbursts of hallucinatory excitement. While the illness has an insidious onset, it progresses rapidly to a state of moderate defect although some capacity for work is retained. One of the two patients was a 39 year old female who had been hospitalized for over 15 years. Her predominant psychopathological symptoms were flat affect, lack of interest and spontaneity with episodic hallucinatory excitement. Neuroleptic treatment did not appear to have any lasting therapeutic effects. She was receiving 40 mg of thiothixene daily when her medication was gradually withdrawn. Discontinuation of medication had no detectable effect even after one year of abstinence. The second patient was a 27 year old male who had been hospitalized for over four years. His predominant psychopathological manifestations were similar to those of the first patient. He was receiving 60 mg of haloperidol daily when his medication was gradually withdrawn. Again, discontinuation of medication had no detectable effect after four drug-free months (Kelwala and Ban, 1981b).

In a survey of 40 chronic hospitalized patients from one of our clinical research wards, it was noted that almost one-half of the patients (49%) manifested signs of tardive dyskinesia. Most important, however, was the observation that the occurrence of tardive dyskinesia seemed to be differentiately present in the different types of patients. Patients with illnesses belonging to one of Leonhard's systematic schizophrenias seemed to manifest tardive dyskinesia three times as often as patients with illnesses belonging to the nonsystematic schizophrenias. Among the systematic schizophrenias, hebephrenic subtypes exhibited tardive dyskinesia three times more often than paraphrenic subtypes. If these findings are sustained in controlled clinical studies, then one would need to consider that maintenance and/or prophylactic therapy is not only ineffective, but may also be harmful for certain patient subgroups of schizophrenic patients subsumed under the general rubric of schizophrenia.

Nonsystematic Schizophrenias

In another study by Prakash, the notion that neuroleptic treatment may not just be ineffective but may also be harmful received further substantiation in a survey of 24 patients treated with lithium/neuroleptic combinations. A common characteristic of these patients was that they had previously shown insufficient therapeutic response to antipsychotic drugs alone. Analyses of data revealed that nine out of 10 patients of the nonsystematic population exhibited a favorable therapeutic response to the combination; while nine out of 14 "systematic" patients showed no response or an unfavorable therapeutic response. Additionally, five of the 24 patients developed neurotoxicity during the course of treatment. Two of the five patients were silly hebephrenics and one each belonged to the expansive, fantastic and confabulatory subtypes of paraphrenia. Thus, while five out of the 14 patients with systematic schizophrenia manifested neurotoxicity, none of the 10 patients with nonsystematic schizophrenia (predominantly affect-laden paraphrenia) developed a similar undesirable response to the lithium/neuroleptic combination (Prakash et al., 1982).

Paraphrenias: Systematic and Nonsystematic

In contrast to the catatonic and some hebephrenic types, patients with the various paraphrenic illnesses seem to respond most favorably to neuroleptic drugs; e.g., among the nonsystematic schizophrenias, patients with affect-laden paraphrenia, and among the systematic schizophrenias, patients with phonemic, hypochondriacal, confabulatory and expansive paraphrenia. There are also some indications that fantastic and incoherent paraphrenics require excessively high dosages of neuroleptics to obtain satisfactory therapeutic effects.

CONCLUSIONS

The several biochemical hypotheses as to the pathophysiology of schizophrenia have been reviewed. Pharmacotherapy of the schizophrenias according to Leonhard's classification has been presented. Whether these relate to different pathophysiology is questioned. Observations on differential responsiveness to neuroleptics have been presented in an attempt to link the different response patterns to clinically different patient populations. The dangers of confounding the action mechanism of a drug with the etiology of an illness have been described in the hope that they will emphasize that neuropharmacology and/or neurochemistry alone are not adequate substitutes for precise clinical psychopathology.

Patients subsumed under the rubric of schizophrenia do not show a uniform therapeutic response to neuroleptics—especially during the maintenance and prophylactic phases of treatment. Patients with illnesses belonging to Leonhard's nonsystematic schizophrenias generally show a more favorable response to neuroleptics than patient belonging to the group of systematic schizophrenias. Within the systematic schizophrenias, patients with illnesses of the paraphrenic type show a more favorable response than patients with illnesses of the hebephrenic type. Catatonic patients (either nonsystematic or systematic) respond least favorably to neuroleptics.

The clinical observations that there may be an increased occurrence of adverse effects when neuroleptics, alone or in combination with lithium, are prescribed to heterogeneous patient populations needs to be verified in well-controlled clinical studies. However, the observations may serve as signals that, for the optimal utilization of new drugs, a reevaluation of traditional nosological concepts in psychiatry is urgently needed. These issues have been discussed by Goldberg in this book.

REFERENCES

Alpert, M. and Friedhoft, A.J.: An un-dopamine hypothesis of schizophrenia. *Schizo. Bull.* 6:387-392, 1980.

Astrup, C: The Chronic Schizophrenias. Universitatsforlaget. Oslo, 1979.

Ban, T.A.: Adverse effects in maintenance treatment: Practical and theoretical considerations. *Prog. Neuro-Psychopharmacol.* 3:231-244, 1979.

Ban TA: Schizophrenia. A Psychopharmacological Approach. Charles C. Thomas, Springfield, 1972.

Ban, T.A. and McEvoy, J.: La esquizoprenia: diagnostico bioquimica y tratamiento. *Salud Mental* 5:30-34, 1982.

Bird, I.D., Barnes, J., Iversen, L. L., Spokes, E.G., MacKay, A.V.P. and Shepherd, M.: Increased brain dopamine and reduced glutamic acid decarboxylate and choline acetyltransferase activity in schizophrenia and related psychoses. *Lancet* II:1157-1158, 1977.

Carlsson, A. and Lindquist, M.: Effect of chlorpromazine or haloperidol on formation of 3-methoxytramine and normetanephrine in mouse brain. *Acta Pharmacol. et Toxicol.* 20:140-144, 1963.

Chouinard, G., Annable, L. and Horrobin, D.F.: An antipsychotic action of penicillin in schizophrenia. *IRCS Journal of Medical Science* 6:187-188, 1978.

Creese, I., Burt, D.R. and Snyder, S.H.: Dopamine receptor binding: Differentiation of agonist and antagonist states with 3H-dopamine and 3H-haloperidol. *Life Sciences* 17:993-1002, 1975.

Delay, J. and Deniker, P.: 38 cas de psychoses traitées par la cure prolongée et continué de 4560 RP. *CR. Congr. Alien. Neurol.* (France) 50:497-502, 1952.

Erlenmeyer-Kimling, L., Nicol, S., Rainer, J.D. and Deming, W.E: Changes in fertility rates of schizophrenic patients in New York State. *Am. J. Psychiat.* 125:916-927, 1969.

Falloon, I., Watt, D.C., Lubbe, K. et al.: N-acetyl-p-aminophenol (paracetamol, acetaminophen) in the treatment of acute schizophrenia. *Psychological Medicine* 8:495-499, 1978.

Feldberg, W.: Possible association of schizophrenia with a disturbance in prostaglandin metabolism: A physiological hypothesis. *Psychological Medicine* 6:359-369, 1976.

Fischman, L.G.: Dreams, hallucinogenic drug states, and schizophrenia: A psychological and biological comparison. *Schizo. Bull.* 9:73-94, 1983.

Fish, F.: The influence of the tranquilizers on the Leonhard schizophrenic syndromes. *Encephale* 1:245-249, 1964.

Fukuda, T. and Mitsuda, H. (eds.): World Issues in the Problems of Schizophrenic Psychoses. Igaku Shoiu, Tokyo, 1979.

Gjessing, T.: Beitrage zur Somatologie der periodischen Katatonie V. *Archiv fur Psychiatrie und Nervenkrankheiten* 191:191-219, 1953.

Hanon, J., Paraire, J. and Velluz, J.: Remarques sur l'action du 4560 RP sur l'agitat on maniaque. *Ann. Medicopsychol.* (Paris) 110:331-335, 1952.

Horrobin, D.F.: Schizophrenia, a prostaglandin deficiency disease. *Lancet* 1:936-937, 1977.

Jacquet, Y.F. and Marks, N.: The C-fragment of β-lipotropin: An endogenous neuroleptic or antipsychotogen. *Science* 194:632-635, 1976.

Janssen, P.A.J.: Structure-activity relations and drug design. In: International Encyclopedia of Pharmacology and Therapeutics, (G. Peters, ed.), Vol. I, Pergamon Press, Oxford, 1973.

Kebabian, J.W. and Calne, D.B.: Multiple receptors for dopamine. *Nature* 277:92-93, 1979.

Kelwala, S., and Ban, T.A.: Febrile catatonia sustained by neuroleptics. *The Psychiatric Journal of the University of Ottawa* 6:135, 1981a.

Kelwala, S., and Ban, T.A.: Is maintenance neuroleptic therapy necessary in shallow hebephrenia? *J. Clin. Psychiatry* 42:482, 1981b.

Kline, N.S., Choh, H.C., Lehmann, H.E. et al.: β-endorphin induced changes in schizophrenic and depressed patients. *Arch. Gen. Psychiat.* 34:1111-1113, 1977.

Lehmann, H.E. and Ban, T.A.: Sex differences in long-term adverse effects of phenothiazines. In: (I.S. Forrest, C.F. Carr and E. Usdin, eds.), The Phenothiazines and Structurally Related Drugs, Raven Press, New York, 1974.

Lehmann, H.E. and Harrahan, G.E.: Chlorpromazine, new inhibiting agent for psychomotor excitement and manic states. *Arch. Neurol. Psychiat.* 71:227-237, 1964.

Leonhard, K.: The Classification of Endogenous Psychoses. English Translation. Irvington, New York, 1979.

Mann, S.A. and Cree, W.: New long-stay psychiatric patients: A national sample survey of fifteen mental hospitals in England and Wales 1972/1973. *Psychol. Med.* 6:603-616, 1976.

Owen, F., Cross, A.J., Crow, T.J., Longden, A., Poulter, M. and Riley, G.J.: Increased dopamine receptor sensitivity in schizophrenia. *Lancet* II:223-224, 1978.

Prakash, R., Kelwala, S. and Ban, T.A.: Neurotoxicity with combined administration of lithium and a neuroleptic. *Compr. Psychiat.* 23:567-571, 1982.

Scheft, T.J.: Schizophrenia as ideology. *Schizo. Bull.* 2:15-19, 1970.

Slater, E. and Cowie, V.: The Genetics of Mental Disorder. Oxford University Press, London, 1971.

Snyder, S.H.: The dopamine hypothesis of schizophrenia. Focus on dopamine receptor. *Am. J. Psychiatry* 133:197-200, 1976.

Staehelin, J.E. and Kielholz, P.: Largactil, ein neues vegetatives Dampfungsmittel bei psychischen Störungen. *Schweiz. Med. Wschr.* 83:581-586, 1953.

Szasz, T.S.: The Myth of Mental Illness. Harper Brothers, New York, 1961.

Tarasov, G.K.: Aminazine. Review of the literature on the psychiatric use of a phenothiazine derivative. *Zh. Nervopat. Psikhiat.* Korsakov 55:296-310, 1955.

Terenius, L., Wahlstrom, A., Lindstrom, L. and Widerlow, E.: Increased CSF levels of endorphines in chronic psychosis. *Neuro-science Letters* 3:157-162, 1976.

Todd, N.A., Bennie, E.H. and Carlisle, J.M.: Some features of new long-stay male schizophrenics. *Brit. J. Psychiat.* 129:424-427, 1977.

Tsuang, M.T. and Vandermay, R.: Genes and the Mind. Oxford University Press, New York, 1980.

Van Kammen, D.P., Docherty, J.P., Marder, S.R., Schulz, S.C., Dalton, L. and Bunney, W.E.,Jr.: Antipsychotic effect of pimoxide in schizophrenia. *Arch. Gen. Psychiat.* 39:261-266, 1982.

Volavka, J., Mallya, A., Gaig, S. and Perez-Cruet, J.: Naloxone in the chronic schizophrenias. *Science* 196:1227-1228, 1977.

Webb, R.R.: "Largactil" in psychiatry. *Med. J. Aust.* 1:759-761, 1955.

Woodruff, R.A. Jr., Goodwin, D.W. and Guze, S.B.: Psychiatric Diagnosis. Oxford University Press, London, 1974.

CHAPTER 7

The Antipsychotic and Neuroleptic-like Action of γ-Type Endorphins

Wim M.A. Verhoeven
Jan M. Van Ree
Frans H.M. Verhey
Vaclav Filip
David De Wied

ENDORPHINS AND PSYCHOPATHOLOGY
Introduction

Since the discovery in the early 1970's of specific opiate binding sites in brain tissue (Terenius, 1973; Simon et al., 1973; Pert and Snyder, 1973) and the subsequent isolation of substances with morphine-like actions from brain extracts or cerebrospinal fluid (Terenius and Wahlström, 1975; Pasternak et al., 1975; Hughes, 1975), several endogenous opioid peptides, endorphins, have been isolated. The known opioid peptides derive from three different precursor proteins, which contain repetitive structures of the different endorphins. Firstly, the pro-enkephalin system, yielding met- and leu-enkephalin, which is located peripherally, particularly in the adrenal modulla, and centrally in nerve terminals of widely distributed short neuronal pathways (Hughes et al., 1975; Watson et al., 1979; Noda et al., 1982; Comb et al., 1982). Secondly, the pro-opiomelano-cortin (POMC) system, which is located predominantly in the pituitary and, to a lesser degree, also in the brain. From the basal hypothalamus, i.e. the nucleus arcuatus, this system spreads to several structures of the limbic system and to the brain stem. POMC is the precursor molecule of ACTH and β-lipotropin (β-LPH) and β-LPH is the precursor molecule of β-endorphin (Mains et al., 1977; Watson et al., 1979; Nakanishi et al., 1979). Proteolytic processing of β-endorphin (BE) yields γ-endorphin (BE 1-17) and α-endorphin (BE 1-16) (Austen et al., 1977; Burbach et al., 1980). Thirdly, the pro-dynorphin system, which is the common precursor of α- and β-neo-endorphin and the dynorphins and which is located in the hypothalamic-hypophyseal neuronal system but also in other brain regions such as the hippocampus (Goldstein et al., 1979; Kakidani et al., 1982; Watson et al., 1981, 1983).

Soon after their discovery, the endorphins have been implicated in chronic pain and various psychopathological syndromes such as psychoses, depressions, mania and addiction. Interest has been focussed mainly on the schizophrenic psychoses. In principle three lines of research have been followed: 1. endorphin excess, evaluated by analyses of endorphin levels in blood and CSF and by treating schizophrenic patients with hemodialysis and opiate-antagonists; 2. endorphin deficiency resulting in the administration of β-endorphin and the synthetic met-enkephalin analogue FK 33-824 to schizophrenic patients; and 3. disturbances in the fragmentation of β-endorphin. The first two research lines are discussed by Doctor Ban in the preceding chapter and will not further be discussed.

Disturbances in β-endorphin fragmentation
Behavioral effects of endorphins

In animal experiments the endorphins related to the POMC system mimic opiates in inducing a variety of behavioral effects e.g. antinociception, hypothermia, excessive grooming, profound immobilisation, muscular rigidity, experimental addiction and development of tolerance and physical dependence. Most, if not all of these effects can be blocked by treatment with opiate antagonists like naloxone and naltrexone (Van Ree et al., 1976, 1979; Bloom et al., 1976; Wei and Loh, 1976; Gispen et al., 1976; Segal et al., 1977; Holaday et al., 1978).

In addition to their morphinomimetric properties, the endorphins induce behavioral effects which are apparently not mediated via opiate receptors, in that these effects persist in the presence of the opiate antagonist naltrexone and after removal of the N-terminal amino acid tyrosine which is essential for opiate-like activity (De Wied et al., 1978a; Van Ree et al., 1980a). Extinction of pole jumping avoidance behavior was delayed by β-endorphin and some of its fragments, e.g. α-endorphin and βE 1-9 (De Wied et al., 1978a). Interestingly, γ-endorphin and, in particular, the non-opiate γ-endorphin fragment, des-Tyr^1-γ-endorphin (DTγE; βE 2-17), had an opposite effect in that these peptides facilitated extinction of pole jumping avoidance behavior, an effect that is similar to that of neuroleptic drugs. Further studies revealed that the effects of DTγE in several aspects are comparable to those of haloperidol and that α-endorphin and its non-opiate fragment, des-Tyr^1-α-endorphin (DTαE; βE 2-16), induced behavioral effects which resemble those observed after administration of psychostimulant drugs like amphetamine (De Wied et al., 1978b; Van Ree et al., 1980a; Van Ree, 1982). In view of this, De Wied (1978) postulated that DTγE, or a closely related neuropeptide, may be an endogenous peptide with neuroleptic-like activity and consequently may be implicated in psychoses, particularly schizophrenia.

Subsequently, several fragments of γ-endorphin were tested on neuroleptic-like activity using facilitation of extinction of pole jumping avoidance behavior, induction of grasping responses and inhibition of apomorphine-induced decreased locomotion as test procedures. These studies revealed that des-enkephalin-γ-endorphin (DEγE; βE 6-17) is the shortest sequence with similar activity as DTγE (De Wied et al., 1980; Van Ree et al., 1982a), suggesting that DEγE rather than DTγE may be the active fragment mediating the neuroleptic-like effects of γ-type endorphins. On the basis of these animal data, it was hypothesized that a balanced generation of α- and γ-type endorphins may be essential for brain homeostatic mechanisms and that consequently an imbalance of these peptides, resulting in a reduced bio-availability of the γ-type endorphins, may be involved in the pathogenesis of schizophrenic psychoses (De Wied, 1978, 1983).

γ-type endorphins and brain dopamine

It has been suggested that a hyperactivity of dopaminergic (DA) systems in specific limbic brain structures, particularly the nucleus accumbens, plays a key role in the pathogenesis of schizophrenia and that the antipsychotic action of neuroleptics is related to their DA-blocking action (Synder, 1972, 1973; Mathhijse, 1974; Crow et al., 1977). Thus, the influence of γ-type endorphins on brain DA-ergic systems was extensively investigated.

It was found that DTγE, like haloperidol, increased the α-methyl-para-tyrosine induced disappearance of DA in some restricted brain areas, while α-endorphin had the opposite effect (Versteeg et al., 1979, 1982). In subsequent animal experiments the interaction of γ-type endorphins with the effects of DA-agonists was studied since neuroleptics attenuate the effects of the directly (apomorphine) or indirectly (amphetamine) acting DA-mimetics. Following systemic administration, DEγE dose-dependently antagonized the hypoactivity induced by low doses of apomorphine but had no effect on the hyperactivity and sterotypy elicited by relatively high doses of apomorphine or amphetamine (Van Ree et al., 1982a,b).

According to the concept of Carlsson (1975), the effect of low doses of apomorphine may result from stimulation of presynaptically located self-inhibiting DA-receptor systems, while the effect of high doses is presumably generated via stimulation of the post-synaptically located DA-receptors. In view of this, it was suggested that γ-type endorphins interfere with presynaptically located DA-receptors. Subsequent studies revealed that the nucleus accumbens may be the site where apomorphine and γ-type endorphins interact. Low doses of γ-type endorphins injected directly into the nucleus accumbens antagonized the decrease of loco-motion induced by intra-accumbal administration of low doses of apo-morphine (Van Ree and Wolterink, 1981; Van Ree et al., 1982b). Inter-estingly, this effect was mimicked by low doses of the classical neuro-leptic haloperidol and the atypical neuroleptic sulpiride (Van Ree et al., 1982b; Serra et al., 1983). Thus, γ-type endorphins like classical and atypical neuroleptics interact with certain presumably presynaptically located DA-receptor systems in the nucleus accumbens. Also other stud-ies on grooming and passive avoidance behavior and electrical self stim-ulation revealed that the nucleus accumbens is an important site of action of γ-type endorphins (Gispen et al., 1980; Kovács et al., 1982; Van Ree and Otte, 1980).

Further studies were focussed on the regulatory influences of these peptides on γ-type endorphin sensitive DA-receptor systems in the nu-cleus accumbens. Subchronic treatment (4 days) with DEγE enhanced the apomorphine induced hypoactivity suggesting alterations in DA-receptor sensitivity (Van Ree et al., 1982a,b). Accordingly, chronic intra-accumbal treatment (10 days) with DEγE resulted in a decreased loco-motion (Van Ree et al., 1982d). On the other hand chronic treatment with γ-type endorphin antiserum into the nucleus accumbens induced hyperactivity, which outlasts the treatment with antiserum (Van Ree et al., (Van Ree et al., 1982d). These data suggest that γ-type endorphins are physiologically involved in the control of the activity of certain DA-ergic systems. It was inferred that γ-type endorphins modulate the set-point for feedback regulation in neurons equipped with γ-type endor-phin sensitive DA-receptor systems. Thus, a chronic deficiency of γ-type endorphins could eventually lead to a subsensitivity of γ-type endorphin sensitive DA-receptor systems resulting in a sustained increase of DA-release and activity. Conversely, chronic treatment with these peptides may lead to a diminished DA-release and consequently to a decreased DA-activity. In this way the hypothesis assuming a deficiency of γ-type endorphins in schizophrenia could be linked in some way to the DA-hypothesis of schizophrenia (Van Ree and De Wied, 1982).

CLINICAL STUDIES WITH γ-TYPE ENDORPHINS
Outline of the studies

To test the hypothesis that the neuroleptic-like γ-type endorphins may have an antipsychotic action in schizophrenic patients, we performed clinical trials in which DTγE or DEγE was administered to patients suffering from different types of schizophrenia or schizo-affective psychoses. So far, we have completed a number of clinical trials including a total of 43 patients treated with DTγE and 17 patients treated with DEγE (Verhoeven et al., 1979, 1981, 1982, 1983). The outline of the studies is mentioned in Table 1. In addition, outside official protocols, 4 patients were treated with 3 mg DEγE i.m. for 10 days following a double-blind design. All patients showed positive psychotic symptoms such as delusions, hallucinations and/or thought disturbances. Most of the patients were relatively resistant to neuroleptic treatment and had relapsed several times despite maintenance therapy with conventional neuroleptic drugs. In the 3rd and 4th study with DTγE, the effects of peptide treatment in neuroleptic-free patients on pituitary function, i.e. hormonal secretion as well as the influences on the metabolism of serotonin, dopamine and noradrenaline were studied.

TABLE 1. Clinical trials with γ-type endorphins in schizophrenia

Study	Number of patients	Design	Neuroleptic medication	Peptide treatment	Scoring of symptoms
DTγE Peptide					
1	6	Open	Discontinued 1 wk before trial	8-14 days; 1 mg i.m. daily	PSSS daily BRPS before and after treatment
2	8*	Double-blind cross-over	Maintained	8 Days; 1 mg i.m. daily	PSSS daily BPRS before and after treatment
3	10	Double-blind cross-over	Discontinued >3 wk before trial	10 Days; 1 mg i.m. daily	PSSS and BPRS daily CGIS after treatment
4	20**	Double-blind cross-over	Discontinued >3 wk before trial	10 Days; 1 mg i.m. daily	PSSS and BPRS daily CGIS after treatment
DEγE Peptide					
1	4	Single-blind	Maintained	10 Days; 1 or 10 mg i.m. daily	BPRS daily CGIS after treatment
2	19***	Double-blind placebo-controlled	Maintained	10 Days; 3 mg i.m. daily (n = 13) placebo only (n = 6)	BPRS daily CGIS after treatment

*One patient was also included in study 1
**Including 2 additional patients
***6 patients were treated with placebo only

The diagnose of the patients was based on 4 criteria: 1. the Present State Examination (PSE) including CATEGO analysis (Wing et al., 1975), 2. the DSM-III (1980) diagnostic criteria, 3. The Research Diagnostic Criteria (RDC; Spitzer et al., 1977, 1978) and 4. the course of illness (Van Praag, 1976). With respect to the criterion of course, the qualification chronic schizophrenia was used when the duration of the patient's last psychotic episode was one year or more. Subtyping of the schizophrenic patients was performed according to the DSM-III criteria in 5 classes: disorganized (hebephrenic), paranoid, catatonic, undifferentiated and residual type of schizophrenia. The qualification residual was restricted to patients who had been hospitalized without interruption for at least five years, while showing predominantly negative and rather stabilized positive psychotic symptoms. In addition, the patients suffering from schizo-affective psychoses were subdivided in depressed and manic type according to the RDC. Symptom assessment was performed among others with the Brief Psychiatric Rating Scale (BPRS), including the 5 subscales (Overall and Gorham, 1962, 1976). The effect of treatment with γ-type endorphins on psychopathological symptoms was assessed by calculating the difference between the total BPRS-score of each individual subject before the experimental treatment (baseline score) and at the end of peptide treatment. When the improvement continued beyond the active treatment period, the lowest BPRS-score in the 15-day posttreatment period was used instead of the score at the end of active treatment. Each subject's response to γ-type endorphins was expressed as percentage decrease of the baseline score. A response to treatment was judged to have occured by a decrease of more than 20% of the total BPRS score. A maximal response of more than 50% was considered to be a clinically significant improvement. The patients were divided among 4 groups according to their individual response: 1. no response (<20%), 2. slight response (20-50%), 3. moderate response (50-80%) and 4. marked response >80%).

The clinical efficacy of peptide treatment was also assessed using a Patient Symptom Specific Scale (PSSS) with items extracted from the data of the PSE of each individual patient. In addition, the Clinical Global Impressions Scale (CGIS, Guy, 1976) was scored at the end or shortly after active treatment in most of the studies.

Clinical Effects
General data

Of the 43 patients treated with DTγE, 10 did not respond and 11 showed a slight response. In the remaining 22 patients a clinically obvious improvement was observed in that 10 patients responded moderately and 12 markedly (table 2). DEγE treatment resulted in a marked improvement in 4 and a moderate improvement in 6 out of 21 patients. In 3 patients

TABLE 2. Maximal decrease (in %) of symptoms according to the BPRS score at the end or during 2 weeks after des-Tyr^1-γ-endorphin (DTγE) or des-enkephalin-γ-endorphin (DEγE) treatment of patients suffering from different types of schizophrenic psychoses

Diagnosis	n	<20	20-50	50-80	>80	Mean ± S.E.M.
DTγE						
Hebephrenic type	9	—	1	4	4	68,3 ± 8,8
Paranoid type	18	—	5	6	7	64,4 ± 5,7
Catatonic type	3	—	3	—	—	39,3 ± 5,5
Undifferentiated type	3	1	2	—	—	22,3 ± 9,7
Residual type	4	4	—	—	—	11,3 ± 4,5
Schizo-affective manic type	1	—	—	—	1	94,0
Schizo-affective depressed type	5	5	—	—	—	13,4 ± 3,1
All diagnoses	43	10	11	10	12	50,3 ± 4,7
DEγE*						
Hebephrenic type	1	—	—	—	1	100,0
Catatonic type	5	1	3	1	—	40,8 ± 5,9
Paranoid type	14	2	4	5	3	55,5 ± 6,6
Schizo-affective depressed type	1	—	1	—	—	37,0
All diagnoses	21	3	8	6	4	53,3 ± 5,3
Placebo all diagnoses	6	6	—	—	—	9,8 ± 3,0

Header spanning columns <20 through >80: Response % BPRS

*Including 4 patients treated outside official protocols

no effect was found, while 8 responded slightly (Table 2). Thus, in half of the patients a clinically significant therapeutic effect was observed which usually started within the first week of active treatment. No obvious differences between DTγE and DEγE treatment could be demonstrated. None of the 6 patients treated with placebo responded more than 20%, neither did any of the patients in whom treatment was started with placebo.

With respect to the antipsychotic efficacy as assessed with the BPRS total and subscales scores, it was found that in patients who responded moderately to markedly upon peptide treatment, all groups of symptoms decreased. No marked differences in the decrease of symptoms were observed either in the degree of improvement shown or in the time course, suggesting that both positive and negative psychotic symptoms may be equally affected by γ-type endorphin treatment. In fact, further analysis of these data revealed that both positive and negative psychotic symptoms similarily decreased during active treatment (Van Ree et al., 1983a). This overall effect on psychotic symptoms can also be inferred from the therapeutic efficacy as assessed with the CGIS in 30 DTγE- and 21 DEγE-treated patients. As indicated in Table 3, a fairly good rela-

TABLE 3. Therapeutic effect of γ-type endorphins in schizophrenic patients as assessed with the clinical global impression scale (CGIS) at the end or shortly after active treatment. This effect is compared to the maximal decrease of symptoms as assessed with the BPRS scoring

CGIS therapeutic effect	BPRS response (%)			
	<20	20-50	50-80	>80
DTγE n = 30				
Worse	—	—	—	—
Unchanged	6	2	—	—
Minimal	—	5	—	—
Moderate	—	1	8	2
Marked	—	—	—	6
DEγE* n = 21				
Worse	—	—	—	—
Unchanged	3	1	—	—
Minimal	—	5	1	—
Moderate	—	2	4	1
Marked	—	—	1	3

*Including 4 patients treated outside official protocols.

tionship was found between the decrease of symptomatology as assessed with the BPRS and the therapeutic efficacy as indicated on the CGIS.

In 11 patients, treatment with γ-type endorphins (DTγE: n = 8; DEγE: n = 3) for one or two consecutive treatment periods resulted in a psychotic-free period of at least 6 months, during which period a substantial improvement in social functioning of the patients was observed, together with a significantly lower level of treatment with neuroleptics as compared to that in the period before peptide treatment. Moreover, the interval between the psychotic periods was extended after peptide treatment (Van Ree et al., 1982c; Verhoeven, 1983).

Also others have investigated the effects of DTγE in schizophrenic patients. A total of 87 patients has so far been treated with DTγE in 9 clinical trials (Table 4). However, only 4 studies were performed using a double-blind design, in which about one-third of the patients responded to DTγE treatment. Thus, in general the responsiveness of the patients to peptide treatment was less marked than in our studies; only 24 of the 87 patients responded to treatment. This reduced responsiveness may be related to the characteristics of the selected patients, in particular the chronicity of their illness. As will be mentioned below, a chronic course of disease among others influences negatively the response to γ-type endorphin treatment.

TABLE 4. Clinical studies with des-tyr¹-γ-endorphin (DTγE; βE 2-17)

Author	Design	Number of patients	Non-responders	Responders*	Remarks**
Bourgeois et al., 1980.	Open	14	12	2	Chronic patients; response in patients with short recent episode
Emrich et al., 1980; 1981.	Double-blind cross-over	13	7	6	More effect in acute than in chronic patients
Manchanda and Hirsch, 1981.	Open	11	9	2	Response in patients with psychotic episode <6 months
Tamminga et al., 1981.	Double-blind	5	5	0	Chronic patients
Casey et al., 1981.	Open	9	9	0	Chronic patients
Fink et al., 1981.	Double-blind	7	3	4	Transient improvement in 3 and longlasting effect in 1 patient
Meltzer et al., 1982a, b.	Open	15	6	9	More effect in younger patients
Korsgaard et al., 1982.	Open	4	4	0	Chronic patients with tardive dyskinesia
Volavka et al., 1983.	Double-blind cross-over	9	8	1	Severe symptoms and using rather high doses of neuroleptics
		87	63	24	

*From the group of responders, 10 patients improved slight to moderate (20-50%) response, while the other patients (14) responded moderate to marked (>50% response).
**No clear definition has been given by the different authors for the terms acute and chronic.

Biochemical and hormonal data

The influence of DTγE on brain monoaminergic systems was analyzed via two strategies. Firstly, the levels of the monoamine metabolites homovanillic acid (HVA), methoxy-hydroxy-phenyl-glycol (MHPG) and 5-hydroxy indole acetic acid (5-HIAA) in the CSF were determined. Secondly, the daily pattern of plasma levels of prolactin, growth hormone and cortisol were measured. Although, initially, a slight effect on HVA levels was observed (Verhoeven et al., 1981), subsequent studies revealed no consistent influence of DTγE treatment on the CSF levels of HVA, 5-HIAA and MHPG, neither did DTγE change the plasma levels of growth hormone and cortisol. However, a small but significant decrease of plasma prolactin levels was observed during DTγE treatment

(Verhoeven et al., 1981, 1983) which effect has also been observed under certain conditions in animal experiments (Lamberts et al., 1982). This interesting effect, which is opposite to that induced by classical and atypical neuroleptics, may be related to some stimulatory effect of DTγE on the tubero-infundibular DA-ergic system.

Also others have investigated the influence of DTγE on biochemical and neurophysiological parameters. Accordingly, Claustrat et al. (1981) reported a stimulatory effect of DTγE on the secretion of melatonin, while a reduction of secondary facilitation of the H-reflex recovery curve and a decreased platelet MAO activity in schizophrenic patients were observed by Metz et al. (1981) and Meltzer et al. (1982b) respectively. Interestingly, the effects of DTγE on the H-reflex and platelet MAO activity are similar to those induced by classical neuroleptics.

Differential responsiveness to γ-type endorphins

Since the response of the patients varied between no response at all to complete remission of psychotic symptoms, we have looked in more detail at the symptomatology and course of illness and the history of the patients in order to analyze whether the degree of responsiveness covaries with these characteristics of the individual patients (Van Ree et al., 1980b, 1981, 1982c; Verhoeven, 1983).

Syndromal characteristics

PSE syndrome profile and subscores. Before the start of the studies, a complete PSE interview was performed in the 30 neuroleptic-free DTγE-treated patients, while in the 19 patients involved in the DEγE studies the PSE interview was restricted to psychotic symptoms and was therefore started with section 11 (derealization and depersonalization). All PSE data were analyzed according to the CATEGO computer program.

With respect to the 30 patients treated with DTγE, analysis of the PSE revealed the following results. One patient was classified in the class of depressive psychosis (D⁺) and the subclass of psychotic depression (PD⁺). According to the DSM-III criteria and the RDC, however, the diagnosis hebephrenic type of schizophrenia with differential diagnosis schizo-affective psychosis, depressed type, was established in this patient. Three patients were classified in the class of borderline and doubtful psychoses (0⁺). Two of them belonged to the subclass of catatonic schizophrenia (CS⁺) and one to the subclass of catatonic schizophrenia/psychotic depression (CSPD). According to the DSM-III criteria and the criterion of course of disease, the 2 patients with CS⁺ were diagnosed as suffering from residual type of schizophrenia and the patient with CSPD as suffering from a paranoid type of schizophrenia. In fact, these three patients showed clear motor disturbances such as catatonic symptoms and motor retardation. The other 26 patients all belonged to the class of schizophrenic psychoses (S⁺) and subclass nuclear schizophrenia (NS$^+$). The PSE syndrome profile of the 30 patients and the 4 subscores as derived from the PSE are depicted in Figure 1. With respect to the classification according to the CATEGO program, the pathology of all patients involved was quantitatively and qualitatively sufficient to justify the classification process since in none of the patients the Index of Definition (ID) appeared to be below the critical point of 5 (ID-5: n = 3; ID-6: n = 6; ID-7: n = 2; ID-8: n = 19). The analysis of the 23 patients involved in the DEγE studies revealed that all patients belonged to the class of schizophrenic psychoses (S$^+$), with subclass nuclear schizophrenia (NS$^+$) in all but one patient. This particular patient was classified into the subclass of nuclear schizophrenia with first rank symptoms, manic type (NSMN), which is in accordance with the diagnosis schizo-affective psychosis, manic type, as assessed with the RDC. The ID appeared to be 8 (n = 21) or 7 (n = 2). The PSE profile of the 23 patients and the 2 subscores as derived from the PSE are presented in Figure 2.

Taken together, in all patients, a fairly good relation was observed between the different diagnostic instruments, in that all patients could be clearly diagnosed as suffering from schizophrenic or schizo-affective psychoses. As can be inferred from Figure 1, the PSE profile of the DTγE treated patient group accords well with those obtained by others (Cooper et al., 1972; WHO, 1973; Verhey, 1981), except that the occurrence of delusions of persecution (PE; syndrome 14) is relatively low, which is due to the fact that patients with such symptoms were excluded from the studies because of extreme paranoid behavior. In particular, the syndrome profiles and subscores of the two patient groups involved in the placebo-controlled DEγE study are quite similar which indicates that both can be compared with respect to the qualitative as well as to the quantitative occurrence of psychopathological symptoms (Figure 2).

Since a more than 50% maximal response to treatment with γ-type endorphins was taken as indicating improvement of clinical significance, the patients were divided among two groups according to the 50% caesure. With respect to the 30 DTγE treated patients, 14 responded less than 50% and in 16 a response of more than 50% was observed, while in the 17 DEγE treated patients, 7 responded less than 50% and 10 more than 50%.

Analysis of the PSE data obtained in the DTγE treated patients revealed that patients with a response of less than 50% showed significantly more symptoms belonging to the syndromes of slowness (SL; 21), catatonic syndrome (CS; 2) and residual syndrome (RS; 4) (Figure 3). Also the BSO subscore appeared to be significantly higher in the group of patients with a response of less than 50% as compared to those who responded more than 50% (Figure 3). The same results were obtained with the PSE data of the DEγE treated patients (Figure 4). In addition,

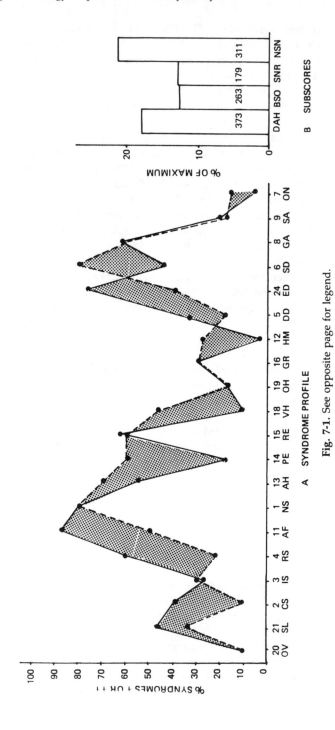

Fig. 7-1. See opposite page for legend.

it was found that the symptoms belonging to the syndrome of depressive delusions and hallucinations (DD;5) occurred significantly higher in the group of DTγE treated patients with a response of more than 50% and that the symptoms belonging to the syndrome of overactivity (OV;20) were significantly more observed in the group of DEγE treated patients with a response of more than 50%. Thus, especially motor symptoms such as retardation and catatonic symptoms as well as non-specific psychotic symptoms which are represented in the BSO subscore seem to influence negatively the response to treatment with γ-type endorphins. It has, however, to be emphasized that the patients involved in our studies showed obviously more motor symptoms as compared to the patients involved in the IPSS project (Figure 1).

However, the significance of the results is difficult to estimate if only the F-values are taken into consideration. Therefore, it is important from a practical point of view to realize that there is a substantial overlap between the subsets selected in the 2 different studies (Table 7). This can be understood as a cross-validation of the results yielded by two separate analyses. As can be inferred from Table 7, the direction in which particular symptoms affect prognosis cannot be explained merely in terms of positive or negative symptoms, since some important positive

---

Fig. 7-1. PSE syndrome profile and subscores of 30 schizophrenic patients treated with des-Tyr¹-γ-endorphin (DTγE; β-endorphin 2-17).
Syndromes involved in the profile are:

20	OV: Overactivity	18	VH: Visual hallucinations
21	SL: Slowness	19	OH: Olfactory hallucinations
2	CS: Catatonic syndrome	16	GR: Grandiose and religious delusions
3	IS: Incoherent speech	12	HM: Hypomania
4	RS: Residual syndrome	5	DD: Depressive delusions
11	AF: Affective flattening	24	ED: Special features of depression
1	NS: Nuclear syndrome	6	SD: Simple depression
13	AH: Auditory hallucinations	8	GA: General anxiety
14	PE: Delusions of persecution	9	SA: Situational anxiety
15	RE: Delusions of reference	7	ON: Obsessional neurosis

A. The 20 syndromes are plotted versus the percentages of the syndromes with a score of + or + + in the group of patients. Solid line represents DTγE-treated patients, broken line represents the syndrome profile of the IPSS-project (WHO, 1973).
B. The 4 PSE subscores of the 30 patients as derived from the PSE and expressed as percentage of the theoretical maximum scores.
Figures in vertical bars indicate absolute values of subscores.
DAH = delusional and hallucinatory syndromes
BSO = behavior, speech and other syndromes
SNR = specific neurotic syndromes
NSN = non specific neurotic syndromes
For details concerning the PSE and CATEGO program see: Wing et al., 1975.

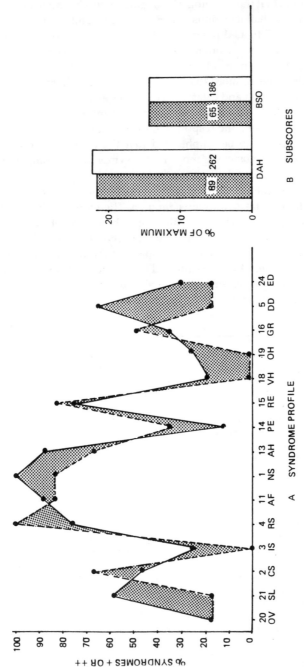

Fig. 7-2. PSE syndrome profiles and subscores of 23 schizophrenic patients involved in the clinical studies with des-enkephalin-γ-endorphin (DEγE; β-endorphin 6-17).

A. The 15 syndromes are plotted versus the percentages of the syndromes with a score of + or + + in both groups of patients.
Solid line: DEγE treated patients (n = 17); broken line: placebo treated patients (n = 6).

B. The 2 PSE subscores (DAH and BSO) of the 23 patients as derived from the PSE expressed as percentage of the theoretical maximum scores. ▨ = placebo treated patients; ☐ = DEγE treated patients. Figures in vertical bars indicate absolute values of subscores.

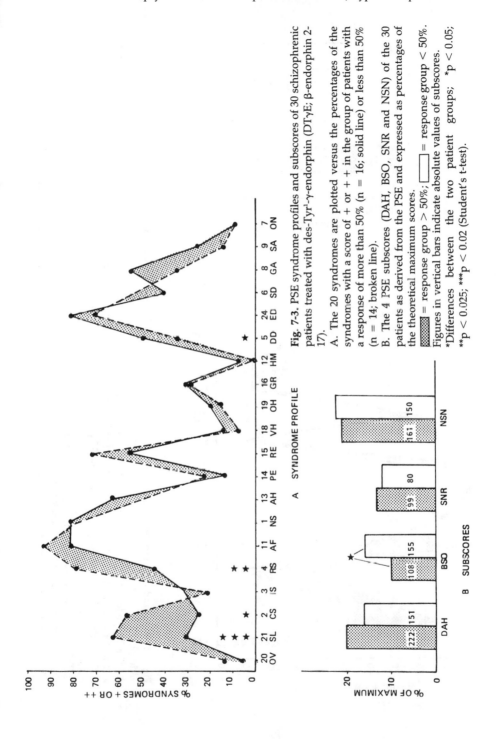

Fig. 7-3. PSE syndrome profiles and subscores of 30 schizophrenic patients treated with des-Tyr¹-γ-endorphin (DTγE; β-endorphin 2-17).

A. The 20 syndromes are plotted versus the percentages of the syndromes with a score of + or ++ in the group of patients with a response of more than 50% (n = 16; solid line) or less than 50% (n = 14; broken line).

B. The 4 PSE subscores (DAH, BSO, SNR and NSN) of the 30 patients as derived from the PSE and expressed as percentages of the theoretical maximum scores.

▨ = response group > 50%; ☐ = response group < 50%. Figures in vertical bars indicate absolute values of subscores.

*Differences between the two patient groups; *p < 0.05; **p < 0.025; ***p < 0.02 (Student's t-test).

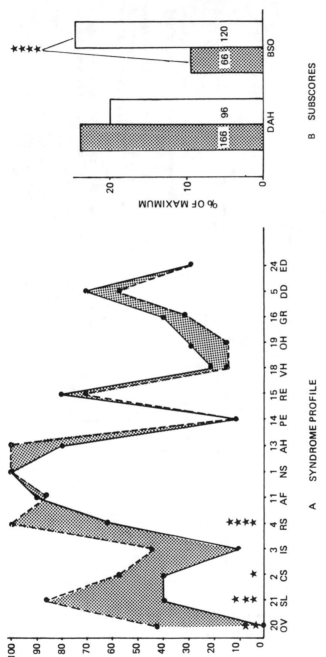

Fig. 7-4. PSE syndrome profiles and subscores of 17 schizophrenic patients treated with des-enkephalin-γ-endorphin (DEγE; β-endorphin 6-17).

A. The 15 syndromes are plotted versus the percentages of the syndromes with a score of + or + + in the group of patients with a response of more than 50% (n = 10; solid line) or less than 50% (n = 7; broken line).

B. The 2 PSE subscores (DAH and BSO) of the 17 patients as derived from the PSE and expressed as percentages of the theoretical maximum scores.

Figures in vertical bars indicate absolute values of subscores.

*Differences between the two patient groups; *p < 0.05; **p < 0.025; ***p < 0.005; ****p < 0.001 (Student's t-test).

symptoms (hallucinations and conceptual disorganization) parallel the negative symptoms in having a negative relationship to the percentage of global improvement. A closer look at the relationship of particular symptoms to the prognosis indicates that the hypothetical dimension along which the symptoms with high predictive power are distributed could be tentatively called "mental organization". Symptoms of "mental disorganization", i.e. fragmentation of a mental function into autonomous, non-related elements, appear to predict poor therapeutic outcome. On the other hand, symptoms of mental "superorganization" i.e. the presence of a complex, rigid and nonadaptive mental structure seem to predict a good therapeutic outcome. To the first group of symptoms belong those rated within the following BPRS items: blunted affect (includes also inappropriate affect), conceptual disorganization (reflects incoherence of speech and thinking), mannerism and posturing (could be interpreted as a disorganization of motoric responses into elementary, autonomous fragments) and hallucinatory behavior (could be interpreted as sensorial disorganization). The second group of symptoms (symptoms of "mental superorganization") consist of two BPRS items: unusual thought content (an item loaded mostly by the presence of a delusional system) and tension (which may be related to the presence of the previous symptom).

Since we were also interested whether it was possible to use a single variable for classification of patients into simple categories like responder/non-responder, a stepwise discriminant analysis was performed using the BMDP7M computer program. The patients were divided among two groups according to the previous mentioned 50% caesure. The discriminant function was computed on the basis of baseline BPRS item scores. In Table 8, the classification matrix and classification function for the item blunted affect is presented. As apparent from this table, the patients taken from the same sample could have been classified a posteriori as clinical responders or non-responders with a average accuracy of 72%, which is a 22% improvement in comparison to the "classification" by chance. Thus, the discrimination function could be used as a balanced assignment of patients to experimental groups in our future studies with γ-type endorphins.

Diagnostic subtypes. Concerning the response of the patients to γ-type endorphins as compared to their diagnostic subtypes of schizophrenia according to the DSM-III criteria and the RDC, there appears to be some relation between the diagnostic subclasses and the response to peptide treatment (Table 2). In fact, patients suffering from hebephrenic (disorganized) type of schizophrenia responded best (mean response ± SEM: 17,5% ± 8,5; n = 10), followed by those suffering from the paranoid type (60,6% ± 4,3; n = 32). Less response was found in patients with a catatonic type of schizophrenia (40,3% ± 4,0; n = 8). Patients with

undifferentiated or residual type of schizophrenia hardly responded
(22,3% ± 9,7; n = 3 and 11,3% ± 4,5; n = 4, respectively). Interestingly, patients suffering from schizo-affective psychosis, depressed type
did not respond to γ-type endorphins (17,3% ± 4,7; n = 6), while in
the patients with a schizo-affective psychosis, manic type, a marked
response to DEγE was observed (94%). Differences between DTγE and
DEγE in this respect were not observed (Table 2). Thus, the differential
response to γ-type endorphins seems to be related to a certain subtype
of schizophrenia. However, it should be kept in mind that the classification in subtypes is rather arbitrary and that the different subtypes can
change over a period of time. Such a classification is based on symp-
tomatological factors, rather than on clearly defined syndromal entities.

Positive versus negative symptoms. Using the baseline CPRS score of
each individual subject, it was analyzed whether special symptoms could
be useful as predictors of responsiveness to γ-type endorphin treatment.
For this purpose a stepwise regression analysis was performed with
baseline BPRS item scores as independent (predictor) variables and maximal response to treatment as the dependent (predicted) variable. The
analyses were performed with the BMDP2R computer program. A fore-
ward stepping followed by backward stepping approach was used. The
"best" subset of predictor variables was selected arbitrarily taking into
consideration both statistical criteria (multiple R^2 value, F-values of the
variables in and out of equation) and practical criteria (minimizing the
number of included variables). The compromise presented here consists
of the smallest subset with no variable having the F-to-enter value greater
than 4.0, left outside the equation.

In the DTγE studies (Table 5), the multiple R^2 of the selected subset
was 0.61, indicating that approximately 60% of the therapeutic response
could have been "predicted" from the baseline values of the included
variables. Three of the variables (blunted affect, mannerism-posturing
and hallucinatory behavior) had a negative regression coefficient, indicating that high scores of these particular items can be considered as a
negative prognostic factor. On the other hand, a high score of the two
variables (tension and unusual thought content) with a positive regression coefficient can be considered as a positive prognostic factor.

In the DEγE studies (Table 6), the multiple R^2 indicated that 69% of
therapeutic response could have been predicted from the baseline values
of the variables in the subset. In fact, the subset consists of two variables
with a negative prognostic value (conceptual disorganisation and
blunted affect), while the variables tension and unusual thought content
have a positive prognostic value.

In addition, the scores of the positive symptoms (conceptual disorganization, grandiosity, suspiciousness, hallucinatory behavior and unusual thought content) and of the negative symptoms (emotional withdrawal, motor retardation and blunted affect) on the baseline BPRS were

TABLE 5. Results of the regression analysis of the DTγE studies (N = 25). The predicted variable was the maximal response to treatment. In order to match with the diagnostic structure of the DEγE studies, 5 patients, diagnosed as schizo-affective psychosis (N = 4) or as residual type of schizophrenia (N = 1), were excluded from the analysis

Variable		Coefficient	St. Err. of coeff.	F to remove
Tension	14	8.33508	3.4637	5.79
Mannerism and posturing	15	-7.41647	3.0075	6.08
Hallucinatory behavior	20	-5.79200	2.5951	4.98
Unusual thought content	23	7.92312	3.2532	5.93
Blunted affect	24	-14.49827	3.8977	13.84
Multiple R		.7785		
Multiple R-square		.6061		

Analysis of variance	Sum of squares	DF	Mean square	F ratio
Regression	10585.488	5	2117.098	5.85
Residual	6880.2998	19	362.1210	

TABLE 6. Results of the regression analysis of the DEγE studies (N = 17). The predicted value was the maximal response to treatment

Variable		Coefficient	St. err. of coeff.	F to remove
Conceptual disorganization	12	-20.87535	4.7120	19.63
Tension	14	24.42994	8.0041	9.32
Unusual thought content	23	11.08340	4.6724	5.63
Blunted affect	24	-17.79352	4.8262	13.59
Multiple R		.8296		
Multiple R-square		.6882		

Analysis of variance	Sum of squares	DF	Mean square	F ratio
Regression	6626.0077	4	1656.502	6.62
Residual	3001.7514	12	250.1459	

TABLE 7. Summary of the results of stepwise regression analysis of the studies with DTγE (N = 25) and DEγE (N = 17). The sets of variables were selected according to the criteria as described in the text. (− or +) = sign of regression coefficient

DTγE		DEγE
Mannerism-posturing (−)	Blunted affect (−)	
Hallucinatory behavior (−)	Unusual thought content (+)	Conceptual disorganization (−)
	Tension (+)	

TABLE 8. Summary of the results of the discriminant analysis with the BPRS item blunted affect in the discriminant function. Analysis was performed with date of 47 patients (DTγE: N = 30; DEγE: N = 17), who were divided among two groups according to the 50% caesure

Classification functions

Variable = blunted affect
Group = nonresp. resp.
Coeff. = 2.28550 1.54287
Constant = −4.48501 −2.42116

Classification matrix

Group:	Percent correct	Number of patients classified into group		
		Nonresp.	Resp.	Total
Nonresp.	77.3	17	6	22
Resp.	68.0	8	17	25
Total	72.3	25	22	47

added for each individual subject. Subsequently, the patients were divided among two groups according to the 50% response caesure. Statistical analysis revealed that the intensity of negative symptoms was more severe in the patients with a response of less than 50% to γ-type endorphin treatment as compared to those with a response of more than 50% (Verhoeven, 1983; Van Ree et al., 1983a). No differences were found between both response groups with respect to the intensity of positive symptoms. In conclusion, these data suggest that the intensity of negative psychotic symptoms, especially blunted affect, may influence negatively the susceptability to treatment with γ-type endorphins. The intensity of positive psychotic symptoms on the other hand seems to influence the efficacy of peptide treatment less profoundly although a relatively high occurrence of unusual thought contents could have a predictive value for good response to peptide treatment.

Other characteristics. It was found that the duration of the last psychotic episode as well as the dosage of neuroleptics the patient received during the last 6 weeks before the start of the trials were negatively correlated with the patient's response. No consistent relation was found between the response and the age of the patients, the duration of the disease and the duration of neuroleptic treatment respectively. Thus, a long duration of the recent psychotic episode and treatment with high doses of neuroleptics may reduce the responsiveness of the patients to treatment with γ-type endorphins (Van Ree et al., 1980b, 1981).

Interestingly, in the patients with a marked and longlasting response to peptide treatment, typing of the lymphocytes for antigens of the HLA system revealed a higher occurrence of the HLA_{B-15} antigen as compared to that found in other patients, suggesting an involvement of genetic factors in their responsiveness to this kind of treatment (De Jongh, et al., 1982). Genetic control of individual response to medication is further discussed in Chapter 4.

CONCLUDING REMARKS

In 32 of the 64 patients treated with γ-type endorphins, a clinically significant antipsychotic effect was observed which appeared to be marked and longlasting in 11 of them. Of the other 32 patients, 13 did not respond while 19 improved only slightly. These data suggest that a subgroup of schizophrenic patients is preferentially sensitive to treatment with γ-type endorphins. The main characteristics of these patients appeared to be a relatively short duration of the last psychotic episode, previous treatment with relative low doses of neuroleptics and a relatively low intensity of negative psychotic symptoms, suggesting that patients responding to peptide treatment may belong to the Type I schizophrenia as proposed by Crow (1980, 1982). The less favourable results with DTγE treatment as observed by others (see: Table 4) may be due to the fact that the patients involved in these studies were suffering predominantly from the Type II schizophrenia which is among others characterized by reduced susceptability to neuroleptic treatment and poor prognosis. Thus, γ-type endorphins resemble closely neuroleptics, in that the response to treatment is most pronounced in patients with relatively less negative psychotic symptoms and belonging particularly to the subclass of hebephrenic and paranoid schizophrenia. According to the hypothesis of Crow, the pathogenesis of Type I schizophrenia could be related to a hyperactivity of DA-ergic systems, particularly in the nucleus accumbens. This is consistent with the data from animal experiments showing that γ-type endorphins may be involved in the control of certain DA-ergic systems in the nucleus accumbens (Van Ree and De Wied, 1982).

Other neuropeptide systems, however, may be also implicated in schizophrenia. It has been demonstrated that cholecystokinine (CCK)-like peptides are present in mesolimbic DA-ergic neurons, e.g. in the nucleus accumbens, where neuroleptics and γ-type endorphins presumably induce their antipsychotic effects. Recently it has been found in animal experiments that the neuroleptic-like activities of γ-type endorphins are comparable to that of CCK-like peptides (Van Ree et al., 1983b). Antipsychotic properties of these neuropeptides have also been observed in a number of schizophrenic patients (Moroji et al., 1982; Nair et al., 1983; Bloom et al., 1983; Van Ree et al., 1983c).

In conclusion, the animal as well as the human data support the hypothesis that disturbances in β-endorphin homeostasis are involved in the pathogenesis of schizophrenia although direct evidence for these disturbances has sofar not been obtained in schizophrenic patients.

REFERENCES

Austen, B.M., Smyth, D.G. and Snell, C.R.: γ-Endorphin, α-endorphin and Metenkephalin are formed extracellularly from lipotropin C fragment. *Nature* 269:619-621, 1977.

Bloom, D.M., Nair, N.P.V. and Schwartz, G.: CCK-8 in the treatment of chronic schizophrenia. *Psychophamacol. Bull.* 19:361-363, 1983.

Bloom, F., Segal, D., Ling, N. and Guillemin, R.: Endorphins: Profound behavioral effects in rats suggest new etiological factors in mental illness. *Science* 194:630-632, 1976.

Bourgeois, M., Laforge, E., Muyard, J., Blayac, J. and Lemoine, J.: Endorphines et schizophrénies. *Ann. Med. Psychol.* 138:1112-1119, 1980.

Burbach, J.P.H., Loeber, J.G., Verhoef, J., Wiegant, V.M., De Kloet, E.R. and De Wied, D.: Selective conversion of β-endorphin into peptides related to γ- and α-endorphin. *Nature* 283:96-97, 1980.

Carlsson, A. Receptor-mediated control of dopamine metabolism. In: Pre- and Postsynaptic Receptors, (E. Usdin and W.E. Bunney, eds.), Marcel Dekker, New York, pp. 49-66, 1975.

Casey, D.E., Korsgaard, S., Gerlach, J., Jørgensen, A. and Simmelsgaard, H.: Effect of Des-Tyrosine-γ-endorphin in tardive dyskinesia. *Arch. Gen. Psychiatry* 38:158-160, 1981.

Claustrat, B., Chazot, C. and Brun J.: Melatonin secretion in man: Stimulating effect of destyrosine gamma endorphin. *Neuroendocrinol. Lett.* 3:35-37, 1981.

Comb, M., Seeburg, P.H., Adelman, J., Eiden, L. and Herbert, E.: Primary structure of the human Met-and Leu-enkephalin precursor and its mRNA. *Nature* 295:663-666, 1982.

Cooper, J.E., Kendell, R.E., Gurland, B.J., Sharpa, L., Copeland, J.R.M. and Simon, R.: Psychiatric diagnosis in New York and London. Oxford University Press, 1972.

Crow, T.J., Deakin, J.F.W. and Longden, A.: The nucleus accumbens—possible site of antipsychotic action of neuroleptic drugs? *Psychol. Med.* 7:213-221, 1977.

Crow, T.J.: Positive and negative schizophrenic symptoms and the role of dopamine. *Br. J. Psychiatry* 137:383-386, 1980.

Crow, T.J.: Two syndromes in schizophrenia? *Trends neurosci.* 5:351-354, 1982.

De Jongh, B.M., Verhoeven, W.M.A., Van Ree, J.M., De Wied, D. and Van Rood, J.J.: HLA, and the response to treatment with γ-type endorphins in schizophrenia. *J. Immunogenet.* 9:381-388, 1982.

De Wied, D.: Psychopathology as a neuropeptide dysfunction. In: Characteristics and Function of Opioids, (J.M. Van Ree and L. Terenius, eds.), Elsevier/North-Holland Biomedical Press, Amsterdam, pp. 113-122, 1978.

De Wied, D., Bohus, B., Van Ree, J.M. and Urban, I.: Behavioral and electrophysiological effects of peptides related to lipotropin (β-LPH). *J. Pharmacol. Exp. Ther.* 204:570-580, 1978a.

De Wied, D., Kovács, G.L., Bohus, B., Van Ree, J.M. and Greven, H.M.: Neuroleptic activity of the neuropeptide β-LPH$_{62-77}$ ((des-Tyr^1)-γ-endorphin; DTγE). *Eur. J. Pharmacol.* 49:427-436, 1978b.

De Wied, D., Van Ree, J.M. and Greven, H.M.: Neuroleptic-like activity of peptides related to (des-tyr^1)-γ-endorphin: structure activity studies. *Life Sci.* 26:1575-1579, 1980.

De Wied, D.: Neuropeptides and adaptive behavior. In: Integrative Neurohumoral L. Angelucci and U. Scapagnini eds.), Elsevier Science Publishers, pp. 3-22, 1983.

DMS III: Diagnostic and Statistical Manual of Mental Disorder. The American Psychiatric Association. 1980.

Emrich, H.M., Zaudig, M., Kissling, W., Dirlich, G., Von Zerssen, D. and Herz, A.: Des-Tyrosyl-γ-endorphin in schizophrenia: a double-blind trial in 13 pa-Mechanisms, (E. Endröczi, D. De Wied, tients. *Pharmakopsychiatrie* 13:290-298, 1980.

Emrich, H.M., Zaudig, M., Von Zerssen, D., Kissling, W., Dirlich, G. and Herz, A.: Action of (Des-tyr¹)-γ-Endorphin in Schizophrenia. *Mod. Probl. Pharmacopsychiatry* 17:279-286, 1981.

Fink, M., Papakostas, Y., Lee, J., Meehan, Th. and Johnson, L.: Clinical trials with des-tyr-gamma-endorphin (GK-78). In: Biological Psychiatry, (C. Perris, G. Struwe and B. Jansson, eds.), Elsevier/North-Holland Biomedical Press, Amsterdam, pp. 398-401, 1981.

Gispen, W.H., Wiegant, V.M., Bradbury, A.F., Hulme, E.C., Smyth, D.G., Snell, C.R. and De Wied, D.: Induction of excessive grooming in the rat by fragments of lipotropin. *Nature* 264:794-795, 1976.

Gispen, W.H., Ormond, D., Ten Haaf, J. and De Wied, D.: Modulation of ACTH-induced grooming by (des-Tyr¹)-γ-endorphin and haloperidol. *Eur. J. Pharmacol.* 63:203-207, 1980.

Goldstein, A., Tachibana, S., Lowney, L.I., Hunkapiller, M. and Hood, L.: Dynorphin-(1-13), an extraordinarily potent opioid peptide. *Proc. Natl. Acad. Sci. USA.* 76:6666-6670, 1979.

Guy, W.: ECDEU Assessment Manual for Psychopharmacology. Rev. ed. National Institute of Mental Health, Rockville, MD, pp. 217-222, 1976.

Holaday, J.W., Loh, H.H. and Li, C.H.: Unique behavioral effects of β-endorphin and their relationship to thermoregulation and hypothalamic function. *Life Sci.* 22:1525-1536, 1978.

Hughes, J.: Isolation of an endogenous compound from the brain with pharmacological properties similar to morphine. *Brain Res.* 88:295-308, 1975.

Hughes, J., Smith, T.W., Kosterlitz, H.W., Fothergill, L.A., Morgan, B.A. and Morris, H.R.: Identification of two related pentapeptides from the brain with potent opiate agonist activity. *Nature* 258:577-579, 1975.

Kakidani, H., Furutani, Y., Takahashi, H., Noda, M., Morimoto, Y., Hirose, T.,

Asai, M., Inayama, S., Nakanishi, S. and Numa, S.: Cloning and sequence analysis of cDNA for porcine β-neoendorphin/dynorphin precursor. *Nature* 298:245-249, 1982.

Korsgaard, S., Casey, D.E. and Gerlach, J.: High-Dose Destyrosine-γ-Endorphin in Tardive Dyskinesia. *Psychopharmacology* 78:285-286, 1982.

Kovács, G.L., Telegdy, G. and De Wied, D.: Selective attenuation of passive avoidance behaviour by micro-injection of β-LPH$_{62-77}$ and β-LPH$_{66-77}$ into the nucleus accumbens in rats. *Neuropharmacology* 21:451-454, 1982.

Lamberts, S.W.J., De Quijda, M., Van Ree, J.M. and De Wied, D.: Non-opiate β-endorphin fragments and dopamine. V. γ-Type endorphins and prolactin secretion in rats. *Neuropharmacology* 21:1129-1135, 1982.

Mains, R.E., Eipper, B.A. and Ling, N.: Common precursor to corticotropins and endorphins. *Proc. Natl. Acad. Sci. USA* 74:3014-3018, 1977.

Manchanda, R. and Hirsch, S.R.: (Des-Tyr¹)-γ-endorphin in the treatment of schizophrenia. *Psychol. Med.* 11:401-404, 1981.

Matthysse, S.: Dopamine and the pharmacology of schizophrenia: the state of the evidence. *J. Psychiatr. Res.* 11:107-113, 1974.

Meltzer, H.Y., Busch, D.A., Tricou, B.J. and Robertson, A.: Effect of (Des-Tyr)-gamma endorphin in schizophrenia. *Psychiatry Res.* 6:313-326, 1982a.

Meltzer, H.Y., Busch, D.A., Lee, J. and Papacostas, Y.: Effect of Des-Tyr-γ-Endorphin in Schizophrenia. *Psychopharmacol. Bull.* 18:44-47, 1982b.

Metz, J., Busch, D.A. and Meltzer, H.Y.: Des-Tyrosine-γ-endorphin: H-reflex response similar to neuroleptics. *Life Sci.* 28:2003-2008, 1982.

Moroji, T., Watanabe, N., Aoki, N. and Itoh, S.: Antipsychotic effects of ceruletide (caerulein) on chronic schizophrenia. *Arch. Gen. Psychiatry* 39:485, 1982.

Nair, N.P.V., Bloom, D.M., Nestoros, J.N. and Schwartz, G.: Therapeutic efficacy of cholecystokinin in neuroleptic-resistant schizophrenic subjects. *Psychopharmacol. Bull.* 19:134-136, 1983.

Nakanishi, S., Inoue, A., Kita, T., Nakamura, M., Chang, A.C.Y., Cohen, S.N. and Numa, S.: Nucleotide sequence of cloned cDNA for bovine corticotropin-β-lipotropin precursor. *Nature* 278:423-427, 1979.

Noda, M., Furutani, Y., Takashashi, H., Toyosato, M., Hirose, T., Inayama, S., Nakanishi, S. and Numa, S.: Cloning and sequence analysis of cDNA for bovine adrenal preproenkephalin. *Nature* 295: 202-206, 1982.

Overall, J.E. and Gorham, D.R.: The Brief Psychiatric Rating Scale. *Psychol. Rep.* 10:797-812, 1962.

Overall, J.E. and Gorham, D.R. B.P.R.S.: Brief Psychiatric Rating Scale. In: ECDEU Assessment Manual for Psychopharmacology, (W. Guy, ed.), Rev. ed, Rockville, MD, National Institute of Mental Health, pp. 157-169, 1976.

Pasternak, G.W., Goodman, R. and Snyder, S.H.: An endogenous morphine-like factor in mammalian brain. *Life Sci.* 16:1765-1769, 1975.

Pert, C.B. and Snyder, S.H.: Properties of opiate-receptor binding in rat brain. *Proc. Natl. Acad. Sci. USA* 70:2243-2247, 1973.

Segal, D.S., Browne, R.G., Bloom, F., Ling, N. and Guillemin, R.: β-Endorphin: endogenous opiate or neuroleptic? *Science* 198:411-414, 1977.

Serra, G., Van Ree, J.M., and De Wied, D.: Influence of classical and atypical neuroleptics on apomorphine-induced behavioral changes and on extinction of a conditioned avoidance response. *J. Pharm. Pharmacol.* 35:255-257, 1983.

Simon, E.J., Hiller, J.M. and Edelman, I.: Stereospecific binding of the potent narcotic analgesic (^{3}H) etorphine to rat brain homogenate. *Proc. Natl. Acad. Sci. USA* 70:1947-1949, 1973.

Snyder, S.H.: Catecholamines in the brain as mediators of amphetamine psychosis. *Arch. Gen. Psychiat.* 27:169-179, 1972.

Snyder, S.H.: Amphetamine psychosis: A "model" schizophrenia mediated by catecholamines. *Am. J. Psychiatry* 130:61-67, 1973.

Spitzer, R.L., Endicott, J. and Robins, E.: Research Diagnostic Criteria (RDC) for a selected group of functional disorders. Biometrics Research, New York, 177.

Spitzer, R.L., Endicott, J. and Robins, E.: Research diagnostic criteria. *Arch. Gen. Psychiatry* 35:773-782, 1978.

Tamminga, C.A., Tighe, P.J., Chase, Th.N., DeFraites, E.G. and Schaffer, M.H.: Des-Tyrosine-γ-endorphin administration in chronic schizophrenics. *Arch. Gen. Psychiatry* 38:167-168, 1981.

Terenius, L.: Characteristics of the "receptor" for narcotic analgesics in synaptic plasma membrane fraction from rat brain. *Acta Pharmacol. Toxicol.* 33:377-384, 1973.

Terenius, L. and Wahlström, A.: Morphine-like ligand for opiate receptors in human CSF. *Life Sci.* 16:1759-1764, 1975.

Van Praag, H.M.: About the impossible concept of schizophrenia. *Compr. Psychiatry* 17:481-497, 1976.

Van Ree, J.M., De Wied, D., Bradbury, A.F., Hulme, E.C., Smyth, D.G. and Snell, C.R.: Induction of tolerance to the analgesic action of lipotropin C-fragment. *Nature* 264:792-794, 1976.

Van Ree, J.M., Smyth, D.G. and Colpaert, F.: Dependence creating properties of lipotropin C-fragment (β-endorphin): evidence for its internal control of behavior. *Life Sci.* 24:495-502, 1979.

Van Ree, J.M. and Otte, A.P.: Effects (Des-Tyr¹)-γ-endorphin and α-endorphin as compared to haloperidol and amphetamine on nucleus accumbens self-stimulation. *Neuropharmacology* 19:429-434, 1980.

Van Ree, J.M., Bohus, B. and De Wied, D.: Similarity between behavioral effects of Des-Tyrosine-γ-endorphin and haloperidol and of α-endorphin and amphetamine. In: Endogenous and Exogenous Opiate Agonists and Antagonists, (E. Leong Way, ed.), Pergamon Press, New York, pp. 459-462, 1980a.

Van Ree , J.M., De Wied, D., Verhoeven, W.M.A. and Van Praag, H.M.: Antipsychotic effect of γ-type endorphins in schizophrenia. *Lancet* II:1363-1364, 1980b.

Van Ree, J.M. and De Wied, D.: Endorphins in schizophrenia. *Neuropharmacology*, 20:1271-1277, 1981.

Van Ree, J.M. and Wolterink, G.: Injection of low doses of apomorphine into the nucleus accumbens of rats reduces locomotor activity. *Eur. J. Pharmacol.* 72: 107-111, 1981.

Van Ree, J.M., Verhoeven, W.M.A., Van Praag, H.M. and De Wied, D.: Neuroleptic-like and antipsychotic effects of γ-type endorphins. *Mode. Probl. Pharmacopsychiatry* 17:226-278, 1981.

Van Ree, J.M.: Non-opiate β-endorphin fragments and dopamine. II. β-endorphin 2-9 enhances apomorphine-induced stereotypy following subcutaneous and intrastriatal injection. *Neuropharmacology* 21:1103-1109, 1982.

Van Ree, J.M. and De Wied, D.: Neuroleptic-like profile of γ-type endorphins as related to schizophrenia. *Trends Pharmacol. Sci.* 3:358-361, 1982.

Van Ree, J.M., Innemee, H., Louwerens, J.W., Kahn, R.S. and De Wied, D.: Non-opiate β-endorphin fragments and dopamine. I. The neuroleptic-like γ-endorphin fragments interfere with behavioural effects elicited by small doses of apomorphine. *Neuropharmacology* 21: 1095-1101, 1982a.

Van Ree, J.M., Caffé, A.M. and Wolterink, G.: Non-opiate β-endorphin fragments and dopamine. III. γ-Type endorphins and various neuroleptics counteract the hypoactivity elicited by injection of apomorphine into the nucleus accumbens. *Neuropharmacology* 21:1111-1117, 1982b.

Van Ree, J.M., Verhoeven, W.M.A., De Wied, D. and Van Praag, H.M.: The use of the synthetic peptides γ-type endorphins in mentally ill patients. *Ann. N.Y. Acad. Sci.* 398:478-495, 1982c.

Van Ree, J.M., Wolterink, G., Fekete, M. and De Wied, D.: Non-opiate β-endorphin fragments and dopamine. IV γ-Type endorphins may control dopaminergic systems in the nucleus accumbens. *Neuropharmacology* 21:1119-1127, 1982d.

Van Ree, J.M., Verhoeven, W.M.A. and De Wied, D.: Antipsychotic actions of the endorphins. In: Antipsychotics, Norman Burrows and ●● Davies eds.), Elsevier/ Amsterdam, 1983a. (In press).

Van Ree, J.M., Gaffori, O. and De Wied, D.: Behavioral profile of CCK-8 related peptides in rats resembles that of antipsychotic agents. *Eur. J. Pharmacol.* 1983b. (In press).

Van Ree, J.M., Verhoeven, W.M.A., Brouwer, G.J. and De Wied, D.: Ceruletide resembles antipsychotics in rats and schizophrenic patients, a preliminary report. *Neuropsychobiology* 1983c. (In press).

Verhey, F.H.M.: Slow brain potentials and measured behavior. Thesis, State University Utrecht, The Netherlands, 1981.

Verhoeven, W.M.A., Van Praag, H.M., Van Ree, J.M. and De Wied, D.: Improvement of schizophrenic patients by treatment with (Des-Tyr¹)-γ-endorphin (DTγE). *Arch. Gen . Psychiatry* 36:294-298, 1979.

Verhoeven, W.M.A., Westenberg, H.G.M., Gerritsen, A.W., Van Praag, H.M., Thijssen, J.H.H., Schwartz, F., Van Ree, J.M. and De Wied, D.: (Des-Tyrosine¹)-γ-endorphin in schizophrenia: clinical, biochemical and hormonal aspects. *Psychiatry Res.* 5:293-309, 1981.

Verhoeven, W.M.A., Van Ree, J.M., Heezius-van Bentum, A., De Wied, D. and Van Praag, H.M.: Antipsychotic properties of (des-enkephalin)-γ-endorphin (DEγE; β-LPH 66-77) in schizophrenic patients. *Arch. Gen. Psychiatry* 39:648-654, 1982.

Verhoeven, W.M.A.: Endogenous Opioids and γ-Type Endorphins in Schizophrenia. Thesis, State University Utrecht, The Netherlands.

Verhoeven, W.M.A., Van Ree, J.M., Westenberg, H.G.M, Krul, J.M., Brouwer, G.J., Thijssen, J.H.H., De Wied, D., Van Praag, H.M., Ceulemans, D.L.S. and Kahn, R.S.: Clinical, biochemical and hormonal aspects of treatment with des-tyr¹-γ-endorphin in schizophrenia. *Psychiatry Res.* 1983. (In press).

Versteeg, D.H.G., De Kloet, E.R. and De Wied, D.: Effects of α-endorphin, β-endorphin and (Des-Tyr^1)-γ-endorphin on α-MPT-induced catecholamine disappearance in discrete regions of the rat brain. *Brain Res.* 179:85-93, 1979.

Versteeg, D.H.G., Kovács, G.L., Bohus, B., De Kloet, E.R. and De Wied, D.: Effect of (des-tyr^1-γ-endorphin and (des-tyr^1)-γ-endorphin on α-MPT-induced catecholamine disappearance in rat brain nuclei: a dose-response study. *Brain Res.* 231:343-351, 1982.

Volavka, J., Hui, K.S., Anderson, B., Nemer, Z., O'Donnell, J. and Lajtha, A.: Short-lived effect of (des-tyr)-gamma-endorphin in schizophrenia. Personal Communication, 1983.

Watson, S.J., Akil, H., Berger, Ph.A. and Barchas, J.D.: Some observations on the opiate peptides and schizophrenia, *Arch. Gen. Psychiatry* 36:35-41, 1979.

Watson, S.J., Akil, H., Ghazarossian, V.E. and Goldstein, A.: Dynorphin immunocytochemical localization in brain and peripheral nervous system: Preliminary studies. *Proc. Natl. Acad. Sci. USA* 78:1260-1263, 1981.

Watson, S.J., Khachaturian, H., Taylor, L., Fischli, W., Goldstein, A. and Akil, H.: Pro-dynorphin peptides are found in the same neurons throughout rat brain: Immunocytochemical study. *Proc. Natl. Acad. Sci. USA* 80:891-893, 1983.

Wei, E. and Loh, H.: Physical dependence on opiate-like peptides. *Science* 193:1262-1263, 1976.

Wing, J.K., Cooper, J.E. and Sartorius, N.: The measurement and classification of psychiatric symptoms. (Cambridge University Press, 1975.

World Health Organisation: The international pilot study of schizophrenia. *Geneva WHO*, I, 1973.

CHAPTER 8

Transmethylation Systems in Schizophrenia and Affective Disorders

John R. Smythies
Lelland C. Tolbert
John A. Monti

HISTORICAL INTRODUCTION

The original transmethylation hypothesis of schizophrenia (Osmond, Smythies, Harley-Mason and Redmill, 1952) was based on the chemical similarity between the hallucinogen, mescaline, and epinephrine and on the clinical similarity between the reaction to mescaline in some people ("bad trips") and acute schizophrenia. The hypothesis suggested that some fault in catecholamine metabolism might lead to the production of mescaline-like metabolites leading to psychotic symptoms. With the discovery of the hallucinogenic methylated tryptamines, such as dimethyltryptamine (DMT) and O-methylbufotenin (OMB), the hypothesis was extended to cover the possible production of methylated psychotoxins as an aberration of tryptamine or 5-hydroxytryptamine (5HT or serotonin) metabolism.

No hallucinogenic derivates of catecholamines have ever been detected in human body fluids, but both DMT and OMB have been shown to be normal, if trace, constituents of human CSF and rat brain by definitive gas chromatographic/mass spectrometric (GC/MS) methods (Smythies et al., 1979). But differences between the level of these compounds in schizophrenics versus normals were only minor, and much higher values were recorded in cases of liver disease without psychotic symptoms. Animal work suggests that DMT and OMB have a role in

99

the brain in stress reactions, since brain levels are significantly increased by stress (Beaton and Morris, 1982).

THE ONE-CARBON CYCLE HYPOTHESIS

In 1963, it was suggested (Smythies, 1963) that the fault in schizophrenia might lie in the *mechanism* of transmethylation itself rather than in any abnormal *products* of transmethylation. This mechanism comprises the one-carbon cycle, of which the essentials are shown in Figure 1. Carl et al. (1978) measured the performance of four enzymes of the one-carbon cycle in erythrocytes from schizophrenic patients diagnosed by the strict Feighner criteria versus normal controls. They found that two enzymes—methionine adenosyltransferase (MAT) and serine hydroxymethyltransferase (SHMT)—were significantly underactive in schizophrenic patients whereas two enzymes (the reductase and dehydrogenase) were normal. MAT and SHMT were low in different subgroups of patients, suggesting two biochemically characterized subtypes of the illness. Since MAT is a key enzyme in the one-carbon cycle that synthesizes S-adenosylmethionine (Adomet), the universal methyl donor in all transmethylation reactions, we concentrated our further studies on this enzyme.

Dunner et al. (1973), using 0.03 µM methionine, reported no difference in Adomet production using erythrocytes from normals or schizophrenic subjects. However, Carl et al. (1978), have reported decreased MAT activity in the erythrocytes from schizophrenic subjects when assayed using 67 µM methionine. The presence of two MAT isozymes in

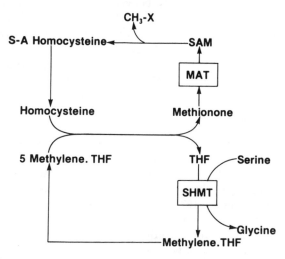

FIG. 8-1. Simplified one-carbon cycle. MAT = methionine adenosyltransferase. SHMT = serine hydroxymethyltransferase. SAM = S-adenosylmethionine. THF = Tetrahydrofolate.

human erythrocytes (Tallan, 1979) could be interpreted as the source of the disagreement between these two reports (Dunner et al., 1978; Carl et al., 1978). In an attempt to resolve this apparent discrepancy, we have performed a kinetic analysis of MAT activity in erythrocytes from schizophrenic subjects and normal controls.

In the earlier study (Kelsoe et al., 1982), Feighner criteria were used. In the present study, Diagnostic and Statistical Manual–3rd edition– (DSM-III) criteria were used to select schizophrenics, depressives, and manic-depressive patients. All patients were medicated. Patients with confounding neurological disorders, history of hallucinogen abuse, or components of organic brain syndrome were excluded. Healthy volunteers without history of psychiatric disorder were selected as controls. All patients were receiving psychotropic medications of various types.

MAT activity was measured using a crude enzyme preparation (partially purified from lysed erythrocytes by Sephadex G-25 column chromatography) and a modification of the assay of Liau et al. (1977). The assay involved incubating radiolabeled methionine (0.6-100 μm) for 1 hours with the enzyme and trapping the radiolabeled Adomet produced on cellulose phosphate paper. The reaction was quantitated by liquid scintillation counting. Vmax and Km were determined by double reciprocal plots of velocity versus substrate concentration after the data for protein concentration were normalized (Kelsoe et al., 1982).

Based on the single pH optimum obtained (7.0) and the lack of an inflection point in the double reciprocal plots of velocity vs. substrate concentration (R^2 for linear regressions were consistently greater than 0.95), kinetic evidence for more than one isozyme in a single subject was not obtained. The apparent Vmax and Km calculated from the double reciprocal plots of individual subjects are reported in Figures 2 and 3, respectively. A Mann-Whitney U test confirmed a significant difference ($P < .002$) in the apparent Vmax of MAT activity between controls and early onset schizophrenics with schizophrenics having a lower Vmax than controls. Significantly lower apparent Km were also observed in samples from schizophrenics when compared to controls ($P < .05$, Mann-Whitney U test). No significant correlations were obtained between the age or sex of the subject and MAT activity.

Because the assays were performed using only partially purified enzyme, our concern was that the observed difference in MAT activity (as measured by differences in ^{3}H-Adomet levels) might reflect differences in Adomet utilization (degradation). For this reason, we conducted the experiments, adding varying concentrations of ^{3}H-Adomet to patient samples and determining percentage recovery as described above. No significant differences in recovery of added ^{3}H-Adomet were observed between subjects. What was more critical, however, was the observation that the percentage of Adomet recovered (range was 9-12%) was inde-

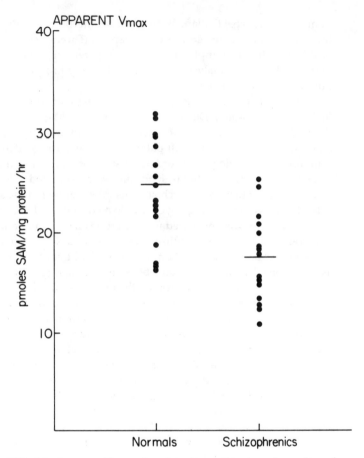

FIG. 8-2. Apparent Vmax of erythrocyte methionine adenosyltransferase.

pendent of both starting Adomet concentrations and time of incubation indicating that the loss of Adomet was due to nonenzymatic associated phenomena. In fact, the losses observed could be accounted for by losses of labeled Adomet from the cellulose phosphate paper during the wash step. Because the recovery was independent of time and concentration, it appears that the various methyltranferases and other Adomet degradative paths are not functioning appreciably under our assay conditions (possibly due to elimination of critical cofactors during the enzyme desalting step) and that our observed differences in ^{3}H-Adomet levels reflect differences in Adomet production (MAT activity) rather than differences in turnover or degradation.

Evaluation of the shape of the kinetic curves for normal and schizophrenic subjects which could be generated from the mean Km and Vmax

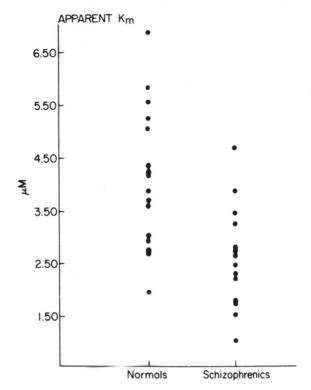

FIG. 8-3. Apparent Km of erythrocyte methionine adenosyltransferase.

for each group (normal x̄ Vmax = 25.4 pmol/mg protein/hr, Km = 3.95 μM; schizophrenic x̄ Vmax = 17.2, Km = 2.94) suggests a possible source of the disagreement between Dunner et al. (1973) and Carl et al. (1978). At the low substrate concentrations Dunner et al. (1973) used (0.03 μM methionine), minimal differences would be expected. However, at 67- μM substrate concentrations (where Carl et al. (1978) conducted their assays) differences in SAM production would be more apparent.

Figure 4 shows the data for Vmax to date in a population of normal controls, schizophrenics, depressives and manics (diagnoses according to DSM III). Note the subgroups of schizophrenics and of depression with low Vmax values and the manics with abnormally high values.

In all such studies the first consideration is to determine whether the findings may be due to medication, i.e. neuroleptics and lithium. To resolve this problem, we studied patients free of all medication for at least one month and then again at two weeks' interval following the start of medication. Table I shows the result for schizophrenics on neu-

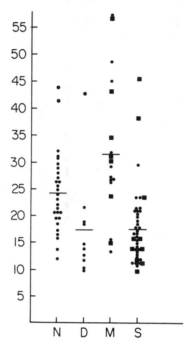

FIG. 8-4. Apparent Vmax of erythrocyte methionine adenosyltransferase. N = normals; D = depressed; S = schizophrenics; M = manics.

TABLE I. Schizophrenics—MAT Vmax

Subject	First	Second
I.O.	13.93	15.07
R.P.	15.57	32.78
R.H.	18.10	22.37
J.S.	11.72	25.19
D.E.	23.42	24.16
A.S.	14.32	15.65
K.G.	38.29	45.10
B.G.	11.9	11.4
J.S.	16.6	29.9
D.K.	45.4	11.2

First = MAT Vmax in blood samples from drug-free
Second = MAT Vmax in blood samples obtained from the same subjects after 2 weeks of neuroleptic therapy.

roleptics and Table II shows the result for manics and lithium. Note in nearly all cases the second Vmax's following neuroleptic medication were *higher* than the initial drug-free level in the case of the schizophrenics. In the case of the manic patients, the second and subsequent levels following the initiation of lithium therapy were *lower*. From these data we can deduce the following: (1) It is improbable that the low Vmax's in our medicated schizophrenics are due to neuroleptic medication. In fact, it is possible that the Vmax would be even lower were it not for the medication. (2) It is improbable that the high Vmax's in our manics medicated with lithium are artifacts of the lithium therapy, since following the start of lithium therapy, the Vmax declined. (3) On the present data one cannot say whether the decline in values for lithium and the increase in values for neuroleptics are straightforward effects of the drug on the enzyme system, or whether they represent changes in Vmax following clinical improvement in the patients. Further clinical data on what occurs in patients who are on medication but who show little or no clinical response are needed. However, *in vitro* experiments may provide enlightenment on this point.

For the *in vitro* approach erythrocytes were obtained from control

TABLE II. MAT Vmax activity in manic subjects under non-drug and drug conditions

| | Samples | | | |
| | Drug-free | Medicated | | |
Subjects	1	2	3	Medication
1	57.21	—	—	—
2	23.98	25.71	—	Hal
3	23.7	12.9	—	Li
4	15.5	12.6	19.2	Hal + Li
5	31.3	23.2	17.06	Li
6	34.6	26.3	18.4	Li
7	—	23.15	—	Hal
8	—	27.03	—	Hal
9	—	27.2	—	Hal
10	—	57.9	—	Hal
11	—	15.22	—	Li
12	—	27.87	—	CPZ + Pro + Art
13	—	29.25	—	Li + CPZ + Thyr
14	—	26.18	—	Nav
15	—	48.55	—	CPZ + Pro

Blood samples were obtained from drug-free manic subjects (1-6) upon admission (Column 1) and at weekly intervals (Column 2 & 3) after being placed on specified medication (Column 3). Additional blood samples were obtained from manic subjects (7-15) who were on medications at the time of admission (Column 2).

TABLE III

Subject	Control		CPZ		Hal		Flu		Thio	
	Vmax	Km	Vmax	Km	Vmax	Km	Vmax	Km	Vmax	Km
H.O.	25.01	1.99	24.87	2.59	25.36	2.87	24.92	3.49	25.42	4.96
J.K.	21.04	3.68	21.23	3.97	20.86	4.08	21.03	4.36	20.95	4.25
L.T.	23.40	5.44	23.61	5.86	24.12	5.73	23.51	6.02	23.46	6.54

CPZ = chlorpromazine, 500 ng/ml
Hal = haloperidol, 30 ng/ml
Flu = fluphenazine, 5 ng/ml
Thio = thioridazine, 500 ng/ml

subjects and aliquoted into five fractions. Four of these fractions were preincubated with high therapeutic plasma levels of neuroleptics (chosen because they represented the predominant medications received by the schizophrenic subject population). All fractions were then treated in a manner strictly analogous to the usual preparation of erythrocytes for MAT assay. This procedure includes a gel filtration step using a Sephadex G-25 column. Using gas chromatographic/mass spectrometric techniques, no neuroleptics were detected in the fractions following this step. The results are summarized in Table III.

The preincubation with neuroleptics resulted in no consistent effect on the Vmax. However, in all trials, all of the neuroleptics tested are associated with an increase in the Km. This lack of effect on Vmax and increase in Km would not support a contention that the decreased MAT activity (decreased Vmax and Km) observed in the schizophrenic patients is caused by the neuroleptics they were receiving.

Our results to date suggest that low Vmax kinetics are not specific for schizophrenia and the marked difference between bipolar depressed and manic patients suggest that Vmax may be a function of the affective state primarily rather than of "psychosis." Moreover, the levels appear to be state rather than trait dependent, although no data are yet available on the same bipolar patient when depressed and when manic. The linkage between Vmax for MAT and the affective state is supported by independent evidence detailed below on the clinical anti-depressant actions of S-adenosylmethionine (Adomet).

ANTI-DEPRESSANT ACTIONS OF ADOMET

In 1976 Agnoli et al. published the results of a double-blind trial of 30 patients on Adomet given intramuscularly at a dosage of 45 mg/day. They noted statistically significant improvements on several items on the Hamilton Rating Scale—namely, depressed mood, suicidal tendencies, work and interests, and psychomotor retardation. Anxiety ratings were not improved. The noted onset of action was rapid (4-7 days), and no side effects were noted except for some possible increased anxiety in some cases. These findings have since been replicated by seven groups of workers (Miccoli et al., 1978; Del Vecchio et al., 1978; Salvadorini et al., 1980; Muscettola et al., 1982; Kufferle et al., 1982; Carney et al., 1983 and Lipinski et al., 1984), and all report an anti-depressant action as good as standard anti-depressant drugs, a rapid onset and very few side effects. Carney et al. (1983) noted that Adomet levels therapy (i.v.i. 200 mg/day) did not increase blood Adomet levels but mean CSF Adomet increased from 48.7 ng/ml to 62.8 ng/ml (p < 0.01). They also noted that the effects of 14 days' therapy (including six cases who otherwise would have merited EST), lasted for at least three months with no relapse in that time, nor need for further Adomet. Three of their patients became hypomanic on Adomet treatment.

The question, therefore, is what is the mechanism of the anti-depressant effect of Adomet? One hypothesis is that Adomet is effective in those cases of depression who have low levels of activity (Vmax) of the enzyme, MAT, which makes endogenous Adomet. This hypothesis is currently under test. This hypothesis also links the high Vmax levels we found in manic patients with the hypomanic responses reported by Carney et al. (1983) in some of their depressed patients being treated with Adomet.

No studies have been reported on the effects of Adomet in mania or in schizophrenia. However, Pollin et al. (1961) reported that the dietary precursor of Adomet—namely, L-methionine—in large doses (20G/day) produced an acute psychotic reaction in some 40% of chronic schizophrenics. This has been confirmed by ten other groups of workers with no reported failures to replicate (see review by Cohen et al., 1974). The "methionine" reaction has always been interpreted as an exacerbation of the schizophrenic process, whereas this new evidence suggests that the reaction may really be an acute manic response superimposed on a chronic schizophrenic illness.

Alterations in the kinetic parameters of MAT would be expected to have widespread effects on neuronal activity because of the range of neuronal functions in which transmethylation plays a part. These include:

(1) Lipid Methylation: Phosphatidylethanolamine in the cell membrane is enzymatically methylated to form phosphatidylcholine (lecithin). It has been suggested that this mechanism plays an important role in coupling receptors for various neurotransmitters, hormones and other agents to adenylate cyclase. For example, Hirata et al. (1979) reported that beta-adrenergic agonists increased phospholipid methylation, membrane fluidity and beta-adrenergic-adenylate cyclase coupling. Prasad and Edwards (1981) reported that vasopressin stimulates rat pituitary phospholipid methyltransferase. Pfenninger and Johnson (1981) reported that nerve growth factor stimulates phospholipid methylation in growing neurites. Epidermal growth factor stimulates phospholipid methyltransferase in hepatocytes from juvenile but not mature rats. Bradykinin increases membrane phospholipid methylation (Dave et al., 1981). Recently, however, negative evidence has been reviewed (Koch et al., 1983) which indicates that lipid methylation is not concerned in many reactions linking receptors to adenylate cyclase, namely in the case of beta-adrenergic receptors in myogenic cells, responses of rat hepatocytes to beta-agonists and glucagon, and mitogen responses in lymphocytes. So it currently remains uncertain what role lipid methylation plays in receptor related events.

If there is a functional relationship between membrane lipid methylation and receptor activity, there exists the possibility of an abnormality in this system in schizophrenia and the affective disorders. Preliminary data on RBC's from manic-depressives suggest lithium effects on phospholipid methyltransferases (PMT's) (Hitzemann and Garver, 1982).

There have been several studies regarding differences in cellular lipid composition in schizophrenia. Stevens (1972) reported that PC and PE levels were reduced in RBC's from schizophrenic patients as compared with normal controls, while PS levels were elevated, and no differences in sphingomyelin (SPH) could be detected. These findings were replicated by Henn and Henn (1983), and recently in our preliminary study. Hitzemann and Garver (1980) have reported similar reductions in the levels of PC, and elevated levels of SPH in RBC's from schizophrenic patients, but no differences in PS, phosphatidylinositol (PI) or ethanolamine plasmalogen. Cordasco et al. (1982) and Lautin (1982) have reported finding no differences in the levels of PC, PE, PS or SPH in erythrocytes from schizophrenic patients as compared with controls, while Sengupta, Datta and Sengupta (1981) have reported data similar to that of Stevens, Henn and our preliminary study, with the exception of an apparent increase in PC in erythrocytes from schizophrenic patients. It is interesting to note that in the latter study, similar differences in lipids were found in both erythrocytes and platelets from schizophrenic patients, which suggests that the lipid abnormality in schizophrenia, if genuine, might be reflected in a number of different types of cells. There are, of course, discrepancies in the results, which we feel might be resolved by: 1) more carefully controlled product isolation and characterization; 2) comparisons of PMT activity, including kinetic studies in lymphocytes and platelets as well as erythrocytes, since in the latter two types of cells, PC biosynthesis can occur via either methylation or by the more general CDP-choline pathway; and 3) examining some of the consequences which might be expected to occur if indeed there are abnormalities in plasma membrane lipids in cells derived from schizophrenic patients. While the data on membrane lipids (abnormal in schizophrenics) is not uniformly consistent, we feel that to date there is sufficient supporting evidence for this hypothesis to warrant further research in the area.

There is the possibility that membrane lipid methylation might be related to the transmethylation and dopamine hypotheses of schizophrenia. As originally enunciated, the transmethylation hypothesis had apparent support from the observation of exacerbation of symptoms in some schizophrenic patients following oral administration of methionine. Methionine, through its conversion to S-adenosylmethionine, might result in abnormal or increased methylation reactions leading to the formation of psychotoxic products. However, studies have indicated that, in fact, administration of high doses of methionine to rats did not lead to increased formation of certain transmethylated products. Further, methionine adenosyltransferase (MAT) activity is decreased in RBC's from schizophrenic patients. Thus, it would appear that the simple explanation of "overmethylation" is insufficient to explain the methionine effect. The hypothesis that two PMT's are involved in phospholipid methylation, which differ in kinetic (Km and Vmax) properties, offers a possible explanation for the methionine effect, the lack of detection of "increased methylated products," and predicts the consequences of low MAT activity. An abnormality in the second PMT (the high Km form) could result in increased accumulation of monomethyl PE (MPE) and a decrease in PE and consequently PC. In schizophrenics the first PMT (low Km form) would, in this hypothesis, function either normally (or perhaps overactively), and would be saturated with respect to Adomet even under conditions where MAT activity was low. Methionine administration might raise the levels of Adomet in schizophrenics, but in this case would tend to exacerbate the condition further, with an even larger buildup of monomethyl PE. It is interesting to note that the first PMT has been described as the rate-limiting step in the phospholipid methylation pathway. Subsequent methylation of MPE is theoretically very rapid. Thus, in order to explain the observed decreases in both PE and PC, an obligatory defect in PMT II (low activity) must be postulated, with the possibility of a defect (high activity) in PMT I. This condition might not be present in all schizophrenics. Indeed, only about 40% of the schizophrenics tested were so-called "methionine responders." It is also important to note that the pool of membrane phospholipids involved in the methylation pathway is quite small compared with the total phospholipid pool. Therefore, in cell types such as lymphocytes, which synthesize PC primarily via the CDP choline pathway, the total amounts of PC and PE might be identical in both normals and schizophrenics. In order to assess possible defects in the methylation pathway, receptor-stimulated phospholipid methylation should be measured. The dopamine theory finds its chief support in the demonstration of the ability of neuroleptics to block dopamine receptors in a manner which is well correlated with their clinical efficacy. We reiterate the recent data which suggests that dopamine stimulates and that certain neuroleptics inhibit (Leprohon et al., 1982) lipid methylation. Again, current hypotheses suggest that lipid methylation, in certain cases, facilitates coupling between receptors and effectors. If in schizophrenia, as proposed in the previous paragraph, the lipid methylation process is locked in an "open" position at the point of MPE, one might expect to see supersensitivity or overactivity of receptor-mediated events. Blockade of the receptors and inhibition of methylation would ameliorate this condition.

(2) Protein Methylation: The methylation of carboxyl groups of protein has been shown to play an important role in neurotransmitter release (Billingsly and Roth, 1983), as well as in the control of chemotaxis in E. Coli (Kehry et al., 1983) and neurite extension (Pfenninger and Johnson, 1981). Other mechanisms affected by protein carboxymethylation are sperm motility, leucocyte chemotaxis, and calmodulin function (Campillo and Ashcroft, 1982). Dopamine agonists stimulate carboxymethylation in striatal synaptosomes, which stimulation is blocked by (+) and not by (−) butaclamol (Billingsly and Roth, 1982). Protein carboxymethylase is found in high concentrations in brain (grey > white), is axonally transported, and rapidly modulates negative charges in protein (by converting the negatively charged carboxyl group to the neutral O-methyl ester) (Diliberto and Axelrod, 1976). There are also high levels in the chromatin granules of the adrenal medulla where it may be concerned in exocytosis. The enzyme also occurs in lens tissue (McFadden et al., 1983). These workers distinguish between two types of carboxymethylase. One enzyme is found only in bacterial chemotactic mechanisms that methylate glutamic acid residues. Another is widely distributed in all tissues and specifically methylates d-aspartic acid in a wide range of proteins. This unusual residue is found in aged proteins as a product of natural racemization as part of a postulated degenerative and racemization-repair pathway. Oden and Clarke (1983) have pointed out that the main function of MAT in red blood cells is carboxymethylation, since these cells contain no nucleic acids or polyamines, and less than 2% of labeled methyl groups are incorporated into lipids.

The methylation of basic groups (e.g. lysine) has been reported to regulate the interactions of proteins with nucleic acids (Hiatt et al., 1982).

(3) Nucleic Acid Methylation is important in gene expression and other related mechanisms.

Biochemical Studies with Adomet and Related Compounds

Andreoli and Maffei (1975) reported that blood levels of Adomet were significantly lower in acute, but not chronic, schizophrenics as compared to normal controls (p = 0.001). They suggested that Adomet should be an effective treatment in acute schizophrenia. This, however, was not reported by Matthysse and Baldessarini (1972). It is noteworthy that both Pollin et al. (1961) and Antun et al. (1971) noted long-term improvement in some of their schizophrenic patients following a "methionine reaction." It should be noted that this reaction followed the administration of 20G L-methionine per day, which may represent a gross overdose. A more controlled and beneficial activation of chronic withdrawn schizophrenics may be obtained if small doses of L-methionine are used.

Iontophoretic injection of Adomet onto neurons in rat sensorimotor cerebral cortex increased the rate of spontaneous firing (Phillis, 1981). This effect was not shared by its precursor–L-methionine–nor the degradation products–L-homocysteine and adenosine. S-adenosyl-L-homocysteine displayed weak Adomet-like activity.

Adomet (i.m. or i.v.) administered to rats caused a rise in brain serotonin and 5HIAA, and in patients treated with Adomet, CSF 5HIAA levels are raised (Curcio et al., 1978).

L-DOPA administration causes a depletion of Adomet concentration by acting as a methyl group receptor (Wurtman et al., 1970; Ovdonez and Wurtman, 1973; Chalmers et al., 1971). Thus depletion can be prevented by Adomet injections (Stramentinoli et al., 1980).

Cimino et al. (1983) have studied lipid transmethylation in the aging process in rats. They find that the brain levels of phosphatidylcholine are reduced in aging rat brain. Fluorescence polarization and electron spin resonance measures revealed a significant decrease in the fluidity of the membrane in aging rats which could be reversed by three months Adomet treatment. This change was confined to the hydrophobic core of the membrane. The same group found that striatal beta-adrenergic binding sites were reduced in aging rat brain, and this too could be partly prevented by Adomet treatment. This effect was also seen in the pineal gland, but not in the cortex, nor in the case of dopamine receptors.

It is of interest that Levi and Waxman (1975) suggested that schizophrenics should have low levels of MAT activity. Their hypothesis was based mainly on the observations that folate-responsive schizophrenia-like syndromes develop in some epileptics treated with anti-convulsant drugs. They further suggest that Adomet should be an effective treatment in these cases. Our present hypothesis postulates that Adomet deficiencies are correlated with an underlying MAT deficiency in depression and an excess in mania, and so this abnormality may be linked to affective disorders rather than schizophrenia. However, it may be the case that stress, of the kind experienced in depression and schizophrenia, via increased levels of catecholamines that are metabolized in part by COMT, leads to a functional depression of MAT activity and Adomet levels, whereas stress of the kind experienced in mania has the opposite effect. Further clinical studies correlating the exact affective condition of the patient with MAT kinetics and Adomet levels may throw further light on this problem.

REFERENCES

Agnoli, A., Andreoli, V., Casacchia, M. and Cerbo, R.: Effect of S-adenosyl-L-methionine (SAMe) upon depressive symptoms. *J. Psychiat. Res.* 13:43-54, 1976.

Andreoli, V.M. and Maffei, T.: Blood levels of S-adenosylmethionine in schizophrenia. *Lancet* ii:922, 1975.

Antun, F.T., Burnett, G.B., Cooper, A.J., Daly, R.J., Smythies, J.R. and Zealley, A.K.: The effects of L-methionine (without MAOI) in schizophrenia. *J. Psychiat. Res.* 8:63-71, 1971.

Beaton, J. and Morris, P.E.: Developmental changes in the levels of N,N-dimethyltryptamine and related indolealkylamines in rat brain. *Soc. Neurosci. Abstracts* 8:176, 1982.

Billingsly, M.L. and Roth, R.H.: Dopamine agonists stimulate carboxymethylation in striatal synaptosomes. *J. Pharm. Exp. Therap.* 223:681-688, 1982.

Campillo, J.E. and Ashcroft, S.J.H.: Protein carboxymethylation in rat islets of Langerhans. *FEBS Letts.* 138:71-75, 1982.

Carl, G.F., Crews, E.L., Carmichael, S.M., Benesh, F.C. and Smythies, J.R.: Four enzymes of one-carbon metabolism in blood cells of schizophrenics. *Biol. Psychiat.* 13:773-776, 1978.

Carney, M.W.P., Martin, R., Bottiglieri, T., Reynolds, E.H., Nissenbaum, H., Toone, B.K. and Sheffield, B.F.: Switch mechanism in affective illness and S-adenosylmethionine. *Lancet* i:820-821, 1983.

Chalmers, J.P., Balesssarini, R.J. and Wurtman, R.J.: Effects of L-Dopa on norepinephrine metabolism in the brain. *Proc. Nat. Acad. Sci., USA* 68(1):662-666, 1971.

Cimino, M., Curatola, G., Pezzoli, C., Stramentinoli, G., Vanini, G. and Algeri, S.: Age-related modification of dopaminergic and beta-adrenergic receptor system: restoration of normal activity by modifying membrane fluidity with S-adenosylmethionine. In: Aging Brain and Ergot Alkaloids, (A. Agnoli, G. Crepaldi, P.F. Spano and M. Trabuchhi, eds.), Raven Press, New York, 1983.

Cohen, S., Nichols, A. and Wyatt, R.: The administration of methionine to chronic schizophrenic patients; a review of ten studies. *Biol. Psychiat.* 8:109-221, 1974.

Cordasco, D.M., Wazer, D., Segarnick, D.J., Lautin, A., Lippa, A. and Rotrosen, J.: Phospholipids and phospholipid methylation in platelets and brain. *Psychopharmacol. Bull.* 18:193-197, 1982.

Curcio, M., Catto, E., Stramentinoli, G. and Algeri, S.: Effect of S-adenosyl-L-methionine on serotonin metabolism in rat brain. *Prog. New Psychopharm.* 2:65-71, 1978.

Dave, J.R., Knazek, R.A. and Leu, S.C.: Arachidonic acid, bradykinin and phospholipase A_2 modify both prolactin binding capacity and fluidity of mouse hepatic membranes. *Biochem. Biophys. Res. Comm.* 103:727-738, 1981.

Del Vecchio, M., Iovio, G., Cocorullo, M., Vacca, L. and Amati, A.: Has SAMe (Adomet) an antidepressant effect? A preliminary trial versus chloroimipramine. *Riv. Sper. Fren.* 102:344-358, 1978.

Di Liberto, E.J., Jr., and Axelrod, J.: Regional and subcellular distribution of protein carboxylase in brain and other tissues. *J. Neurochem.* 26:1159-1165, 1976.

Dunner, D.L., Cohn, C.K., Weinshilboum, R.M. and Wyatt, R.J.: The activity of dopamine-beta-hydroxylase and methionine-activating enzyme in blood of schizophrenic patients. *Biol. Psychiat.* 6:215-220, 1973.

Henn, F.A. and Henn, S.W.: Phospholipids as markers for schizophrenia. In: Biological Markers in Psychiatry and Neurology, (E. Usdin and I. Hanin, eds.), Pergamon Press, New York, pp. 183-185, 1982.

Hiatt, W.R., Garcia, R., Merrick, W.C. and Sypherd, P.S.: Methylation of elongation factor 1 alpha from the fungus Mucor. *Proc. Nat. Acad. Sci., USA* 79:3433-3437, 1982.

Hirata, F., Strittmatter, W.J. and Axelrod, J.: Beta-adrenergic receptor agonists increase phospholipid methylation, membrane fluidity, and beta-adrenergic-adenylate cyclase coupling. *Proc. Nat. Acad. Sci., USA* 76:368-372, 1979.

Hitzemann, R. and Garver, D.: Membrane abnormalities in schizophrenia. *Psychopharmacol. Bull.* 18:190-193, 1982.

Kehry, M.R., Bond, M.W., Hunkapiller, M.V. and Dahlquist, F.W.: Enzymatic deamidation of methyl-accepting chemotaxic proteins in *Escherichia coli* catalyzed by the *cheB* gene product. *Proc. Nat. Acad. Sci., USA* 80:3599-3603, 1983.

Kelsoe, J.R., Tolbert, L.C., Crews, E.L. and Smythies, J.R.: Kinetic evidence for decreased methionine adenosyltransferase activity in erythrocytes from schizophrenics. *J. Neurosci. Res.* 8:99-103, 1982.

Koch, T.K., Gordon, A.S. and Diamond, I.: Phospholipid methylation in myogenic cells. *Biochem. Biophys. Res. Comm.* 114:339-347, 1983.

Kufferle, B. and Grunberger, J.: Early clinical double-blind study with S-adenosyl-L-methionine: a new potential anti-depressant. In: Typical and Atypical Antidepressants: Clinical Practice, (E. Costa and C. Racagni, eds.), Raven Press, New York, 1982.

Lautin, A., Cordasco, D.M., Segarnick, D.J., Wood, L., Mason, M.F., Wolkin, A. and Rotrosen, J.: Red cell phospholipids in schizophrenia. *Life Sci.* 31:3051-3056, 1982.

Leprohon, C.E., Blusztajn, J.K. and Wurtman, R.: Monoamines stimulate phosphatidylethanolamine methylation in rat brain. *Proc. Soc. Neurosci.* (abstract #197.8), 1982.

Levi, R.N. and Waxman, S.: Schizophrenia, epilepsy, cancer, methionine and folate metabolism. *Lancet* ii:11-13, 1975.

Liau, M.C., Lin, G.W. and Hurlbert, B.B.: Partial purification and characterization of tumor and liver S-adenosylmethionine synthetases. *Cancer Res.* 37:427-435, 1977.

Lipinski, J.F., Cohen, B.M., Frankenburg, F., Tohen, M., Waterhaux, C., Altesman, R., Jones, B. and Harris, P.: Open trial of S-adenosylmethionine for treatment of depression. *Amer. J. Psychiat.* 141:448-450, 1982.

McFadden, P.N., Horwitz, J. and Clarke, S.: Protein carboxymethyltransferase from cow eye lens. *Biochem. Biophys. Res. Comm.* 113:418-424, 1983.

Matthysse, S. and Baldessarini, R.J.: S-adenosylmethionine and catechol-O-methyltransferase in schizophrenia. *Amer. J. Psychiat.* 128:1310-1312, 1972.

Miccoli, L., Porro, V. and Bertolino, A.: Comparison between the antidepressant activity of S-adenosylmethionine (SAMe) and that of some tricyclic drugs. *Acta Neurologica* 33:243-255, 1978.

Muscettola, G., Golzenati, M. and Balbi, A.: SAMe versus placebo: a double-blind comparison in major depressive disorders. In: Typical and Atypical Antidepressants: Clinical Practice, (E. Costa and G. Racagni, eds.), Raven Press, New York, 1982.

Oden, K.I. and Clarke: S-adenosyl-L-methionine synthetase from human erythrocytes: role in the regulation of cellular S-adenosylmethionine levels. *Biochemistry* 22:2978-2986, 1982.

Osmond, H., Smythies, J.R., Harley-Mason, J. and Redmill, J.: Schizophrenia. A new approach. *J. Ment. Sci.* 98:309-315, 1952.

Ovdonez, L.A. and Wurtman, R.J.: Folic acid deficiency and methyl group metabolism in rat brain: effects of L-Dopa. Reversal effect by S-adenosyl-L-methionine. *Arch. Biochem. Biophys.* 160:372-376, 1974.

Pfenninger, K.H. and Johnson, M.: Nerve growth factor stimulates phospholipid methylation in growing neurites. *Proc. Nat. Acad. Sci., USA* 78:7797-7800, 1981.

Phillis, J.W.: S-adenosylmethionine excites rat cerebral cortical neurons. *Brain Res.* 25:223-226, 1981.

Pollin, W., Cardon, P.V., Jr. and Kety, S.S.: Effects of amino acid feedings in schizophrenic patients with iproniazid. *Science* 133:104-105, 1961.

Prasad, C. and Edwards, R.M.: Stimulation of rat pituitary phospholipid methyltransferase by vasopressin but not oxytocin. *Biochem. Biophys. Res. Comm.* 103:559-564, 1981.

Salvadorini, F., Galeone, F., Saba, P., Tognetti, G. and Mariani, G.: Evaluation of S-adenosylmethionine (SAMe) effectiveness in depression. *Curr. Therap. Res.* 17:908-918, 1980.

Sengupta, N., Datta, S.C. and Sengupta, D.: Platelet and erythrocyte membrane lipid and phospholipid patterns in different types of mental patients. *Biochem. Med.* 25:267-275, 1981.

Smythies, J.R.: Biochemistry of schizophrenia. *Postgrad. Med. J.* 39:26-33, 1963.

Smythies, J.R.: Recent advances in the biochemistry of schizophrenia. *Guy's Gazette* May 14, 2-7, 1966.

Smythies, J.R., Morin, R.D. and Brown, G.B.: Identification of dimethyltryptamine and O-methylbufotenin in human ce-

rebrospinal fluid by combined gas chromatography/mass spectrometry. *Biol. Psychiat.* 14:549-556, 1979.

Stevens, J.D.: The distribution of the phospholipid fractions in the red cell membranes of schizophrenics. *Schizophr. Bull.* 6:60-61, 1972.

Stramentinoli, G., Cato, E., Algeri, S. and Agnoli, A.: Effetto di un trattamento con L-Dopa o con L-Dopa piu' inibitori della Dopa-decarbossilasi sui livelli cerebrali di S-adenosil-L-mentionlna nel topo. Atti della 6th Riunione della Lega Italiana per la lotta Contro il Morbo di Parkinson, 221-225, 1980.

Tallan, H.H.: Methionine adenosyltransferase in man: evidence for multiple forms. *Biochem. Med.* 21:129-140, 1979.

Wurtman, R.J., Rose, C.M., Matthysse, A., Stephenson, J. and Baldessarini, R.J.: L-dihydroxyphenalanine: effect on S-adenosylmethionine in brain. *Science* 169: 395-397, 1970.

CHAPTER 9

Blood Levels of Neuroleptic Drugs and their Relevance for Clinical Practice

Joseph Zohar
David Greenberg
R.H. Belmaker

INTRODUCTION

The attention that has been devoted to the measurement of blood levels of therapeutic agents has resulted in a significant improvement in the quality of care in several areas of medicine (Shannon et al, 1944; Jelliffe et al, 1972). In routine clinical use today, monitoring of blood levels of drugs is used with the cardiac glycoside group, various cardiac antiarrhythmics (lidocaine, quinidine and procainamide), anticonvulsants (primidone, phenobarbitone, phenytoin and carbamazepine), antibiotics (gentamicin and chloramphenicol), theophyline and methothrexate.

Montoring of blood levels provides the physician with an important facility for the following: adjusting the dose to reach the optimal level for a particular patient, assessment of patient compliance, early warning and confirmation of toxicity.

Two decades of research involving thousands of patients have demonstrated that neuroleptic agents produce a clear and valuable clinical improvement in schizophrenia (Casey et al, 1960; Adelson and Epstein, 1962; Lasky et al, 1962; NIMH-PSC Collaborative Study Group, 1964; Engelhardt et al, 1967). Few would deny that neuroleptic agents are a significant component in the treatment of psychoses (Davis and Cole, 1975; Klein et al, 1980; Gaind and Barnes, 1981). The obvious advantages of repeated measurement of therapeutic blood levels plus the existence of a large population of schizophrenics who are either noncompliant (Van-Putten, 1974) or unresponsive to neuroleptic therapy (Davis and Cole, 1975) have resulted in great interest in the monitoring of blood levels of neuroleptic agents.

Unlike the topic to be discussed, blood levels of antidepressant medication have been the subject of review articles for several years (Risch et al, 1979; Friedel, 1982). Presumably the association between antidepressant blood levels and the clinical state is clearer and the state of knowledge more complete than in the case of antipsychotic medication. Among the reasons for this discrepancy are that antidepressants have fewer active metabolites in comparison with the majority of neuroleptics (Kutz and Davidson, 1977) and that the recommended dose range of antidepressants is a factor of 2 - 3, while the dose range with neuroleptics is a factor of up to 100 (Davis and Cole, 1975). Nevertheless, of late, there has been progress in the measurement of neuroleptic blood levels.

ASSESSMENT METHODS OF NEUROLEPTIC PLASMA LEVELS

Fluorimetry is based on the photosensitivity of a compound at a specific wavelength and absorption of light at another wavelength. The method is not specific and the values are relatively high, so that it is now obsolete. It is important nowadays that clinicians should not use values based on the results of studies using this method (Gottschalk et al, 1976; Smith et al, 1977), unless the research was replicated using more reliable methods (Gottschalk et al, 1976).

Gas chromatography (G.C.) is based on the passage of a compound along a column and its identification according to the speed with which it separates within the column (McNair and Bonelli, 1969). It is necessary to devise a method of extraction for each compound and to ascertain its characteristic rate of passage.

As early as 1968, Curry and Marshall investigated the levels of chlorpromazine and some of its metabolites using G.C. In 1971, Zingaler (1971) and Marcucci et al (1971) developed methods for measuring the blood levels of haloperidol, but these methods are lengthy and inaccurate. In 1974, Forsman et al published a rapid and relatively accurate method of measurement of haloperidol blood levels. This new method, with minor modifications, is used today to measure levels of this drug using G.C. It has a high reliability; for example, about 10 percent for haloperidol (Forsman et al, 1974). (Test-retest reliability is the extent to which the same procedure will yield the same result in repeated tests of the same specimen.) Using G.C., the range of sensitivity to haloperidol is 0.5-20 ng/ml of plasma (Forsman et al, 1974). Its validity, however, could be questioned. (Validity is the extent to which a particular test is measuring what it claims to be measuring.) The validity of measurements using G.C. is particularly problematic with compounds such as chlor-promazine, which have many metabolites, as invariably only a small portion of them are measured in the test; and, it may well be that other psychoactive metabolites are not being measured. This method is capable of measuring a variety of metabolites on an individual basis. If, on the basis of animal experiments, we knew which were the metabolites which had an effect on behavior, which did not, and the interaction between them, then G.C. would be a highly reliable method (Snyder and Kirland, 1974). However, even then the majority of the proteins of the blood would have to be extracted as they impede column function, and every metabolite would require a specific extraction process based on its chem-ical properties. Economically, G.C. requires expensive equipment and technical expertise and has a low output—the column can only be used for one specimen at a time, taking over 10 minutes. The operation, maintenance and calibration also consume time and expertise. However, unlike radioimmunoassay techniques (see below), G.C. does not require expensive substances that deteriorate rapidly, so that once the equip-ment is available it is relatively inexpensive to run.

In High Performance (Pressure) Liquid Chromatography, air pres-sure at several thousand pounds per square inch facilitates the separation process. By adding sensitive detectors that monitor the compound as they leave the column, it can be used to measure blood levels of neu-roleptics. In contrast to G.C., extraction/isolation of the fragments prior to introduction into the column is a simpler process: it is more specific, more rapid and capable of a higher output. In all other respects, it is similar to G.C.

Radioimmunoassay (RIA) was initially developed for immunogenic polypeptide hormones and is based on the production of antibodies to the test compound (Berson and Yalow, 1968). Antibody production is stimulated in animals, usually a rabbit or a goat, by repeated injection of large molecules (Playfair et al, 1974). RIA method is available for a variety of neuroleptics: chlorpromazine (Kawashima et al, 1975), pi-mozide (Michiels et al, 1975), flupenthixol (Robinson and Risby, 1977), fluphenazine (Wiles and Franklin, 1978) and haloperidol. There are two forms of antibody to haloperidol available: one that cross-reacts with several metabolites (Michiels et al, 1976) and one that is specific to halo-peridol alone (Clark et al, 1977). RIA requires only minute specimens (micolitres of plasma or serum) and has a high output—one technician can perform dozens of tests daily. Its reliability and sensitivity are de-pendent on several factors, including the characteristics and specificity of the antibodies. The setting up of this assay in a particular laboratory is also dependent on the regular supply of antibodies. Furthermore, different goats can produce differing qualities of antibodies, which can result in variations in the absolute results between tests and give rise to difficulties in fixing normal values. Occasionally, the antibody does not bind to a particular metabolite, necessitating an additional test specifically for that metabolite. At the start of an assay, an ampoule of antibodies is opened which, when dissolved, deteriorates within days. It is possible to test scores of specimens of blood simultaneously with the dissolved antibody. The cost of twenty simultaneous tests is, therefore, almost identical to a single test, so that it is only really economical if a group of specimens is to be tested together, i.e. once a week in a hospital. When a large number are carried out on one day, the simplicity and economy of the techniques are such as to make it less expensive than G.C.

The advantage of the radioreceptorassay (RRA), developed by Creese and Snyder (1977), is that it measures the medication and its metabolites' capacity to block dopaminergic receptors (Lader, 1980). There is much support for the hypothesis that the mode of action of neuroleptic and medication involves blocking dopamine receptors (Carlsson and Lindquist, 1963). The ability of all neuroleptic drugs to block dopamine receptors in the brains of laboratory animals is directly proportional to the mean neuroleptic dosage used in psychoses in humans (Creese et al, 1976). It would, therefore, seem reasonable to consider that RRA is a bioassay that measures the potency of the medication at its pharmacological target. The method is based on the competition between the unknown concentration of neuroleptic medication in the sample with a known quantity of radioactively-labelled neuroleptic compound (3H-haloperidol or 3H-spiroperidol) which is bound to a dopaminergic receptor. The method essentially parallels radioimmunoassays that measure the binding of a radioactive compound to an antibody that binds the radioactive compound. In the case of RRA, the medication in the patient's plasma competes with the radioactive material and decreases the quantity of medication bound to the receptor. The advantages of the method are: a) it measures all active components [chlorpromazine and thioridazine, for example, have over one hundred active metabolites (Sakalis et al, 1972), and it would be very difficult to measure them all using G.C. or RIA]; b) unlike G.C., but similar to RIA, specimens of plasma are usable without extraction or any additional preparation, which simplifies and accelerates the procedure; c) the method is uniformly applicable to all neuroleptics as all antipsychotics are dopaminergic receptor blockers. When a variety of types of neuroleptics are tested, the results are presented as equivalents of 1 mg chlorpromazine (Tune, 1980).

The main flaw of RRA is its relatively low sensitivity. In an average outpatient population receiving maintenance medication equivalent to 10 mg haloperidol, the blood levels of the majority of the patients will be below the threshold of sensitivity of this method (Tune, 1980).

THE PHARMACOKINETICS OF NEUROLEPTIC MEDICATION

The factors that determine the levels of neuroleptic medication in the blood include the degree of absorption into the blood (Bianchelli et al, 1980), the rate of breakdown in the body (Curry et al, 1970), and the general physical condition of the patient (Axelsson, 1976). The level of neuroleptic in the blood following oral administration is approximately 50 percent less than the level following intramuscular or intravenous administration (Cressman et al, 1974; Forsman and Ohman, 1976; Bianchelli et al, 1980). Chlorpromazine, for instance, is metabolized into inactive fragments in the mucosal wall during digestion (Curry et al, 1971), while haloperidol is metabolized in the "first pass" in the liver (Forsman and Ohman, 1976). Active charcoal, antacid and kaopectate decrease the absorption of neuroleptics by absorption (Forrest et al, 1970; Fann, 1973; Fann et al, 1973).

Neuroleptic medication has a high affinity for fats (Gothel and Karczmar, 1963; Oldendorf and Dewhurst, 1978), is concentrated in fatty tissue, such as brain, and crosses the blood-brain barrier without difficulty (Ohman et al, 1977). The levels of neuroleptic medication in brain tissues are several times higher than in the blood. This fact may confound any attempt to find an association between blood levels and the psychoactivity of the medication. On the other hand, it is possible that a significant proportion of the medication concentrated in the brain is dissolved in fats that are not related to the dopaminergic system. The dopaminergic receptor is thought to be the pharmacological target of neuroleptic medication (Carlsson and Lindquist, 1963). This receptor is a huge molecule that faces out from the cell membrane towards the extracellular fluid. Therefore, it is reasonable to assume that the level in the plasma (extracellular fluid) may reflect the level of drug in the vicinity of the dopaminergic receptor, even though the drug level in the entire brain, including the fat-bound drug, is much higher.

More than 90 percent of a neuroleptic drug in plasma is protein bound (Rubin et al, 1980). The level of neuroleptics in the cerebrospinal fluid (CSF) is 3-10 percent of the level in the blood (Forsman and Ohman, 1977), presumably a consequence of the low level of proteins in the CSF (Forsman and Ohman, 1977). Neuroleptic drugs in the CSF are in a state of equilibrium with the free fraction of the drug in the blood. Furthermore, there is a high correlation ($r = .84$) between the total neuroleptic blood level and the level of free drug (Rubin et al, 1980). A correlation of this magnitude should permit us to deduce the concentration at the brain-binding sites from the total blood drug level. This can, of course, lead to erroneous conclusions, as in the case of an undernourished patient with a low serum albumin, who would have low blood levels with a marked behavioral response. In such a case, there is a large fraction of unbound drug because of the diminished binding capacity.

Pharmacokinetic research has been carried out on normal volunteers following a single dose of neuroleptic medication. The levels of chlorpromazine following a single intramuscular injection vary widely between individuals (Curry and Marshall, 1968). Similar peak level times (4 hours) and half-life (5 hours) have been demonstrated with mesoridazine (Gottschalk et al, 1976). Following a single intramuscular injection, haloperidol peaks in 2-6 hours (Ohman et al, 1977), although its half-life is longer, about 14 hours (Ohman et al, 1977), and similar to butaperazine (Casper et al, 1980). The half-life and time to reach peak levels following a single injection, however, are of no significance in prolonged therapy with these drugs. As these drugs are highly lipophilic, they penetrate all fatty tissues for storage. The rate of elimination from blood following a single injection is a consequence both of penetrating the body fat and of being metabolized. It is only after the loading of fatty tissues is completed that the half-life will reflect the rate of leaving the fatty tissue and their metabolism. In the case of haloperidol, it takes six days to achieve stable blood levels, a state of equilibrium between the blood and the body's fatty tissues (Forsman and Ohman, 1977). In a patient terminating prolonged treatment, the half-life of haloperidol is 12-38 hours (Forsman and Ohman, 1977).

Once neuroleptic drugs have been stored in fatty tissues, including brain, they need only be prescribed once daily (Klein et al, 1980). The presence of a reservoir of medication in the fatty tissues will prevent sharp changes in blood levels even while receiving a single daily dose, although such a situation only exists once the stores have been loaded. For this reason, it is necessary to give a neuroleptic drug several times a day at the start of treatment in order to prevent large variations in blood levels. The time required for the loading of fatty stores and the achievement of steady-state equilibrium in about 6-10 days. Until the steady state equilibrium is achieved, the blood level is primarily determined by the period of time since the last dose of medication. The level in the blood may be used as an index of the drug level at the dopaminergic site only after a steady-state equilibrium has been reached, since it is only then that the level in the blood is in equilibrium with the drug concentration in other body tissues. From this, it follows that after any alteration in dose of medication, about 10 days must be allowed to elapse until a new steady-state is reached and only then can the blood test be considered a reflection of the level in the brain. Neuroleptic drugs have side effects such as fainting after peripheral vasodilatation which are directly related to blood levels and not brain levels. Patients who are sensitive to such side effects should not be given a large single daily dose of a drug that may produce a peak level in the blood, even though there is no necessity on the basis of its antipsychotic action.

When chronic administration of neuroleptic medication is terminated, the medication gradually leaves the fatty stores. Several days later, there will no longer be a significant concentration in the blood (Goldman et al, 1981). The clinical state of schizophrenic patients does not necessarily deteriorate during this period in the same way that it can take several weeks for improvement to occur when therapy is started (Klein et al, 1980). Single assessment performed throughout this period, therefore, may well fail to reveal an association between the clinical state and the blood level. The only conditions under which a significant correlation could be expected are if both blood levels and the clinical assessment are measured after equilibrium has been attained. The drug levels should be related to the changes in the clinical state of the particular patients and not to a single evaluation of their condition.

THE ASSOCIATION BETWEEN CLINICAL RESPONSE AND BLOOD LEVELS

The pioneer of blood levels of neuroleptic medication was Curry, whose first publication on the subject appeared in 1968 (Curry, 1968). Subsequent work from the same group found neither a correlation between oral dosage and blood levels (Curry and Marshall, 1968) nor between clinical response and blood levels (Sakalis et al, 1972). They considered this a consequence of the many metabolites of the drug (Curry et al, 1972) [chlorpromazine has in excess of one hundred (Sakalis et al, 1972)]. It is not clear which metabolites to measure and what relative weighting should be given to each product in arriving at a total measure of blood drug level—a problem now resolved by using RRA.

Sakalis et al (1973) tried to discover an association between the clinical response and the blood level of the main metabolites of chlorpromazine. Using quantitative thin layer chromatography on the plasma of eight schizophrenic patients, the patients who improved were found to have high levels of chlorpromazine and 1-hydroxy chlorpromazine, while those who did not improve had high levels of sulphoxide-chlorpromazine. These findings were not statistically significant and have not been replicated.

Using G.C., Rivera-Calimlim et al (1973) found an association between blood level and clinical response in 12 schizophrenic patients: unresponsive patients had a low blood level (30 ng/ml); responsive patients had an intermediate blood level (150-300 ng/ml); while patients with side effects had a high blood level (700-1000 ng/ml). This study measured chlorpromazine alone and not other metabolites, which may be equally psychoactive, and it should be noted that the patients received other medication in addition to chlorpromazine. In contrast, Simpson et al (1973) reported that 4 out of 8 patients, who had a good clinical response to chlorpromazine, had blood levels below 15 ng/ml.

A further attempt to find a correlation between the blood levels of the many metabolites of chlorpromazine and the clinical response was made by MacKay et al (1974). In an investigation of 86 schizophrenic patients receiving an average daily dose of 280 mg. chlorpromazine, the ratio of 7-hydroxy-chlorpromazine to sulphoxide chlorpromazine in the blood was related to three distinct clinical subgroups: there was a good clinical response when the ratio was high and a poor clinical response when the ratio between these two metabolites was low. To date, this has not been replicated.

In 1976, Rivera-Calimlim et al (1976) used G.C. to investigate the relationship between the clinical state and the blood level in 29 acute and 21 chronic schizophrenics. They found an association between thought disorder and delusions and the drug level in the blood, but no correlation between oral dose and blood level. The only substance measured was chlorpromazine, and no metabolites were included. The absence of a correlation between dose and blood level implies that it is practically impossible to estimate the blood level on the basis of a given dose, and this emphasizes the importance of blood levels.

If there is an association between clinical response and blood level, but not between blood level and oral dose, then the only satisfactory way of knowing if an adequate blood level has been reached is by a direct measurement of that blood level. This finding was supported by the research published in 1978 by Wode-Helgodt et al (1978). Forty-four acutely-psychotic patients were divided into three different dosage groups receiving 200, 400 or 600 mg chlorpromazine daily as a fixed dose. The drug levels in the CSF and the plasma were correlated with clinical improvement after two and four weeks' treatment. The correlation between drug plasma level and clinical improvement after two weeks only just reached statistical significance. The correlation of clinical improvement and drug level in the CSF was more significant while there was no correlation between improvement and dosage group. The chlorpromazine was measured by a combination of G.C. and mass spectrometry, and the following active metabolites were included: 1-desmethyl-chlorpromazine and 7-hydroxy-chlorpromazine. In 1981, using the same combination of G.C. and mass spectrometry, May et al (1981) measured the blood and saliva levels of 48 acute schizophrenics. At the end of four weeks on a fixed dose of chlorpromazine, they found no correlation between blood level and clinical improvement. The discrepancies between the studies could be attributed to the inclusion or exclusion of metabolites in the test: Wode-Helgodt et al (1978) included metabolite and demonstrated a correlation between blood level and clinical improvement, while May et al (1981) did not include metabolites and found no such correlation.

Despite promising reports (Rivera-Calimlim et al, 1973; Sakalis et al,

1973; MacKay et al, 1974; Rivera-Calimlim et al, 1976; Wode-Helgodt et al, 1978), there would not seem to be a straightforward correlation (Sakalis et al, 1972; Simpson et al, 1973; May et al, 1981) between the blood level of chlorpromazine and the clinical response. The studies that did report a correlation measured differing compounds: metabolites alone (Sakalis et al, 1973), chlorpromazine alone (Rivera-Calimlim et al, 1973; Rivera-Calimlim et al, 1976; Wode-Helgodt et al, 1978) and the ratio between metabolites (MacKay et al, 1974). At this stage, the absence of a clear outcome is, in our opinion, more indicative of the methodological and technical difficulties involved in such studies rather than proof of there being no such correlation. The complications arise from the multiple metabolites of chlorpromazine and the methodology employed in the studies. Therefore, further work on the blood levels of neuroleptic medication should initially be carried out on drugs with fewer metabolites, such as haloperidol.

Research on fluphenazine has been impeded by technical problems—either the method used was not reliable (Sakalis et al, 1978) or its specificity was questionable (Chien et al, 1976). The research that has been done has recorded levels of a few ng/ml plasma (Tjaden et al, 1976). As with all depot neuroleptics, the doses given are so low that their measurement in blood is not within the range of chemical methods such as G.C., but requires more sensitive techniques such as RIA or a combination of HPLC and RIA (Langone et al, 1975). The concentrations of this medication are just within the sensitivity threshold of RRA [equivalent to 5 ng/ml of haloperidol (Tune et al, 1980)]. An additional problem that pertains to all depot neuroleptics is the rate of release of the drug from its site. It would appear that this rate is not a fixed one and is influenced by many factors including external pressure on the injection site. This means that a single blood sample may not have been taken at a time of equilibrium and may be a random high level that gives an unreliable impression of the concentration of the medication. For these reasons, studies of this subject have been beset by technical and pharmacokinetic difficulties so that their results cannot be considered conclusive. A possible method of investigating the relationship between blood level and clinical response in patients receiving this medication is by using the functional method of RRA. It may be hypothesized that it is only when blockade of dopaminergic receptors has occurred (which implies that the neuroleptic level is above the sensitivity threshold of the method) that there will be a clinical response. In this way, the apparent weakness of RRA—its low sensitivity threshold—can be utilized as a solution to the problem of the relatively low blood levels of depot medication.

Although it is not a commonly-used neuroleptic, butaperazine has been investigated by a number of researchers (Garver et al, 1977; Smith et al, 1977) because it has a reliable fluorometric test available, enabling blood levels to be measured using relatively simple equipment. In a double-blind trial, Garver et al (1977) measured butaperazine levels in 10 schizophrenics after twelve days of medication. They compared clinical improvement with drug levels in the blood and in erythrocytes. They found a curvilinear correlation, i.e., a "therapeutic window" ($r^2 = 0.58$) between blood level and clinical response.

A "therapeutic window" implies that there is a particular range of concentrations of a known drug within which its clinical effect is maximal and that above or below that range its effectiveness is decreased. The implication of finding a "therapeutic window" effect of a drug is relevant to the field of blood levels as it means that drug administration should have accompanying facilities for measurement of blood levels. Further work by the same group (Smith et al, 1977) measured plasma levels after a single 40 mg dose of butaperazine was given to 17 treatment-resistant chronic schizophrenics and 25 treatment-resistant acute schizophrenics. Both groups were found to have significantly low peak levels (p .001) compared to the peak plasma levels of treatment-responsive acute schizophrenics who received the same dose. No correlation was found between the dose of neuroleptic required in the past and the current blood level, so that the difference in plasma levels in this sample could not be attributed to differences in the rate of metabolism of the drug in the liver following prior exposure to neuroleptics (Loga et al, 1975). What does emerge, however, is that the patients who did not respond to the recommended dosage had lower plasma levels than patients who did respond at that dosage. This suggests that measurement of the blood level after a single dose could be used to predict the dose necessary for optimal therapeutic activity.

The research on blood levels of haloperidol will be reviewed separately in chronic and acute patients.

At the Jerusalem Mental Health Center, the "drug holiday" of twelve chronic schizophrenics provided an opportunity to find the lowest blood level compatible with therapeutic activity (Goldman et al, 1981). All twelve patients had shown some response to neuroleptics. Blood levels of haloperidol were measured using RRA while the dose was decreased by 10 mg every 10 days from an initial dose of 60 mg. The sample for measurement was taken at the end of each 10-day period when equilibrium should have been reached. The correlation between dose and blood level was high in each patient ($r = .72$), but low between patients ($r + .38$). Whereas a decrease in dose lead to a drop in the plasma level of a particular patient, the same dose gave a wide range of drug levels in different patients. During the step-wise reduction of medication, there was no definable blood level at which patients deteriorated, so that it was also not possible to discover an optimal maintenance blood level.

Clinical states deteriorated only several weeks after there was no measurable drug in the plasma, exemplifying the discrepancy between pharmacokinetic findings and behavior. This means that periods of at least a month at each dose and at each state of equilibrium will be necessary to find an association between blood level and optimal maintenance dose. Although pharmacokinetic equilibrium is reached in 6-10 days, clinical improvement can take two weeks in an acute state and two months in a chronic state.

Bjorndal et al (1980) also found no correlation between blood levels of haloperidol and clinical response in 23 chronic schizophrenics. Using a double-blind design, they gave one group of patients high doses of haloperidol (on average, 103 mg daily) and one group low doses of haloperidol (on average, 15 mg daily). A significant positive correlation was found between dose and blood level ($r = .9$, $p < 0.001$), although there was no correlation between blood level and clinical state. Itoh et al (1982) also found no association between clinical state, as measured by the Brief Psychiatric Rating Scale (BPRS) (Overall and Gorham, 1962), and blood level of haloperidol, as measured by RRA, in a sample of 20 chronic schizophrenics. Rama-Rao et al (1980) used RIA to measure blood levels of haloperidol in 30 chronic schizophrenics treated over six months with tailored dosages of haloperidol that produced the maximal clinical improvement, and they also failed to find a correlation between blood level and clinical state.

In contrast to these negative results in research with chronic schizophrenics are the positive results found in research with acute schizophrenics. Tune et al (1980) investigated the association between blood level and clinical response in 30 acute schizophrenics two to four weeks after admission. They measured blood levels with RRA and clinical response with a modified version of the Present State Examination (PSE). Eighteen patients received haloperidol, and the remainder were prescribed other neuroleptics. The specimen was taken 4-6 hours after drug administration. Their findings indicate that if the drug concentration is below 50 ng/ml (the units were expressed as equivalents of chlorpromazine), there is no clinical response, while in the range of 100-200 ng/ml there is a good response ($t = 2.75$, $p < .02$). In this study, they did not find an association between the dose administered and the level in the blood or between dose and clinical response. The absence of such an association emphasizes the need for blood level measurement in clinical practice as dose is no predictor of clinical response, while blood level is a possible indicant.

Magliozzi et al (1981) also found an association between clinical improvement and blood levels of haloperidol. They found that maximal improvement occurred among 17 acute schizophrenics when plasma levels of haloperidol were in the range of 8-18 ng/ml (units of haloperidol). This "therapeutic window" was noted after 3-12 weeks of therapy. The blood levels were measured using G.C. Clinical state was measured on the BPRS by two independent raters who were blind to the blood levels. Improvement was measured by subtracting the average final BPRS score from the average initial BPRS score. Their findings achieved statistical significance (p < .001).

A similar trend, a "therapeutic window" of the plasma levels of haloperidol in acute schizophrenics, was noted by Smith et al (1982). Using RRA in 26 subjects, they found the range of 5-14 ng/ml (units of haloperidol) to be associated with improvement. Although their results failed to reach statistical significance, they were practically identical with those of Magliozzi et al (1981). This means that two separate groups using different methods (G.C. and RRA) have achieved the same results.

Additional support for a probable link between blood level and clinical response emerged in the prospective study of Brown et al (1982). They found that out of 61 schizophrenics receiving maintenance medication of a variety of neuroleptics, 10 patients deteriorated. Using RRA, they found that these 10 patients had blood levels significantly lower than the remaining patients (t = 2.66, p < 0.01). The importance of this research lies in its implication of a possible additional use of blood level measurement. This function would be a refinement of clinical capacity in preventing relapse in patients on maintenance neuroleptic medication, in addition to achieving the maximal clinical response in acute patients.

The publications of various groups (Garver et al, 1977; Tune et al, 1980; Magliozzi et al, 1981; Smith et al, 1982) over the last two years on the association between haloperidol levels and clinical response in acute schizophrenics would appear to be promising. That such an association could be found with haloperidol, but not with chlorpromazine, may be a consequence of the former having no active metabolites, so that its blood levels have a better validity. The absence of such a correlation in chronic patients (Bjorndal et al, 1980; Rama-Rao et al, 1980; Goldman et al, 1981; Itoh et al, 1982) may be attributed to there being less room for short-term improvement. A long-term study in chronic schizophrenics remains to be carried out to ascertain the lowest blood level that is capable of preventing relapse.

THE ASSOCIATION BETWEEN SIDE-EFFECTS AND BLOOD LEVELS OF NEUROLEPTIC MEDICATION

Kolakowska et al (1976) investigated the blood levels of chlorpromazine in 18 schizophrenics, taking one sample during treatment on a fixed dosage and a further sample during treatment on increasing doses. In this design, there was no association between blood levels, Parkinsonism and tardive dyskinesia during prolonged treatment. Chlorpromazine levels were measured by G.C. Calil et al (1979) who reported that in a group of 58 patients receiving different neuroleptics for at least two weeks there was no association between blood levels and parkinsonian side-effects. Blood levels were measured by RRA and expressed in equivalents of chlorpromazine.

Van Putten et al (1980) found no correlation between chlorpromazine levels and akinesia in 43 acute schizophrenics using G.C. Rama-Rao et al (1980) reported that in 30 chronic patients treated with haloperidol there was no correlation between extra-pyramidal symptoms and blood levels of haloperidol measured by RIA, although there was a correlation between extra-pyramidal symptoms and prolactin levels. Itoh et al (1982) found no significant correlation between blood level and the frequency of tardive dyskinesia in 20 schizophrenics on long-term treatment with haloperidol. Despite this, they reported that below 10 ng/ml of haloperidol in the blood, extra-pyramidal symptoms did not appear.

Rosenblatt et al (1981) found relatively high levels of thioridazine or mesoridazine in 8 patients with tardive dyskinesia compared with 5 dose-matched patients who had not developed tardive dyskinesia. Blood levels were measured by RRA. In a study performed on 152 patients (Smith et al, 1983), the opposite results emerged. Patients with symptoms of tardive dyskinesia had plasma levels of neuroleptics, measured by RRA, which were 40 percent lower than patients without symptoms of tardive dyskinesia. It is known that the symptoms of tardive dyskinesia can be "covered up" by raising the neuroleptic dose (Jeste and Wyatt, 1982). So it is possible that for some of this population the association between tardive dyskinesia and blood level is not a real one, and the syndrome only "surfaces" at low doses.

From these studies, it would appear that once equilibrium has been reached, the blood level is not a factor that determines the emergence of the main side effects in schizophrenic patients. It is possible, however, that the last word on the matter remains to be said. Jeste and Wyatt (1982) reported a higher frequency of tardive dyskinesia in patients who had received neuroleptics on an irregular basis compared with patients who had received regular medication. A possibility for future research arising out of this finding would be to relate the incidence and severity of side effects of fluctuations in blood levels and not the blood level per se.

THE INFLUENCE OF ANTIPARKINSONIAN DRUGS ON BLOOD LEVELS OF NEUROLEPTIC MEDICATION

The methods of measuring levels of neuroleptics have made it possible to investigate the problems of interaction between conbinations of various drugs with respect to blood levels. Most attention has been devoted to the combination of neuroleptic and antiparkinsonian drugs. Such a combination is very common, arising out of the need to treat the parkinsonian side effects of neuroleptic medication.

Rivera-Calimlim et al performed two studies (Rivera-Calimlim et al, 1973; Rivera-Calimlim et al, 1976) suggesting that trihexyphenidyl reduces the level of chlorpromazine. In their first study, they compared the blood levels of two patients whose trihexyphenidyl was stopped, with three patients whose antiparkinsonian medication was maintained. In their second study, they investigated 15 patients who received a combination of chlorpromazine and trihexyphenidyl with blood samples for chlorpromazine levels taken before and after the addition of trihexyphenidyl. In the statistical analysis, the authors excluded three patients whose blood levels were raised after adding trihexyphenidyl. Two patients' blood levels were zero after the addition of trihexyphenidyl. Such results are suggestive of noncompliance in taking medication, rather than being a consequence of the addition of the trihexyphenidyl.

Loga et al (1975) investigated the interaction of orphenadrine and phenobarbitone on chlorpromazine and found that orphenadrine reduced chlorpromazine levels. Furthermore, Gautier et al (1977) reported that stopping antiparkinsonian drugs was followed by a rise in blood levels of neuroleptics. They used a variety of neuroleptics and three different antiparkinsonian drugs (trihexyphenidyl, procyclidine and benztropine). Chouinard et al (1977) concluded that procylidine reduces blood levels of penfluridol, having found a negative correlation between the dose of procyclidine and the blood level of penfluridol in 14 patients, 12 of whom required antiparkinsonian medication. Despite these findings, Kolakowska et al (1976) found an elevation in chlorpromazine levels following the addition of trihexyphenidyl in 13 patients, while Tune et al (1980) found that anticholinergic drugs did not influence the blood levels of neuroleptics. In an open study on five patients, El-Yousef and Manier (1974) also noted that benztropine had no effect on levels of butaperazine.

Simpson et al (1980) were the only group to use patients as their own controls. They used only two drugs, chlorpromazine and trihexyphenidyl, and only after pharmacokinetic equilibrium had been reached did they take several samples of blood. They concluded that antiparkinsonian drugs have no effect on chlorpromazine levels.

The contradictory results in these studies indicate that if there is an influence of anticholinergic drugs on neuroleptic drug levels, then it is both slight and inconsistent. In some patients, however, the influence of anticholinergic drugs on neuroleptic blood levels could be a result of their reduced absorption following suppression of gastrointestinal activity by the anticholinergic activity of these drugs. It follows that patients who do not respond to neuroleptics, or who have a low blood level, may benefit from stopping their anticholinergic drugs. The results reported above do not justify a general distrust in the use of anticholinergic drugs combined with neuroleptics nor do they imply that doses of neuroleptics should be raised whenever anticholinergic medication is added.

THE ASSOCIATION BETWEEN BLOOD LEVELS OF NEUROLEPTICS AND PROLACTIN LEVELS

Any treatment that blocks dopamine receptors raises the levels of prolactin in the blood, as these receptors inhibit the secretion of prolactin from the pituitary. The first to report such an association were Winnik and Tennenbaum (1955). Kolakowska et al (1976) published findings based on blood measurement on 18 schizophrenics receiving long-term treatment with chlorpromazine: they found no association between the blood levels of chlorpromazine and prolactin.

Using G.C. and RIA, Rubin et al (1980) found a correlation ($r = .83$) between plasma haloperidol levels and prolactin levels. They concluded that prolactin provided an in-vivo measure of plasma haloperidol levels. This claim is supported by earlier studies (Meltzer and Fang, 1976; Gruen et al, 1978).

It would appear, therefore, that there is a positive correlation between levels of haloperidol and prolactin. Reports are contradictory, however, concerning the range of the correlation. It has been maintained (Ohman and Axelsson, 1978; Rubin and Hays, 1978) that the dopaminergic receptors are already completely blocked with consequent maximal secretion of prolactin at very low doses of antipsychotic compounds. Others (Meltzer and Fang, 1976; Bjorndal et al, 1980), however, have also reported a correlation between haloperidol and prolactin levels at therapeutic dosages. If the range of the correlation does indeed include therapeutic dosages, then the prolactin levels can be used as an index of the dopaminergic activity of untested drugs or as a physiological measure of the dopaminergic activity of drugs in-vivo.

THE MEASUREMENT OF LEVELS OF NEUROLEPTIC MEDICATION IN CEREBRO-SPINAL FLUID (CSF), ERTHROCYTES AND SALIVA

With the exception of sulpiride, neuroleptic medications are lipophilic, implying that they can penetrate into the brain. It is only the portion of the drug that is not protein bound that can affect behavior, as it is in equilibrium across the blood-brain barrier with drug levels surrounding brain cells. Only 8-10 percent of haloperidol and 3 percent of chlorpromazine are in a free state in plasma. The measurement of drug levels in body tissues other than plasma (erythrocytes, saliva, CSF) has been proposed as a possible alternative way of gaining information of greater validity on the effective concentration of medication by measuring levels that are in equilibrium with the unbound fraction. The concentration of medication in erythrocytes, being tissues with lipophilic membrane, may reflect the absorption in lipophilic tissues such as brain. Neuroleptics are more concentrated in saliva, which may resemble what occurs in certain fatty sites in the brain after storage and concentration of the drug. CSF is near the central nervous system and across the blood-brain barrier, so that its drug level may reflect the drug levels in the brain.

In a study carried out in our own unit (Rimon et al, 1981), we investigated the hypothesis that poor response to medication in a group of chronic schizophrenics was attributable to the medication not reaching the brain. Plasma and CSF levels of haloperidol were measured in 12 chronic schizophrenics who did not respond to the routine dosage of neuroleptics. Plasma and CSF levels were repeated after the dose was doubled. After one month of 60 mg haloperidol daily, the CSF level was 3 ± 1 ng/ml. Following one month of 120 mg haloperidol daily, the level in the CSF rose to 6.3 ± 2 ng/ml. This rise produced no clinical improvement in the patients. There was a correlation (r) of .55 ($p < 0.01$) between the plasma level and the CSF level. These findings support the hypothesis that levels in the CSF and, possibly, in the brain are related to levels in the plasma. They also demonstrate that for this particular population the cause of treatment nonresponsiveness is not inadequate levels of medication.

Sedvall et al (1977) investigated 15 acute schizophrenics who received a fixed dose of chlorpromazine for four weeks. They found a correlation between the medication level in the CSF and the clinical state ($r = .64$, $p < 0.01$), but no correlation with the plasma blood level. They used a combination of G.C. and mass spectrometry and included two active metabolites of chlorpromazine: 1-desmethyl-chlorpromazine and 7-hydroxy-chlorpromazine. It would appear that in certain cases the concentration of medication in the CSF is a more relevant pharmacokinetic means of measurement than in the plasma. The different results that have been reported in studies on CSF levels of neuroleptics (Sedvall et al, 1977; Rimon et al, 1981) could be a consequence of the different populations used—in one study a chronic population not responsive to neuroleptics (Rimon et al, 1981) and in the other study acute psychotics who responded well to medication (Sedvall et al, 1977).

Casper et al (1980) found a "therapeutic window" when measuring red blood cell butaperazine levels in 18 patients on a fixed dose of butaperazine ($r = .52$, $p < .01$). Patients who responded to treatment had red blood cell levels between 30-70 ng/ml, while those whose levels were higher or lower than the range showed less marked improvement. Measurement of butaperazine levels in plasma showed a correlation with a similar tendency which did not reach statistical significance. Erythrocyte and plasma levels were measured using the fluorometric method. Using the same method, Garver et al (1977) found a similar but even more striking correlation (r^2 = 0.90) between red blood cell butaperazine and clinical response. Smith et al (1982) also found a "therapeutic window" with concentrations of haloperidol in erythrocytes using G.C. The range of the "window" was 2.4-5.4 ng/ml of red blood cells. These exciting findings are consistent with the reports of a "therapeutic window" using plasma levels (Garver et al, 1977; Magliozzi et al, 1981; Smith et al, 1982).

Saliva is another body fluid where the level of medication can be measured. For example, by measuring the levels of lithium in saliva (Creese and Snyder, 1977; Ben-Arey et al, 1980), it is possible to monitor patients who refuse to give blood samples but are taking lithium. The concentration of chlorpromazine in saliva is 4-50 times that in plasma (Chien et al, 1976), which means that it is possible to use RRA, a relatively insensitive method, to measure the levels in the saliva of patients receiving comparatively low doses. May et al (1981) found a significant correlation between blood levels and saliva levels of chlorpromazine (r = .62) using G.C. in 48 acute schizophrenics. They found no correlation between clinical improvement and blood or saliva levels after reaching a state of pharmacokinetic equilibrium. On the other hand, there was a correlation between saliva and blood levels 24 hours after taking medication and the clinical improvement measured after 28 days of medication. This confusing finding may be attributed to the test dose level reflecting the quantity of medication taken during the majority of the trial, while compliance may have decreased prior to the first assessment.

In our department, research is currently being carried out on the correlation between blood and saliva levels in patients receiving low doses of a variety of neuroleptics. The aim is to discover if neuroleptics other than chlorpromazine are concentrated in saliva and if there is a fixed relationship between the levels in blood and saliva. If such a relationship exists, it should be possible to monitor the compliance of patients receiving neuroleptic medication by measuring saliva levels with RRA.

METHODOLOGICAL ISSUES IN CLINICAL RESEARCH ON MEDICATION LEVELS

In studies in which the dose is varied according to clinical judgment, a higher dose is given to patients who do not respond to the usual dose. This creates an artifact whereby lower levels will be found in those patients whose clinical response is, in part, a feature of the benign natural history of their illness. A correlation based on a research design such as this is, in fact, measuring the association between blood level and the severity of the illness and not the correlation between blood level and clinical response. For example, Rama-Rao et al (1980) found that the sicker the chronic schizophrenic, the higher the dose and blood level of neuroleptic he received in a study where clinicians could freely adjust dosages. It is essential to investigate the association between the distribution of blood levels and clinical response by giving a dose of neuroleptic medication that is standard and fixed to different patients.

From a pharmacokinetic viewpoint alone, a valid blood level is that which is measured after the patient has been on a fixed dose for 6-10 days (Goldman et al, 1981; Itoh et al, 1982). From a clinical viewpoint, however, a patient receiving neuroleptics requires two to three weeks for optimal clinical improvement (Davis and Cole, 1975; Klein et al, 1980). It seems appropriate that this discrepancy should be taken into consideration in clinical research on blood levels by waiting up to three weeks before finally assessing the impact of a particular level on the clinical response, rather than assessing the response immediately after pharmacokinetic equilibrium has been reached. This may be done by measuring the change in the clinical state; in other words, the clinical state at the time of blood sampling compared with the pretreatment clinical state. Single point assessment may well obscure real correlations between plasma level and clinical response. For example, the blood level in an acute patient who has improved somewhat may well be the same as the blood level of a chronic patient who has not improved. If the clinical state is measured on a single-point basis, it may well be identical in both cases; and one's improvement and the other's treatment-resistance are not apparent in the correlation then measured. If, instead, we measure the change in clinical state, then we can relate the particular level found in a given patient to the corresponding therapeutic effect.

CONCLUSIONS

The significant contribution of RRA to the field of blood levels of neuroleptic medication is apparent in the area of research. All studies based on this method (Rivera-Calimlim et al, 1973; Rivera-Calimlim et al, 1976; Garver et al, 1977; Wode-Halgodt et al, 1978, Magliozzi et al, 1981) on acute patients have demonstrated a correlation between blood level and clinical response (Tune et al, 1980; Brown et al, 1982; Smith et al, 1982).

Studies carried out on chronic populations (Bjorndal et al, 1980; Rama-Rao et al, 1980; Goldman et al, 1981; Itoh et al, 1982) have either found no correlation between blood level and clinical response or found it to be marginal. It is likely that when treating chronic patients the main issue is not to find the optimal dose for the maximal change in the clinical state, but to find the minimal dose that will prevent relapse.

The current state of knowledge in the field supports the use of blood levels of neuroleptic medication for limited clinical purposes:

    1. Assessment of compliance. Noncompliance among psychiatric patients is a formidable problem. About 50 percent do not take

their drugs as prescribed (Amdur, 1979). The ability to monitor such patients with confidence and modify their therapy accordingly may well improve the course of the illness.

2. Aid in dose adjustment in treatment-resistant patients. The present state of the art provides the physician with preliminary options of therapeutic range. Measurement of blood levels in resistant patients may help to distinguish those patients who, despite taking an average dose of a neuroleptic, have plasma levels that are either very high or very low and to alter the dose accordingly. Dunlop et al (1982) have recently reported that, with the aid of blood level measurement, they succeeded in improving the condition of three chronic patients.

3. Diagnosis in cases of suspected intoxication. Measurement of blood levels can help in the differential diagnosis of sudden change in the physical state of a patient: if the blood level is in the usual range, then the alteration is presumably related to a physical illness; while if the level is very high, the alteration may be a product of intoxication by neuroleptic medication.

Monitoring plasma levels of neuroleptic medication may have a further benefit in that the optimal dose of medication may be ascertained for each patient. This additional indication is as yet unproven. It could, perhaps, be directly investigated by dividing the population of patients on neuroleptic medication into two groups. The prescribing physician of one group is informed of the blood levels of that group, while the other is not. If the group, whose prescribing doctor was told the blood levels, is different from the other group with respect to the course of illness, then this would prove the clinical importance of the measurement of blood levels. This study is currently being carried out in our department at the Jerusalem Mental Health Center.

REFERENCES

Adelson, D. and Epstein, L.J.: A study of phenothiazines with male and female chronically ill schizophrenic patients, *J. Nerv. Ment. Dis.* 134:543-554, 1962.

Amdur, M.A.: Medication compliance in outpatient psychiatry, *Compr. Psychiatry* 20:339-346, 1979.

Axelsson, R.: Antipsychotic Drugs: Pharmacodynamics and Pharmacokinetics (G. Sedvall, B. Uvnas and Y. Zotterman, eds.), *Pergamon Press* Oxford, pp. 353-358, 1976.

Ben-Arey, H., Naon, H., Szargel, R., Gutman, D. and Hefets, Z.: Salivary lithium concentration—a tool for monitoring psychiatric patients, *Oral Surgery, Oral Medicine, Oral Pathology* St. Louis, 50:127-129, 1980.

Berson, S.A. and Yalow, R.S.: General principles of radioimmunoassay, *Clin. Chim. Acta* 22:51-69, 1968.

Bianchelli, G., Zarifian, E., Poirier-Litlre, M.F., Morselli, P.L. and Deniker, P.: Influence of route of administration on haloperidol plasma levels in psychotic patients, *International Journal of Clinical Pharmacology, Therapy and Toxicology* 18: 324-327, 1980.

Bjørdnal, N., Bjerre, J., Gerlach, P., Kristjansen, P., Magelund, G., Oestrich, I.H.

and Waehrens, J.: High dosage haloperidol therapy in chronic schizophrenic patients: a double-blind study of clinical response, side-effects, serum haloperidol and serum prolactin, *Psychopharmacology* 67:17-23, 1980.

Brown, W.A., Laughren, T., Chisholm, E. and Williams, B.W.: Low serum neuroleptic levels predict relapse in schizophrenic patients, *Arch. Gen. Psychiatry* 39:998-1000, 1982.

Butler, V.P. Jr. and Beiser, S.M.: Dixon and Kunkel Adv. Immunol. Academic Press, New York, p. 255, 1973.

Calil, H.M., Avery, D.H., Hollister, L.E., Creese, I. and Snyder, S.H.: Serum levels of neuroleptics measured by dopamine radioreceptor assay and some clinical observations, *Psychiatry Research* 1:39-44, 1979.

Carlsson, A. and Lindquist, M.: Effect of chlorpromazine or haloperidol on formation of 3-methoxytyramine and normetanephrine in mouse brain, *Acta Pharmacol. Toxicol.* 20:140-144, 1963.

Casey, J.F., Lasky, J.J., Klett, C.J. and Hollister, L.E.: Treatment of schizophrenic reactions with phenothiazine derivatives, *Am. J. Psychiatry* 117:97-105, 1960.

Casper, R., Graver, D.L., Dekirmenjian, H., Chang, S. and Davis J.M.: Phenothiazine levels in plasma and red blood cells, their relationship to clinical improvement in schizophrenia, *Arch. Gen. Psychiatry* 37:301-305, 1980.

Chien, C.P., Chan, T.L., Daniano, D. et al: Abstracts 10th Congress CINP, Quebec, Canada, 1976.

Chouinard, G., Annable, L. and Cooper, S.: Antiparkinsonian drug administration and plasma levels of penfluridol, a new long-acting neuroleptic, *Comm. Psychopharmacol.* 1:325-331, 1977.

Clark, B.R., Tower, B.B. and Rubin, R.T.: Radioimmunoassay of haloperidol in human serum, *Life Sci.* 20:319-326, 1977.

Creese, I. and Snyder, S.H.: A simple and sensitive radioreceptor assay for antischizophrenic drugs in blood, *Nature* 270:180-182, 1977.

Creese, I., Burt, D.R. and Snyder, S.H.: Letter to editor, in response to Dopamine

receptors and average clinical doses, *Science* 194:546, 1976a.

Cressman, W.H., Bianchine, J.R., Slotnick, V.B., Johnson, P.C. and Plostnicks, J.: Plasma level profile of haloperidol in man following intramuscular administration, *Europ. J. Clin. Pharmacol.* 7:99-103, 1974.

Curry, S.H.: Method for the estimation of nanogram quantities of chlorpromazine and some of its relatively non-polar metabolites in plasma using gaschromatography with an electron capture detector, *Analyt. Chem.* 40:1251-1256, 1968.

Curry, S.H. and Marshall, J.H.L.: Plasma levels of chlorpromazine and some of its relatively non-polar metabolites in psychiatric patients, *Life Science* 7:9-17, 1968.

Curry, S.H., Marshall, J.H., Davis, J.H. and Janowsky, D.S.: Chlorpromazine plasma levels and effects, *Arch. Gen. Psychiat.* 22:289-296, 1970.

Curry, S.H., D'Mello, A. and Mould, G.P.: Destruction of chlorpromazine during absorption in rat in vivo and in vitro, *Br. J. Pharmacol.* 42:403-411, 1971.

Curry, S.H., Lader, M.H., Mould, G.P. and Sakalis, G.: Clinical pharmacology of chlorpromazine, *Brit. J. Pharma.* 44:370-371, 1972.

Davis, J.M. and Cole, J.O.: American Handbook of Psychiatry (S. Arieti, ed.), Basic Books Inc., New York, pp. 441-475, 1975.

Dunlop, S.R., Shea, P.A. and Hendrie, H.C.: The relationship between plasma and red blood cell neuroleptic levels, oral dosage, and clinical par-meters in a chronic schizophrenic population, *Biological Psychiatry* 17:929-936, 1982.

El-Yousef, M.D. and Manier, D.H.: Letter to the editor: the effect of benztropine mesylate on plasma levels of butaperazine maleate, *Am. J. Psychiatry* 131:471-472, 1974.

Engelhardt, D.M., Rosen, B., Freedman, N. and Margolis, R.: Phenothiazines in prevention of psychiatric hospitalization, *Arch. Gen. Psychiatry* 16:98-101, 1967.

Fann, W.E.: Some clinically important interactions of psychotropic drugs, *South Med. J.* 66:661-665, 1973.

Fann, W.E., Davis, D.S., Janowski, D.S.

and Schmidt, S.: The effects of antacids on the blood levels of chlorpromazine, *Clin. Pharmacol. Ther.* 14:135, 1973.

Forrest, F.M., Forrest, I.S. and Serra, M.T.: Modification of chlorpromazine metabolism by some other drugs frequently administered to psychiatric patients, *Biol. Psychiatry* 2:53-58, 1970.

Forsman, A. and Ohman, R.: Pharmacokinetic studies on haloperidol in man, *Curr. Therap. Res.* 20:319-336, 1976.

Forsman, A., and Ohman, R.: Applied pharmacokinetics of haloperidol in man, *Curr. Ther. Res.* 21:396-411, 1977.

Forsman, A., Martensson, E., Nyberg, G. and Ohman, K.: A gas chromatographic method for determining haloperidol. A sensitive procedure for studying serum concentration and pharmacokinetics of haloperidol in patients, *Arch. Pharmacol.* 286:113-124, 1974.

Friedel, R.O.: The relationship of therapeutic response to antidepressant plasma level: an update, *J. Clin. Psychiatry* 43:37-42, 1982.

Gaind, R.N. and Barnes, T.R.: Handbook of Biological Psychiatry (H.M. Van-Praag, M.H. Lader, O.J. Rafaelson and E.J. Sachar, Eds.), Marcel Dekker Inc., New York and Basel, vol. IV, p. 152, 1981.

Garver, D.L., Dekirmenjian, H., Davis, J.M., Casper, R. and Ericksen, S.: Neuroleptic drug levels and therapeutic response: preliminary observations with red blood cell bound butaperazine, *Am. J. Psychiatry* 134:304-307, 1977.

Gautier, J., Jus, A., Villeneuve, A., Jus, K., Pires, P. and Villeneuve, R.: Influence of antiparkinsonian drugs on the plasma level of neuroleptics, *Biological Psychiatry* 12(3):389-399, 1977.

Goldman, Z., Ebstein, R.P., Lerer, B., Zohar, J., Hermoni, M. and Belmaker, R.H.: Haloperidol blood levels during dosage reduction in chronic schizophrenic patients, *Neuropsychobiology* 7:281-284, 1981.

Gothelf, B., Karczmar, A.G. and Kaufman, M.: Distribution of intravenously administered chlorpromazine in cat tissues, *Int. J. Neuropharmacol.* 2:39-49, 1963.

Gottschalk, L.A., Dinovo, E., Biener, R., Birch, H., Syben, M. and Noble E.P.: Plasma levels of mezoridazine and its metabolites and clinical response in acute schizophrenia after a single intramuscular drug dose, in: Pharmacokinetics of Psychoactive drugs (L.H. Gottschalk and S. Merlis, eds.), Spectrum, New York, pp. 171-189, 1976.

Gruen, P.H., Sachar, E.J., Langer, G., Altman, N., Leifer, M., Frantz, A. and Halpern, F.S.: Prolactin response to neuroleptics in normal and schizophrenic patients, *Arch. Gen. Psychiatry* 35:108-116, 1978.

Itoh, H., Yagi, G., Ohtsuka, N. and Ichikawa, K.: Clinical significance of measuring plasma level of haloperidol, Abstract 13th CINP Congress, Jerusalem, p. 344., 1982.

Jelliffe, R.W., Buell, J. and Kalaba, R.: Reduction of digitalis toxicity by computer-assisted glycoside dosage regimens, *Ann. Intern. Med.* 77:891-906, 1972.

Jeste, D.V. and Wyatt, R.J.: Therapeutic strategies against tardive dyskinesia, *Arch. Gen. Psychiatry* 39:803-815, 1982.

Jeste, D.V., Potkin, G.A., Shubha, S., Feder, S. and Wyatt, R.J.: Tardive dyskinesia reversible and persistent, *Arch. Gen. Psychiatry* 36:585-590, 1070.

Kawashima, K., Dixon, R. and Spector, S.: Development of radioimmunoassay for chlorpromazine, *Eur. J. Pharmacol.* 32: 195-202, 1975.

Klein, D.F., Gittelman, R., Quitkin, F. and Rifkin, A.: Diagnosis and Drug Treatment of Psychiatric Disorders, 2nd ed., Williams & Wilkins Co., Baltimore, pp. 149-155, 1980.

Kolakowska, J., Wiles, D.H., Gelder, M.G. and McNeilly, A.S.: Clinical significance of plasma chlorpromazine levels II. Plasma levels of the drug, some of its metabolites and prolactin in patients receiving long-term phenothiazine treatment, *Psychopharmacology* 49:101-107, 1976.

Kutz, A. and Davidson, S.: Tricyclic antidepressant medication: pharmacodynamic aspects and clinical implications, *Harefuah* 93:209-213, 1977.

Lader, S.R.: A radioreceptor assay for neuroleptic drugs in plasma, *J. Immunoassay* 1:57-75, 1980.

Langone, J.J., Van Vunakis, H. and Bachur, N.R.: Perphenazine and fluphenazine. Adriamycin and metabolites: separation by high-pression liquid chromatography and quantitation by radioimmunoassay, *Biochem. Med.* 12:283-289, 1975.

Lasky, J.J., Klett, C.J., Caffey, E.M., Bennett, J.L., Rosenblum, M.P. and Hollister, L.E.: Drug treatment of schizophrenic patients, *Dis. Nerv. Syst.* 23:698-706.

Loga, S., Curry, S.H. and Lader, M.: Interactions of orphenadrine and phenobarbitone with chlorpromazine: plasma concentrations and effects in man, *Brit. J. Clin. Pharmacol.* 2:197-208, 1975.

MacKay, A.V.P., Healey, A.F. and Baker, J.: The relationship of plasma chlorpromazine to its 7-hydroxy and sulphoxide metabolites in a large population of chronic schizophrenics, *Brit. J., Clin. Pharmacol.* 1:425-430, 1974.

Magliozzi, J.R., Hollister, L.E., Arnold, K.V. and Earle, G.M.: Relationship of serum haloperidol levels to clinical response in schizophrenic patients, *Am. J. Psychiatry* 138:365-367, 1981.

Marcucci, F., Airoldi, L., Mussini, E. and Garattini, S.: A method for the gas chromatographic determination of butyrophenones, *J. Chromatogr.* 59:174-177, 1971.

May, P.R.A., Van Putten, T., Jenden, M.D., Coradee, Y. and Dixson, W.J.: Chlorpromazine levels and the outcome of treatment in schizophrenic patients, *Arch. Gen. Psychiatry* 38:202, 1981.

McCormick, W., Ingelfinger, J.A., Isakson, G. and Goldman, P.: Errors in measuring drug concentrations, *New England J. of Medicine* 299:1118-1121, 1978.

McNair, H.M. and Bonelli, E.J.: Basic Gas Chromatography, Varian Aerograph Col., Walnut Creek, pp. 1-7, 1969.

Meltzer, H.Y. and Fang, V.S.: The effect of neuroleptics on serum prolactin in schizophrenic patients, *Arch. Gen. Psychiatry* 33:279-286, 1976.

Michiels, L.J.M., Heykants, J.J.P., Knaeps, A.G. and Janssen, P.A.J.: Radioimmunoassay of the neuroleptic drug pimozide, *Life Sci.* 16:937-944, 1975.

Michiels, M., Hendricks, R. and Heykantz,

J.: Antibody to Haloperidol: A Very Sensitive Tool for the Radioimmunologic Determination of Some Butyrophenones—Preclinical Research Report, Janssen Pharmaceutica, Beerse, Belgium, 1976.

NIMH-PSC Collaborative Study Group, Phenothiazine treatment in acute schizophrenia, *Arch. Gen. Psychiatry* 10:246-261, 1964.

Ohman, R. and Axelsson, R.: Relationship between prolactin response and antipsychotic effect of thioridazine in psychiatric patients, *Eur. J. Clin. Pharmacol.* 14:111-116, 1978.

Ohman, R., Larsson, M., Nilsson, I.M. et al: *Arch. of Pharmacology* 299:105, 1977.

Oldendorf, W.H. and Dewhurst, W.G.: The blood-brain barrier and psychotropic drugs, in: Principles of Psychopharmacology (W.G. Clark and J. del-Guindice, eds.), Academic Press, New York, 2nd edition, pp. 183-191, 1978.

Overall, J.E. and Gorham, D.R.: The brief psychiatric rating scale, *Psychological Reports* 10:799-812, 1962.

Playfair, J.H.L., Hurn, B.A.L. and Schulster, D.: Production of antibodies and binding reagents, *Br. Med. Bull.* 30:24-31, 1974.

Rama-Rao, V.A., Bishop, M. and Coppen, A.: Clinical state, plasma level of haloperidol and prolactin: A correlation study in chronic schizophrenia, *Brit. J. Psychiat.* 137:518-521, 1980.

Rimon, R., Averbuch, I., Rozick, P., Fijman-Danilovich, L., Kara, T., Dasberg, H., Ebstein, R.P. and Belmaker, R.H.: Serum and CSF levels of haloperidol by radioimmunoassay and radioreceptor assay during high-dose therapy of resistant schizophrenic patients, *Psychopharmacology* 73:179, 1981.

Risch, S.C., Huey, L.Y., and Janowsky, D.S.: Plasma levels of tricyclic antidepressants and clinical efficacy: a review of the literature. Part I and II, *J. Clin. Psych.* 40:6-58, 1979.

Rivera-Calimlim, L., Costanceda, L. and Lasagna, L.: Effects of mode of management on plasma chlorpromazine in psychiatric patients, *Clin. Pharmacol. Ther.* 4:978-986, 1973.

Rivera-Calimlim, L., Nasrallah, H., Straus, J. and Lasagna, L.: Clinical response and plasma levels: effect of dose, dosage schedules and drug interactions on plasma chlorpromazine levels, *Am. J. Psychiatry* 133:646-652, 1976.

Robinson, J.D. and Risby, D.: Radioimmunoassay for flupenthixol in plasma, *Clin. Chem.* 23:2085-2088, 1977.

Rosenblatt, J.E., Pary, R.J. Bigelow, L.B., Delisi, L.E., Wagner, R.L., Klienman, J.E., Weinberger, P.R., Potlein, S.G., Shiling, D., Jeste, D.V., Alexander, P. and Wyatt, R.J.: Measurement of serum neuroleptic concentrations by radioreceptor assay, concurrent assessment of clinical response and toxicity, in: Neuroreceptors: Basic and Clinical Aspects (E. Usdin, W.E. Bunney and J.M. Davis, eds.), John Wiley & Sons, New York, pp. 165-188, 1981.

Rubin, R.T. and Hays, S.: Profiles of prolactin response to antipsychotic drugs: some methodologic considerations, *Psychopharmacol. Bull.* 14:9-11, 1978.

Rubin, R.T., Forsman, A., Heykantz, J., Ohman, R., Tower, B. and Michiels, M.: Serum haloperidol determinations in psychiatric patients, *Arch. Gen. Psychiatry* 37:1069-1074, 1980.

Sakalis, G., Curry, S.H., Mould, G.P. and Lader, M.H.: Physiologic and clinical effects of chlorpromazine and their relationship to plasma level, *Clin. Pharmacol. and Ther.* 13:931-946, 1972.

Sakalis, G., Chan, T.L., Gershon, S. and Park, S.: The possible role of metabolites in therapeutic response to chlorpromazine treatment, *Psychopharmacologia* 32:279-284, 1973.

Sakalis, G., Sadilovsky, A., Traficante, L.J. et al: Depot Fluphenazines: Twelve Years of Experience (F.J. Ayd, ed.), Ayd Medical Communications, Baltimore, p. 72, 1978.

Sedvall, G., Alfredson, G., Bjerkenstedt, L., Eneroth, P., Fyro, B., Harnryd, C. and Wode-Helgodt, B.: Central biochemical correlates to antipsychotic drug action in man, in: The impact of Biology in Modern Psychiatry (E.S. Gershon, R.H. Belmaker, S.S. Kety and M. Rosenbaum, eds.), Plenum Press, New York and London, p. 41-54, 1977.

Shannon, J.A., Earle, D.P., Brodie, B.B., Taggart, J.V. and Berliner, R.W.: The pharmacological basis for the rational use of atabrine in the treatment of malaria, *J. Pharmacol. Exp. Ther.* 81:307-330, 1944.

Simpson, G.M., Varga, E., Reiss, M., Copper, T.B., Bergner, P.E. and Lee, J.H.: Bioequivalency of generic and brand-named chlorpromazine, *Clin. Pharm. & Thera.* 15:631-641, 1973.

Simpson, G.M., Cooper, T.B., Bark, N., Sud, I. and Lee, H.: Effect of antiparkinsonian medication on plasma levels of chlorpromazine, *Arch. Gen. Psychiatry* 37:205-208, 1980.

Smith, R.C., Dekirmenjian, H., Davis, J.M., Crayton, J. and Evans, H.: Plasma butaperazine levels in long-term chronic non-responding schizophrenics, *Communication in Psychopharmacology* 1:319-324, 1977.

Smith, R.C., Vroulis, G., Shvartsburd, A., Allen, R., Lewis, N., Schoolar, J.C., Chojnacki, M., Johnson, R.: RBC and plasma levels of haloperidol and clinical response in schizophrenia, *Am. J. Psychiatry* 139:1054-1056, 1982.

Smith, R.C., Misra, C.H., Allen, R. and Gordon, J.: Dosage and blood levels of neuroleptics in tardive dyskinesia, In: New Directions in Tardive Dyskinesia Research (J. Bennet and R.H. Belmaker, eds.), S. Karger, Basel, pp. 87-96, 1983.

Snyder, L.R. and Kirkland, J.J.: Introduction to Modern Liquid Chromatography, Wiley & Sons, New York, pp. 2-4, 1974.

Tjaden, U.R., Lankelma, J., Poppe, H. and Muusze, R.G.: Anodic coulometric detection with a glass carbon electrode in combination with reversed-phase high performance liquid chromatography: determination of blood levels of perphenazine and fluphenazine, *J. Chromatogr.* 125:275-286, 1976.

Tune, L.E.: Haloperidol drug level monitoring: Pharmacokinetic and methodologic considerations on radioreceptor assay techniques, in: Ayd Haloperidol Update: 1958-1980, Ayd Medical Communications, Baltimore, pp. 220-230, 1980.

Tune, L.E., Creese, I., Depaulo, J.R., Slavney, P.R., Coyle, J.T. and Snyder, S.H.: Clinical state and serum neuroleptic levels measured by radioreceptor assay in schizophrenia, *Am. J. Psychiatry* 137:187-190, 1980.

Van-Putten, T.: Why do schizophrenic patients refuse to take their drugs? *Arch. Gen. Psychiatry* 31:67-72, 1974.

Van-Putten, T., May, P.R. and Wilkins, J.N.: Importance of akinesia: plasma chlorpromazine and prolactin levels, *Am. J. Psychiatry* 137:1446-1448, 1980.

Wiles, D.H. and Franklin, M.: Radioimmunoassay for fluphenazine in human plasma, *Br. J. Clin. Pharmacol.* 5:265-268, 1978.

Winnik, H.Z. and Tennenbaum, L.: Apparition de galactorrhee au cours du traitement de largactil, *Presse Med.* 63: 1092, 1955.

Wode-Helgodt, B., Borg, S., Fyro, B. and Sedval, G.: Clinical effects and drug concentrations in plasma and cerebrospinal fluid in psychotic patients treated with fixed doses of chlorpromazine, *Acta. Psychiatr. Scand.* 58:149-173, 1978.

Zingales, I.A.: A gas chromatographic method for determination of haloperidol in human plasma, *J. Chromatogr.* 54:15-24, 1971.

CHAPTER 10

Neuropsychopharmacology of the Childhood Psychoses: A Critical Review

Wayne H. Green
Stephen I. Deutsch
Magda Campbell
Lowell T. Anderson

MAJOR AFFECTIVE DISORDERS WITH PSYCHOTIC FEATURES
Diagnostic Criteria

DSM-III (1980) subsumes under the Major Affective Disorders those psychiatric conditions whose essential feature is a full affective syndrome (mood disturbance) accompanied by a full manic or depressive syndrome and not caused by other physical or mental disorders.

If a patient has ever had, or is having at present, a manic episode, a diagnosis of Bipolar Disorder (mixed, manic, or depressed) is made. If the patient has had only major depressive episodes, the condition is diagnosed Major Depression (single episode or recurrent).

According to DSM-III both Bipolar Disorder and Major Depression exist along a continuum from nonpsychotic to psychotic. Other than the presence of psychotic symptoms, diagnostic criteria are identical. DSM-III suggests that "with psychotic features" be added when the manic episode is characterized by delusions or hallucinations or grossly bizarre behavior . . . or flight of ideas without apparent awareness of the individual that the speech is not understandable" (DSM-III, 1980, p. 209) and that, in addition, it be specified whether the psychotic features are mood congruent or mood-incongruent. Likewise, "with psychotic features" should be added when the major depressive episode shows "apparently . . . gross impairment in reality testing, as when there are delusions or hallucinations, or depressive stupor," (DSM-III, 1980, pp. 214-215) and it should be noted if the psychotic features are mood congruent or mood-incongruent.

Just as DSM-III does not distinguish between psychotic and neurotic major affective disorders, so too, it does not distinguish between endogenous and non-endogenous (reactive) affective Major Affective Disorders.

It should be noted that there are no studies of brain function, neurotransmitters, metabolic products, or psychopharmacological treatments where psychotic affective disorder was treated as an independent group.

Biological Investigations and Theories of Major Affective Disorder
Neurotransmitters and Metabolites

The existence of endogenous affective illness in children would be best corroborated by the demonstration of biological abnormalities. Altered central noradrenergic transmission has been implicated in the etiology of endogenous major depressive disorders in adults. In a preliminary investigation, Cytryn and associates (1974) studied the 24-hour urinary excretion of norepinephrine and 2 of its major metabolites (vanillylmandelic acid and 3-methoxy-4-hydroxyphenylethyl glycol) in 9 hospitalized children (aged 6 to 12 years) in an attempt to determine whether a similar abnormality could be demonstrated in affectively disturbed children. Their sample was sufficiently impaired to warrant hospitalization and depressive symptoms persisted for at least 2 months prior to study. The sample included 4 children with chronic depressive reactions, 3 children with acute depressive reactions, 1 child with a masked depressive reaction and 1 child with a hypomanic reaction. Urinary collections obtained from a control sample of 18 normal 10-year old boys were used for comparisons. All of the participants were maintained on low catecholamine and indoleamine diets and the patients were medication-free for at least 2 weeks prior to entry into the study. In this study, individual patients showed lower 24-hour urinary excretion of norepinephrine, vanillylmandelic acid (VMA), and 3-methoxy-4-hydroxyphenylethyl glycol (MHPG). However, no consistent pattern of differences existed between the patient group and control sample. The authors considered the possibility that urinary excretion of norepinephrine and VMA may more accurately reflect activity level and peripheral pools of this catecholamine. However, the dissociation between patterns of norepinephrine and VMA excretion in individual patients could not be explained by this consideration. Of special interest, was the dramatic reduction of MHPG excretion in the one hypomanic child. Urinary excretion of

MHPG is felt to be a reflection of norepinephrine turnover in brain. Although a definite relationship between urinary excretion of norepinephrine or a specific metabolite and diagnostic category was not shown, alterations of noradrenergic metabolism in at least some affectively disturbed children were suggested. The authors emphasized that their finding of no consistent noradrenergic abnormality was not dissimilar from what has been observed in affectively disordered adults.

McKnew and Cytryn (1979) pursued their interest in noradrenergic metabolism in affectively disturbed children by examining the 24-hour urinary excretion of norepinephrine, VMA and MHPG in a uniform group of 9 children (ages 6-12) with chronic depressive reactions. Urinary collections from two reference groups were used for comparison; the original control sample of 10-year old boys (n = 18) and 9 children (ages 6-12) free of psychopathology but bedridden for at least 3 weeks secondary to a fractured lower limb. The orthopedic reference sample was selected to control for the possible effect of activity level on these measures. All measures were expressed per body surface area to account for differences in age, size and weight. Despite probable differences in activity levels among the 3 groups, there were no differences in the urinary excretion patterns of norepinephrine and VMA. The depressed sample showed variability in its range of MHPG values which was felt to indicate a lack of diagnostic homogeneity. However, as a group, the depressed children excreted significantly less MHPG than the control sample of 18 normal 10-year old boys. Thus, these data suggest that diminished central norepinephrine turnover occurs in at least a subgroup of depressed children. An unexpected finding was that the bedridden, orthopedic reference group showed the least variability and lowest urinary excretion of MHPG. The authors hypothesized that this might reflect despair and suppression of arousal in this immobilized group of children. The normal urinary excretion values of norepinephrine and VMA for this group of children argue against diminished activity as the causative factor.

Lowered 24-hour urinary excretion of MHPG and blunting of the plasma growth hormone (GH) response to insulin-induced hypoglycemia in prepubertal depressives support hypotheses of impaired noradrenergic, and possibly serotonergic, transmission in these patients (Cytryn et al, 1974; McKnew and Cytryn, 1979; Puig-Antich et al, 1981). These data support pharmacotherapeutic interventions designed to facilitate noradrenergic and serotonergic transmission. Imipramine, a tertiary tricyclic antidepressant, and its principal demethylated metabolite, desipramine, prevent the presynaptic reuptake of serotonin and norepinephrine in brain. Imipramine has been shown to have salutary effects in prepubertal children with major depressive disorders (Puig-Antich et al, 1979b). This will be reviewed below.

Hormonal Relationships and Influences

The neuroendocrine strategy assumes that the secretion of pituitary hormones into the blood can reflect the influence of central neurotransmitter systems upon the hypothalamus. The rise in growth hormone (GH) secretion in response to a variety of provocative tests has been reported to be abnormal in subgroups of adults with major depressive disorders. Growth hormone hyporesponsivity in adult depressives has occurred following challenges with insulin-induced hypoglycemia, desmethylimipramine (DMI), and clonidine. These data suggest a diminished sensitivity of postsynaptic noradrenergic receptors in hypothalami of some adult depressives. The demonstration of blunted GH responses to provocative tests in depressed children would provide similar evidence for a biological abnormality involving noradrenergic mechanisms in these children.

Using unmodified adult RDC criteria (Spitzer et al, 1978) for major depressive disorder (MDD) to select their samples, Puig-Antich and associates (1981) studied GH secretion in response to an intravenous bolus of insulin (0.1 units/kg) in 27 children aged 6-12 years with endogenous MDD (n = 10), nonendogenous MDD (n = 10), and nondepressed neurotic disorders (n = 7). The children in the endogenous sample showed significantly lower plasma GH concentrations at 30, 45 and 60 minutes post-insulin; a lower total GH release for up to 60 minutes post-insulin as determined by area under the concentration curves; and lower maximal GH peak. There were no significant differences in any of these measures between the children with nonendogenous MDD and nondepressed neurotic disorders. In this study, about 90% of children with endogenous MDD were correctly classified using a cutoff of 4.0 ng/ml for peak plasma GH concentration in a 60-minute period post-insulin. No child with a neurotic disorder showed a peak plasma GH concentration below this value. However, this single criterion cannot be used to resolve the endogenous from nonendogenous samples as about 50% of nonendogenous children showed peak plasma concentrations below this value. Using area under the GH curve for 0 to 60 minutes post-insulin as a criterion for resolving these 3 groups provided similar results. In this sample of children with endogenous MDD, the sensitivity of the GH response to insulin-induced hypoglycemia (about 90% using 4 ng/ml as cutoff for peak plasma GH concentration) was greater than that found with adult endogenous depressives (about 50%). These data strongly suggest the existence of endogenous MDD as a distinct diagnostic category in children.

Hyposecretion of GH in response to insulin-induced hypoglycemia persisted in a recovered sample of prepubertal children with the endogenous subtype of major depressive disorder (Puig-Antich et al, 1984c). These patients showed a blunted GH response post-insulin infusion after at least a 4-month period of sustained recovery and one month of medication-free status. Therefore, persistence of an abnormal GH response may be a genetic trait marker of the endogenous subtype of major depressive disorder reflecting abnormal neuroregulatory mechanisms.

Prepubertal major depressives also showed another abnormality of GH secretion. A sample of these patients hypersecreted GH during the first 180 and 300 minutes of sleep (Puig-Antich et al, 1984a). Moreover, GH hypersecretion during the first few hours of sleep occurred during both a depressive episode and full recovery in a sample of children studied in both states (Puig-Antich et al, 1984b). Thus, regulation of GH secretion in prepubertal major depressives displays many features of a genetic trait marker.

The Dexamethasone Suppression Test

An insensitivity of the hypothalamic-pituitary-adrenal axis to inhibition by dexamethasone (1 mg, p.o.) occurs in about 50% of adult patients with endogenous or primary depression (Carroll et al, 1981). These patients display a failure to suppress serum levels of cortisol below 5 μg/dl at some time during the day following an 11:00 p.m. oral administration of dexamethasone. In adult patients, the dexamethasone suppression test (DST) may serve as a useful state marker for the prediction of relapse and the assessment of treatment efficacy before the appearance of clinical improvement (Greden et al, 1983).

Poznanski et al (1982) reported the results of DSTs performed in a series of 18 dysphoric children (ages 6-12 years) diagnosed according to the RDC (Spitzer et al, 1978). Nine children in this sample fulfilled criteria for major depressive disorder and 8 of these children qualified for endogenous subtype. The other 9 children served as the comparison group and received a variety of nondepressive diagnoses. In their DST procedure, Poznanski et al (1982) administered a 0.5 mg dose of dexamethasone at 11:00 p.m. on the evening before blood sampling to yield the same ratio of steroid to body weight as in adults. Using a serum cortisol concentration of 5 μg/dl as the cutoff, 5 out of 9 children with major depressive disorders were nonsuppressors following dexamethasone administration. The sensitivity of the procedure improved to 63% when the 8 patients with the endogenous subtype were considered as a group. Moreover, the specificity of the test in prepubertal children remained high (about 90%) as only 1 child in the comparison group failed to suppress. In addition to providing nosologic validity for the category of major depressive disorders in children, the authors argue that the DST may serve as a useful diagnostic aid. The syndrome of major depressive disorders is less well appreciated in children than in adults.

Robbins and associates (1983) reported the DST results of 28 adolescent psychiatric inpatients (ages 13 to 18 years) who were diagnosed according to the Research Diagnostic Criteria after administration of the

Schedule for Affective Disorders and Schizophrenia (SADS) (Endicott and Spitzer, 1978). Nine of these 28 patients satisfied criteria for major depressive disorder-endogenous subtype and, of these 9 patients, 4 showed escape from cortisol suppression by dexamethasone. None of 7 patients with major depressive disorder-nonendogenous subtype or 3 patients with minor depressive disorder showed an abnormality of their DST. In this study of adolescent inpatients, the sensitivity of the DST for the endogenous subtype of major depressive disorder was about 44 percent and there were no false positives. These data were viewed as further corroboration of the existence of an endogenous subtype with a biological abnormality. Of note is the fact that patients with less than 80% of ideal body weight were excluded from this study to avoid the possibility of a false positive result.

Hsu and associates (1983) presented their DST results on 101 consecutive admissions (ages 13 to 19 years) to an adolescent psychiatric inpatient service over a one-year period. The patients were diagnosed according to DSM-III criteria and 9 of 14 patients with major depressive disorders showed nonsuppression (64%). The incidence of nonsuppression in 27 patients with affective disorders, irrespective of DSM-III diagnostic category, was 48 percent. With the exception of 4 out of 5 patients with bulimia (80%), the percentage of patients from nonaffective diagnostic categories showing nonsuppression was significantly lower. Although bulimia may be related to affective disorders, the fact that all of the bulimic patients had lost weight prior to admission confounds interpretation of this result. Three of the 14 patients with major depressive disorders had first-degree relatives with depression, but without mania, alcoholism or sociopathy, and would qualify for the classification of familial pure depressive disease (FPDD) (Winokur et al, 1978). All 3 of these patients showed a nonsuppression of serum cortisol by dexamethasone. Thus, this category of FPDD may reflect a more homogeneous subgroup of depressive patients. In this study by Hsu and associates (1983) the specificity of the DST for major depressive disorders in adolescents was not as high as suggested in the report by Robbins and associates (1983). For example, 25% of patients with conduct disorder showed nonsuppression. The relationship, if any, of nonsuppressors with nonaffective disorder diagnoses to nonsuppressors with depressive diagnoses is unclear at this time. In any event, the DST may serve as an aid in differential diagnosis and as a prognostic guide to relapse and treatment response in some adolescent patients with depressive disorders.

Psychopharmacological Treatment: Review of the Literature
Major Depressive Disorder, Psychotic

Chambers et al (1982) reported that about ⅓ of 58 prepubertal children fulfilling Research Diagnostic Criteria (RDC) for major depressive disorder, exhibited psychotic symptoms: 36% reported auditory hallucinations, 16% had visual or tactile hallucinations and 7% had delusional ideas.

Puig-Antich et al (1978) reported 13 prepubertal depressed children who fit unmodified RDC criteria for major depressive disorder. Of these, 4 were psychotic. Eight of these 13 children were treated with imipramine in an open, clinical trial. Six of the 8 improved after 4 continuous weeks on maximum dosage. Therapeutic effects were noted between the third and fourth weeks of drug therapy. The authors did not specify how many psychotic children were among the 6 that improved. Of the 2 cases that did not respond, one was a psychotic subtype. Her dosage was 4 mg/kg and blood level was 100 ng/ml. When the dosage was increased to 5 mg/kg, blood level increased to 304 ng/ml and she met criteria for a responder. Untoward effects of mild somnolence and dry mouth required lowering dosage to 4.5 mg/kg and the child retained her clinical gains without side effects. Puig-Antich et al (1979, b) reported on 13 prepubertal children with major depressive disorder treated with imipramine in a double-blind placebo controlled study. Mean maintenance dosage was 105 mg/day (range 50-145 mg/day) or 3.98 mg/kg/day (range 1.5-5 mg/kg/day). Six children were responders and 7 nonresponders. Responders had significantly higher plasma levels (mean 231 ng/ml ± 66) than non-responders (mean 128 ng/ml ± 87) (p < 0.05). There was no significant correlation between maintenance doses and plasma levels. The only subject specifically identifiable as psychotic was the only child among the 13 who was delusional. He had the second highest plasma level (314 ng/ml) and the worst clinical response. This parallels results in several adult studies where adult delusional depressives do not respond to dosage or plasma levels of imipramine associated with response in nondelusional adult depressives (Puig-Antich et al, 1979b).

In a later communication, Puig-Antich et al (in press) studied the relationship of plasma imipramine plus desmethylimipramine levels to clinical response in 30 prepubertal children (including the above 13) with major depressive disorder diagnosed by RDC criteria. The mean age of the 18 boys and 12 girls was 9.56 ± 1.46 years. Twelve subjects were rated psychotic on at least 1 pretreatment interview. Three children had auditory depressive hallucinations and one was delusional on both pretreatment interviews. This was a double-blind fixed dosage protocol. Maximum dosage was 5 mg/kg/day. After 5 weeks, children were classified responders if both depressed mood and anhedonia were rated "slight, of questionable clinical significance" and as non-responders if either of these was rated as mild or worse. Untoward side effects prevented the maximum maintenance dosage in 17 (56.7%) of the subjects; however, weight corrected imipramine dosage was not significantly related to clinical response.

Plasma maintenance levels of imipramine plus desmethylimipramine were significantly higher in the 20 responders (mean 283.85 ± 224.89 ng/ml) than in the 10 non-responders (mean 144.7 ± 80.16 ng/ml) (p < 0.007). Eighty-five percent of responders had total levels over 155 ng/ml whereas only 30% with total levels less than 155 ng/ml responded; the difference was significant (p < 0.009).

The psychotic subgroup was significantly less likely to improve than the nonpsychotic children. Only 5 (42%) of the 12 psychotic children vs. 15 (83%) of the 18 nonpsychotic children were responders (p < 0.05). The authors concluded that those prepubertal children with major depressive disorder who are most likely to respond to imipramine have (1) the least severe depressive symptoms and (2) develop higher plasma levels of imipramine and desmethylimipramine. Conversely, "the more severe the picture of major depression, the higher the plasma level necessary to induce a clinical response," (Puig-Antich et al, in press).

Puig-Antich (1983) reported that among 32 depressed adolescents many failed to show significant response to imipramine and that this was unrelated to plasma levels. The 15 (47%) who responded received mean doses of 240 mg/day of imipramine and had plasma levels of 378 ng/ml. The 17 (53%) who failed to respond received mean doses of 249 mg/day of imipramine and had plasma levels of 301 ng/ml; this is near the upper limit of the therapeutic range for adults.

Petti and Wells (1980) described a 12½ year old who developed a psychotic depression with delusions and hallucinations after he shot and killed his twin brother. He was treated with imipramine which was raised to 200 mg/day (3.5 mg/kg/day) with rapid remission of the psychotic symptoms, but an increase in hostility and anger. Aggression has been reported as a side effect of imipramine in the treatment of childhood depression (Pallmeyer & Petti, 1979).

Bipolar Disorder, Psychotic

Baron et al (1983) collected data on 142 bipolar probands (61 males, 81 females) and 110 siblings. They noted the following ages of onset for probands and siblings during childhood and adolescence in non-cumulative percents:

> Ages 0-9 years: 1% of female probands
> Ages 10-14 years: 3% of male probands
> 3% of female probands
> Ages 15-19 years: 20% of male probands
> 8% of female probands
> 3% of male siblings.

A total of 2% of siblings and probands under 15 and 11% under age 20 had major affective illness. The authors noted that bipolar siblings did not differ from bipolar probands in age of onset, nor did unipolar siblings differ from the bipolar probands or siblings. This supports the hypothesis that "bipolar and unipolar affective disorders in biological relatives of bipolar probands are phenotypic manifestations of the same underlying disease," (p. 15).

As Baron et al (1983) have demonstrated Bipolar Disorder is rare in prepubertal children, but becomes increasingly common as adolescence proceeds.

Several authors (e.g. Horowitz, 1977; Carlson and Strober, 1978; Bowden and Sarabia, 1980) have noted that bipolar disorder is underdiagnosed, particularly in adolescence chiefly because of confusion with schizophrenic disorder. In their discussion of differential diagnosis of manic-depressive illness and schizophrenia, Pope and Lipinski (1978) have emphasized schizophrenic symptoms such as hallucinations, delusions, and even catatonia, are present in many cases of carefully diagnosed manic-depressive illness. This is of particular therapeutic importance as manic episodes often respond poorly to neuroleptics while appropriate therapy with lithium carbonate will usually effect remission of the psychosis.

Horowitz (1977) reported 8 cases (5 females, 3 males) of psychotic adolescent manic-depressive illness ages 15-18 all of whom were hospitalized with an initial diagnosis of acute schizophrenic reaction. All 8 were treated with unspecified neuroleptics and failed to respond. Upon reassessment all were found to meet Feighner et al's (1972) criteria for primary affective disorder. All had symptoms of mood disturbance, mood lability, pressured speech and delusions. Seven had elevated mood and flight of ideas. Five had auditory and 2 visual hallucinations. Neuroleptics were discontinued and lithium was begun. All 8 patients had complete remission of their psychoses. Dosage of lithium carbonate ranged from 1350-2400 mg/day and serum lithium levels from 0.5 to 1.2 mEq/L. The author emphasized that a symptom constellation of mood disturbance with marked lability and prominent elevation and depression, grandiosity and flight of ideas, and pressured speech, hyperactivity and distractibility predict lithium responsive manic-depression even when massive alterations of thinking and hallucinations are present.

In their 1980 report, Bowden and Sarabia described 3 psychotic manic-depressive adolescents ages 15 to 16 years who had been incorrectly diagnosed as schizophrenic. All 3 failed to respond to neuroleptics (chlorpromazine or thiothixene). Two showed complete remission and the third marked improvement within a week following initiation of lithium carbonate. Serum lithium levels were 0.8-1.0 mEq/L.

Carlson and Strober (1978) reported retrospectively 6 psychotic manic-depressive adolescents all of whom were initially misdiagnosed schizophrenic at ages of 12.7 to 16.5 years. Psychotic delusions and thought disorder were present in all 6 patients and auditory hallucinations in 3 during one or more of the 23 episodes of mania or depression they experienced from onset through follow-up at a mean interval of 54 months later.

In what appears to be the same 6 patients, Carlson (1979) noted she usually prescribed an average dose of 1500 mg lithium daily with a range of 900 to 2700 mg and that higher dosages are usually required to maintain therapeutic serum levels during manic phases. Four of these patients responded well to lithium, one of them after a period of non-compliance. The other two had recurrences of mania while on maintenance lithium therapy, however, upon discontinuation during a non-manic period, both became acutely manic suggesting that some recurrences were being suppressed by lithium.

Strober and Carlson (1982) conducted a prospective 3- to 4-year follow-up of 60 adolescents (47 females, 13 males) ages 13 to 16 years who were hospitalized for the first time for a major depressive episode. Psychotic features (mood congruent delusions or hallucinations) were rated present in 12 (20%) by both independent raters during the first week of hospitalization; the raters agreed 85% of the time on the presence of psychotic features. Nine of the psychotic group (75%) developed mania during the follow-up period and were designated Bipolar Disorder while only 3 of the non-psychotic group (6%) did so. This is a highly significant difference (p < .000).

Of the 60 adolescents, a total of 12 (20%) developed mania (Bipolar Disorder). This included 8 (17%) of the 47 females and 4 (31%) of the 13 males. Bipolar outcome was predicted by (1) a symptom cluster of precipitous onset, psychomotor retardation and mood-congruent psychotic features, (2) specifics of family history for affective and bipolar disorder and (3) drug-induced hypomania.

A total of 56 patients (45 with nonbipolar outcomes and 11 with bipolar outcomes) were treated daily with at least 150 mg of amitriptyline hydrochloride or imipramine hydrochloride for a minimum of 2 weeks. Eleven of these were also given neuroleptics initially to manage agitation and psychotic symptoms. Twenty-four (53%) of the nonbipolar outcomes and two (18%) of the bipolar outcomes had unequivocally positive responses to antidepressant therapy. The authors suggested "the comparatively lower rate of improvement in the bipolar-outcome group stems from the high incidence of psychosis in these patients, a clinical factor known to moderate antidepressant response in adult depressives," (p. 553). The average dosage levels between the two groups were not significantly different; serum levels were not given.

Two of the 56 patients developed hypomanic episodes, one on day 9 and one on days 12-15 of antidepressant therapy. Both were in the bipolar-outcome group and hypomanic symptoms subsided following dosage reduction. This concurs with Akiskal et al's (1979) finding in adult depressives that a transient hypomanic episode during treatment with antidepressants predicts a bipolar outcome in every case.

McKnew et al (1981) reported two girls ages 9 and 12 who were diagnosed bipolar affective disorder, mixed. One's mother had bipolar affective disorder, mixed; the other's paternal grandmother and uncle had episodic affective disorders. Both girls appeared psychotic from the author's descriptions. Lithium was administered in a double-blind cross-over design and both girls responded well, however, the 12-year old's mother made statistical analysis impossible by occasionally giving her daughter the grandmother's lithium during a placebo period. Both children were strong augmenters on evoked potentials on EEG to light stimulation. There was a significant increase in amplitude for the N120 component in the occipital lead which was similar to that previously described in adult lithium responders.

Kelly et al (1976) reported a single case study of a 15-year old mildly retarded manic depressive. She had a history of seizures and was maintained on anticonvulsants. The patient fit 8 of the 10 criteria of Anthony and Scott (1960) for manic depressive illness in childhood. Her "highs" did not respond well to neuroleptics (chlorpromazine—up to 1000 mg/day or haloperidol—4 mg/day). Lithium carbonate, however, in doses of 600 to 900 mg/day (maintenance serum level 0.7 mEq/L) controlled symptoms remarkably well. During a 4-year period, there was a single acute exacerbation of behavioral symptoms which was successfully treated by adding 6 mg of haloperidol daily.

Berg et al (1974) reported a 14-year old girl with "typical bipolar manic-depressive psychosis." She was initially unresponsive to lithium and required ECT. It was found she required unusually high doses of lithium; 2400 mg of lithium daily was necessary to maintain a plasma level of 1.0 mEq/L. Interestingly, her father had bipolar manic-depression and also required similar high doses of lithium to achieve therapeutic plasma levels.

A 15-year old manic-depressive adolescent with borderline IQ responded promptly to a combination of neuroleptic and lithium (1200-1800 mg/day; serum level 1.0 mEq/L) (White and O'Shanick, 1977).

Psychopharmacological Treatment of Major Affective Disorders
Imipramine Hydrochloride

Criteria for Use of Imipramine Hydrochloride. The drug of choice in treating Major Depression and Bipolar Disorder, Depressed based on clinical experience and the review of the literature is imipramine.

It should be noted that imipramine is approved by the FDA for use in children under age 12 only for the treatment of enuresis and not for major depressive disorder or other conditions.

Laboratory Evaluation and Monitoring. Prior to administration, a baseline EKG should be obtained because of known cardiotoxicity at higher dosage levels. It is suggested periodic EKG monitoring be performed until a maintenance level is reached. Routine laboratory studies including liver function tests (SGOT, SGPT, alkaline phosphatase) CBC and urinalysis are also recommended.

Dosage of Imipramine. The Physicians' Desk Reference (PDR) (1984) states dosage of 2.5 mg/kg/day should not be exceeded in children. The FDA will approve research protocols only if imipramine dosage does not exceed 5.0 mg/kg/day (Hayes et al, 1975).

Untoward Effects. Potential side effects are those of the tricyclic antidepressants and the same as in adults. They include cardiovascular, behavioral and anticholinergic effects. A complete listing of untoward effects is in the latest edition of the Physicians' Desk Reference (PDR) (1984).

Two studies in particular have bearing on side effects in children. In order to assess the relationship between plasma drug levels of imipramine and desipramine and side effects, Preskorn and associates (1983) measured steady state plasma tricyclic levels in 22 children (aged 7 to 12 years), each of whom fulfilled DSM-III criteria for major depressive disorder receiving a fixed bedtime dose of 75 mg of imipramine for 3 weeks. They related these levels to alterations in pulse rate, blood pressure, and EKG, as well as the emergence of unpleasant subjective side effects. A fixed dose was employed to permit an assessment of interindividual variability in plasma drug concentrations. On this fixed dose of imipramine, there was marked interindividual variability between the 22 children with a sevenfold difference in total plasma tricyclic concentration. Furthermore, the ratio of plasma levels of desipramine to imipramine ranged from 0.86 to 6.4. The emergence of unpleasant side effects was unrelated to plasma concentrations of parent drug or metabolite, either individually or combined. In this study, significant effects on prolongation of the QT interval and reduction of T-wave amplitude occurred at plasma levels of total drug above 225 ng/ml. In addition, first-degree heart block due to prolongation of the PR interval appeared in 3 patients with total drug levels above 350 ng/ml. A positive association was also found between blood levels and increases in diastolic blood pressure and standing heart rate. These data emphasize the importance of blood levels to assess the adequacy of a clinical antidepressant trial. Plasma total imipramine and desipramine levels should be maintained below 225 ng/ml to avoid possible serious cardiovascular toxicity. Reliance upon subjective complaints, often mediated by peripheral anticholinergic effects, is an insensitive guide to dosage regulation and can result in under- or overdosage (Preskorn et al, 1983).

Puig-Antich et al (in press) found untoward effects prevented further increases of imipramine before the maximum dose of 5 mg/kg/day was reached in 17 (56.7%) of their 30 subjects. Untoward cardiac effects accounted for 10 children (33%); nine had increased PR interval limit (≥0.18 sec) and one had increased heart rate (≥130 beats/min) above the acceptable limit. The authors noted, however, that minor EKG changes from baseline occurred in nearly all the children. The non-cardiac untoward effects preventing the other 7 children from dosage increases or requiring decrease in dose included 2 with orthostatic hypotension, 2 with marked irritability, 2 with forgetfulness and perplexity and one with chest pain.

Lithium Carbonate

Criteria for Use of Lithium Carbonate. The use of lithium in childhood and adolescent psychiatric conditions, including bipolar and major depressive disorders has been recently reviewed by Campbell et al (1984a). Lithium's effectiveness in treating manic episodes in adult bipolar disorder and in the prophylaxis of recurrent manic and depressive episodes is well established. The available literature suggests that lithium is the drug of choice for children and adolescents with mania as well. Although some children with depression appear to respond, no methodologically adequate studies exist. It appears those children whose parents or close relatives have episodic disorders and who are lithium-responders, are more likely to be responders themselves.

At present, lithium is not approved by the FDA for administration to children under age 12. In adolescents age 12 years or over, it is approved only for the treatment of manic episodes of bipolar disorder and maintenance therapy in bipolar disorder.

Lithium is contraindicated in patients with renal, hepatic, thyroid, or cardiac disorders. It should be administered with caution to adolescents at risk for pregnancy as cardiac teratogenicity has been reported (Kallen and Tandberg, 1983).

Laboratory Evaluation and Serum/Saliva Monitoring. A reasonable work-up prior to lithium administration should include routine blood studies (SMA 12, CBC), thyroid studies (T_3, T_4, TSH), and kidney function (urinalysis, BUN, serum creatinine and, if possible, a creatinine clearance test). An EEG within the past year would also be desirable. It is essential that laboratory facilities to monitor serum and/or saliva lithium levels be readily available during titration of medication and for periodic monitoring during maintenance. Untoward effects and lithium toxicity in particular are related to high serum levels. Blood samples should be drawn in the morning 8-12 hours after the last dose and before the morning dose when serum lithium levels are relatively stable.

Dosage of Lithium. Therapeutic doses and serum levels of lithium in children and adolescents do not differ from those in adults. Therapeutic serum levels range from 0.32 to 1.5 mEq/L and usually require 500 to 2100 mg of lithium intake daily to be maintained (Campbell et al, 1984a). As noted by Carlson (1979) during manic episodes higher than usual doses may be required to maintain serum levels in the therapeutic range.

Initial dose should be low: 300 mg q.d. or 300 mg b.i.d. and increments should be in divided doses and gradual with careful monitoring of serum or saliva levels—twice weekly is recommended. (Saliva levels are about 2.5 times greater than serum values (Perry et al, 1984). Lithium should be gradually titrated upward until therapeutic values and remission of symptoms occur—or until untoward effects prevent this. Desirable maintenance levels of serum lithium are usually between 0.6-1.2 mEq/L. The PDR (1984) recommends lithium not be allowed to exceed 2.0 mEq/L during the acute treatment phase.

Untoward Effects and Toxicity. Untoward effects and toxicity are usually related to the serum lithium levels. Untoward effects do not appear qualitatively different among children, adolescents and adults nor among the various disorders treated with lithium. Quantitatively, however, there may be some differences. For example, higher serum levels may be tolerated during the treatment of manic episodes with reduction of dosage and serum level necessary during the maintenance period. Although the PDR (1984) suggests adverse reactions are seldom encountered below serum levels of 1.5 mEq/L, this does not appear to be the case in children. The only reports in the literature on children treated with lithium where correlations between serum and saliva lithium levels and untoward effects are detailed are those of Campbell and her colleagues (Campbell et al, 1984a, b Perry et al, 1984). Although the 21 children treated in this double-blind, placebo controlled study were conduct disorders, many developed side effects with serum levels below 1.5 mEq/L and many when serum levels were below 0.5 mEq/L. A total of 19 different untoward effects (decreased appetite, stomach ache, nausea, vomiting, headache, dizziness, pallor, decreased verbal production, tearfulness, fatigue, subdued, "glazed look," decreased motor activity, feeling sleepy, falling asleep, fidgetiness, tremor, ataxia and dysarthria) occurred a total of 42 times in 17 of the 21 patients. On optimal dose (mean 1166 mg; range 500-2000 mg/day) and with serum levels of 0.32-1.51 mEq/L and saliva levels of 0.81-5.05 mEq/L, 11 patients experienced 13 untoward effects (Campbell et al, 1984b). Thus, future studies will be needed to determine whether children, as a group, tend to develop untoward effects at lower serum levels than most adults, or whether it is only nonpsychotic children or a nonpsychotic subgroup who do so.

For a review of other untoward effects, the current PDR is recommended.

SCHIZOPHRENIC DISORDER IN CHILDREN AND ADOLESCENTS
Diagnostic Criteria

DSM-III (1980), for the first time, does not distinguish between schizophrenic disorder in childhood and adulthood. Diagnostic criteria are identical for both. DSM-III does distinguish clearly between infantile autism and schizophrenic disorder. Prior to this, there had been considerable diagnostic confusion and many studies either contained a heterogeneous mixture of psychotic children, or the exact makeup of the samples cannot be ascertained (Green et al, 1984).

Rutter (1967) and Kolvin (1971) were particularly important in separating infantile autism (early onset psychosis) from schizophrenic disorder (late-onset psychosis).

Biological Investigations and Theories of Schizophrenic Disorder

The ability to identify prepubertal schizophrenic children with unmodified DSM-III criteria (Green et al, 1984) suggests a possible continuity between childhood and adult forms of this disorder.

The dopamine hypothesis and endorphine investigations with adult schizophrenic populations have been reviewed in previous chapters. There are no specific additional data from studies of children and adolescents.

Neuroendocrine Abnormalities

Different neuroendocrine measures in schizophrenia may be useful as either state markers of the illness (e.g., exacerbation vs. remission) or genetic trait markers for a subgroup of patients. Growth hormone (GH) secretion is stimulated by the intravenous infusion of luteinizing hormone-releasing hormone (LRH) and thyrotropin hormone-releasing hormone (TRH) in subgroups of adolescent schizophrenic patients (Gil-Ad et al, 1981; Weizman et al, 1982). GH rise in response to LRH may be a state marker as this response was blunted in 4 patients who had shown a marked elevation prior to treatment, following a 3-month period of neuroleptic administration (Gil-Ad et al, 1981). GH responses to TRH administration may be a genetic trait marker in a subgroup of adolescent schizophrenic patients as this measure remained elevated despite up to 1 year of neuroleptic administration (Weizman et al, 1982). Moreover, there is the suggestion of a higher incidence of positive family history in those patients showing a plasma GH elevation in response to TRH. The application of these measures to wider samples of schizophrenic patients, including prepubertal subjects, should further refine our nosology and understanding of pathophysiology.

Neurostructural Abnormalities

The advent of computerized tomography (CT), a noninvasive tool for the structural examination of the brain, prompted a series of studies in schizophrenia and other functional disorders. Several of these studies suggested the existence of a subgroup of schizophrenic patients with neurostructural abnormalities (i.e., enlarged lateral ventricles, sulcal prominence, cerebellar atrophy and brain-density deficits), cognitive impairment, negative symptoms (e.g., affective flattening, impoverished speech and thinking), and poor response to neuroleptic treatment (Deutsch and Davis, 1983). In the initial reports, the incidence of neurostructural abnormalities in subchronic and chronic samples of schizophrenic patients approached 50 percent. However, subsequent CT studies, which addressed the effects of sample selection, including the selection of controls, definition of ventricular abnormalities and techniques for measurement of these abnormalities, have led to a downward revision (to about 20%) of the incidence of ventricular enlargement in samples of chronic schizophrenic patients (Deutsch and Davis, 1983; Rieder et al, 1983). Moreover, the specificity of these CT findings for schizophrenia is uncertain as similar rates of abnormality have been reported in samples of patients with schizoaffective and bipolar disorders (Rieder et al, 1983). Clearly, the application of these CT measures to samples of prepubertal schizophrenic patients would help to resolve the issue of whether ventricular enlargement in some schizophrenic patients is an incidental finding, a consequence of chronicity of illness or effect of treatment, or an early neurostructural accompaniment of a unique subgroup.

Psychopharmacological Treatment: Review of the Literature

The only double-blind, placebo controlled study in children or adolescents is that of Pool et al (1976). They compared the efficacy of loxapine, haloperidol and placebo over a 4-week period in 75 adolescents (ages 13 to 18 years) who were diagnosed schizophrenia and all of whom had a gross disorder of thought associations and/or hallucinations. Average daily doses were 87.5 mg for loxapine (maximum dose was 200 mg), 9.8 mg for haloperidol (maximum dose was 16 mg), and 5.4 capsules of placebo. Loxapine and haloperidol were both significantly better than placebo on some specific clinical items associated with schizophrenia on both the Brief Psychiatric Rating Scale (BPRS) and the Nurses' Observation Scale for Inpatient Evaluation (NOSIE). All 3 groups improved, however. On the Clinical Global Ratings of Improvement (CGI), there were no significant differences among the 3 groups although there was a trend ($p = 0.06$) for more patients rated "severely" or "very severely ill" to improve on haloperidol or loxapine than on placebo.

The most common side effect in the entire group of 75 adolescents was sedation in 40 (53.3%). This occurred in 21 of 26 (80.8%) of those on loxapine; 13 of 25 (52%) of those on haloperidol; and 6 of 24 (25%) of those on placebo. Extrapyramidal side effects, the most common of which was muscular rigidity of the parkinsonian type, were present in 38 subjects (50.7%). This included 19 (73.1%) of those on loxapine; 18 (72%) of those on haloperidol, and 1 patient on placebo (Pool et al, 1976).

Simeon et al (1973) treated 10 children, 4 of whom were diagnosed childhood schizophrenia, with a course of placebo for 3-9 weeks (mean 5.2 weeks), then trihexyphenidyl 2.0 mg daily for 1-3 weeks (mean 1.6 weeks) to which thiothixene was then added. Thiothixene was given for 6 to 46 weeks (mean 16.5 weeks). In the 4 schizophrenic children, maximum daily dosage ranged from 10 to 50 mg (average 27.5 mg) and optimal dosage ranged from 6 to 20 mg/day (average 12.75 mg/day). On Clinical Global Improvement ratings compared to baseline placebo, one child showed moderate improvement and the other 3 slight improvement. In the 10 patients, motor activity, speech, thought content, social relationship, mood, emotion, feeding and attention improved significantly. Untoward effects were mild and transient, except for weight gain in 5 patients, and did not interfere significantly with the patients' functioning.

LeVann (1969) administered haloperidol in an open study to 100 (54 retarded and 46 non-retarded) hospitalized psychiatric children and adolescents. Of these, 46 were diagnosed childhood schizophrenia. Sixteen (ages 10-21, mean 15.1 years) were retarded and 30 (ages 9-20, mean 13.5 years) were non-retarded. Maximum doses for both groups ranged from 0.75 to 12.0 mg/day. Average maximum dose for the retarded group of 54 patients was 3.0 mg/day and for the non-retarded group of 46 patients, it was 3.1 mg/day. Although LeVann did not analyze the results according to diagnostic category, 95% of the non-retarded group and 78% of the retarded group showed some improvement. Haloperidol was significantly effective ($p = 0.05$) in reducing each of 6 symptoms: hyperactivity, assaultiveness, self-injury, excitability, insomnia, and poor appetite. Of importance, there was little or no evidence of loss of mental alertness.

The relationship of responsivity of psychotic and other symptoms to serum levels of haloperidol was described in a 13½ year old schizophrenic male described as "preadolescent" (Meyers et al, 1980). In this clinical report, symptoms (i.e., delusions, hallucinations, affective disturbance, social withdrawal) persisted in spite of a total daily oral dose of 20 or 25 mg of haloperidol. A remission of symptoms was observed when the dose was increased to 30-40 mg/day coinciding with serum neuroleptic levels of about 100 ng/ml well above the 50 ng/ml of chlorpromazine (CPZ) equivalents felt to be therapeutic. When dosage was progressively lowered to 20 mg/day, serum levels fell to only 12 ng/ml and psychotic symptoms including auditory hallucinations, persecutory delusions and inappropriate affect, reemerged. Following an increase in dosage to 30 mg/day and serum levels of 68 ng/ml hallucinations and delusions again remitted. In this child, abatement of psychotic symptoms was accompanied by a 13-point increase in full-scale IQ (WISC). This clinical report suggests that psychotic symptoms in prepubertal schizophrenia are sensitive to neuroleptics and interfere with intellectual functioning. Moreover, a failure of symptoms to remit could be due to lack of attainment of an adequate serum neuroleptic level.

A single case report described a positive synergistic interaction between methylphenidate and chlorpromazine, of at least two and one-half years duration, in a prepubertal 11-year old schizophrenic boy (Rogeness and Macedo, 1983). In addition to psychotic symptoms, the symptom profile of this patient included hyperactivity, impulsivity and poor attention. However, from one single case one cannot make generalizations.

Psychopharmacological Treatment of Schizophrenic Disorder in Children and Adolescents
Neuroleptics (Major Tranquilizers)

Criteria for the Use of Neuroleptics. It has been well established that neuroleptics are the drugs of choice in adult schizophrenic disorder. There is increasing evidence that children and young adolescents diagnosed schizophrenic disorder according to strict DSM-III criteria are on a continuum with adult schizophrenic disorder (Green et al, 1984).

As shown above, there is a paucity of literature on the use of neuroleptics in children and adolescents. The one major study in adolescence shows that they are effective in reducing symptoms although the development of excessive sedation and parkinsonian untoward effects detract from their therapeutic value (Pool et al, 1976).

The literature is scant on children under twelve. One reason is that this is a rather rare condition in this age group. In our clinical experience children with schizophrenic disorder respond much less favorably to neuroleptics than do adults. Administration of neuroleptics rarely produces changes of sufficient magnitude to permit them to go home and function on their premorbid levels.

Laboratory Tests. Prior to initiation of medication, routine laboratory studies including CBC and liver function tests are recommended.

Dosage of Neuroleptics. Unless the schizophrenic child is truly an immediate danger to himself or others, it is recommended that inpatient hospitalization be followed by a medication-free period for baseline observation as well as assessment of the effects of hospitalization per se. Drug administration should then begin at a low, possibly ineffective dose, and be gradually titrated upward. The above principles may be more difficult to carry out in adolescents.

Table I lists the major classes of neuroleptics, a typical drug from each class and gives the usual range of dosages for children and adolescents. It is recognized that clinically severely disturbed psychotic youngsters may require higher doses to control their symptoms.

Polypharmacy is not recommended. In our clinical experience and research, we do not use antiparkinsonian drugs when extrapyramidal side effects occur. Rather, we prefer to reduce the dosage as there is some evidence that antiparkinsonian agents reduce serum concentrations of neuroleptics (Rivera-Calimlim et al, 1976). Moreover, these anticholinergic/antihistaminic agents themselves can cause sedation, cognitive dulling, thought disorganization and toxic psychosis.

Untoward Effects. Campbell and her associates (1983a) have recently reviewed the neuroleptic-induced dyskinesias in children and adolescents.

In our experience, acute dystonic reactions are less frequent when neuroleptics are begun in low doses and very gradually titrated upwards, especially with high-potency drugs. If they occur, diphenhydramine (Benadryl) 25 mg p.o. or i.m. is usually a rapidly effective treatment.

Untoward effects are as in adults although because of the relatively small amount of data available for children, less is known and not all those reported in adults have been reported in children. The current PDR is recommended for review. Parkinsonian side effects are much less frequent in very young children than in older children, adolescents or adults. On the other hand, behavioral toxicity is more frequent in younger children and may often appear before extrapyramidal side effects.

INFANTILE AUTISM
Diagnostic Criteria

Infantile Autism was considered a discrete diagnostic syndrome for the first time in 1980 by the American Psychiatric Association's official nomenclature (DSM-III, 1980). Prior to this, children who would now be diagnosed infantile autism were called "schizophrenic reaction, childhood type" in the first edition of DSM (1952) and "schizophrenia, childhood type" in DSM-II (1968) (Campbell and Green, 1985; Green et al, 1984). Because of this nosological confusion, the exact diagnostic makeup of the subjects in many of the earlier studies of childhood schizophrenia is difficult or impossible to determine. Hence, only those studies in which subjects can clearly be identified as infantile autistics will be reviewed.

Infantile Autism is the only pervasive developmental disorder for which we have a useful body of reliable data. Childhood Onset and Atypical Pervasive Developmental Disorders are rarely seen. Their existence and relationship to infantile autism remains to be validated by further research and they will not be considered here (Campbell and Green, 1985).

Biological Investigations
Neurotransmitters and Their Metabolites

Neurochemical studies of infantile autism have focused upon enzymes and metabolites associated with indoleamines and catecholamines. To date, no consistent abnormality has been found in all autistic patients examined and no single abnormality can differentiate samples of these patients from children with other psychiatric disorders or normal subjects (Young et al, 1982). However, abnormalities of these measures in some children may permit identification of homogeneous subgroups of autistic patients.

Approximately one-third of autistic children show hyperserotonemia in blood due to an elevation of serotonin in platelets (Campbell et al, 1974, 1975; Young et al, 1982). Moreover, lowered levels of 5-hydroxyindoleacetic acid (5-HIAA), the major central metabolite of serotonin, have been reported in spinal fluid obtained from autistic patients. This dissociation between increased platelet serotonin levels and lowered CSF 5-HIAA levels suggests that at least some autistic patients may have an impairment in the release and turnover of serotonin. Lowered CSF 5-HIAA levels have also been reported in other psychiatric disorders and may be related to deficient impulse control irrespective of diagnosis (Träskman et al, 1981). Hyperserotonemia has low specificity and has been reported to occur in a heterogeneous group of patients with severe mental retardation (Campbell et al, 1974, 1975; Young et al, 1982). The mechanism of hyperserotonemia in infantile autism does not seem to be due to decreased oxidative deamination as the activity of platelet monoamine oxidase (MAO) is normal in these children (Campbell et al, 1976a).

Increased levels of homovanillic acid (HVA) in CSF (Cohen et al, 1977) and the salutary effects of haloperidol, a potent dopamine antagonist (Campbell et al, 1978a, 1982a) implicate hyperdopaminergic activity in at least some patients with infantile autism. Haloperidol reduces stereotypies, withdrawal, hyperactivity and fidgetiness at doses which do not cause sedation and promote learning in the laboratory. Higher CSF HVA levels are observed in those autistic patients with greatest locomotor activity and stereotypies (Cohen et al, 1977). Therefore, haloperidol may be most effective in a subgroup of patients characterized by high turnover and release of dopamine.

A preliminary study of 24-hour urinary collections of norepinephrine equivalents and 3-methoxy-4-hydroxyphenethylene glycol (MHPG), the principal CNS metabolite of norepinephrine, in 5 autistic boys suggested a diminished noradrenergic activity in these patients (Young et al, 1982). Reduction of urinary MHPG excretion has a low specificity as it has been also reported in hyperactive, depressed and bedridden, orthopedic patients. The low specificity of this measure suggests that a reduction of noradrenergic activity may not reflect a primary deficiency of a specific disorder but rather a suppression of arousal in subgroups of patients with various disorders (Young et al, 1982). However, alterations of dopamine-β-hydroxylase (DBH) activity, the enzyme which converts dopamine to norepinephrine and is an index of noradrenergic activity, in serum in some autistic patients suggest that subgroups of patients with primary noradrenergic abnormalities may exist (Coleman et al, 1974; Young et al, 1982). These patients may manifest problems with discrimination and regulation of arousal and anxiety (Redmond and Huang, 1979).

The selection of homogeneous subgroups according to specific neurotransmitter abnormalities should encourage the development of more neurotransmitter-specific interventions.

Neuroendocrine Abnormalities

There have been a few reports of neuroendocrine approaches applied to infantile autism. Although basal levels of specific hormones in autistic children may be within normal limits, alterations in rhythms of secretion or response to stressors may be abnormal (Maher et al, 1975; Yamazaki et al, 1975). Plasma concentrations of growth hormone (GH) and cortisol were measured in 11 autistic and 11 subnormal children (ages 4-13 years) in response to insulin-induced hypoglycemia (Maher et al, 1975). The group means of the pre-insulin levels of glucose, GH and cortisol did not differ significantly between the 2 groups. Insulin was infused (0.15 units/kg, i.v.) 30 minutes after cannula insertion and blood was sampled over the subsequent 3-hour period. The autistic group of children showed a slower recovery of basal levels of glucose post-insulin infusion than the control group of subnormal children. They also showed a faster rise and sustained higher concentrations of plasma cortisol for the entire 3-hour period post-insulin infusion. Differences post-insulin GH secretion between the 2 groups were not detected but this could have been due to large between-subject and between-sample variances in this measurement. Despite normal basal levels of cortisol, the autistic children showed a more robust cortisol response to insulin-induced hypoglycemia. Also, the dissociation between slower recovery of basal levels of glucose and higher concentrations of cortisol post-insulin infusion in the autistic group is contrary to prediction. These data suggest that some aspects of the stress response might be impaired in autistic children. The focus of this impairment could be the regulation of hypothalamic secretion of corticotropin releasing factor (CRF). These data require replication and a future study should avoid inclusion of a heterogeneous diagnostic group of subnormal children as controls.

The circadian rhythm of corticosteroid hormone secretion in humans appears to be established at the age of 2 years and is similar to that found in adults (see for discussion Yamazaki et al, 1975). Variations in the normal circadian rhythm could reflect abnormalities in the cerebro-hypothalamic system. Yamazaki and associates (1975) examined the circadian rhythm of plasma 11-hydroxycorticosteroids (11-OHCS) in 7 autistic children (ages 6-10 years) and their plasma 11-OHCS response to intravenous pyrogen administration. Circadian rhythms were established by obtaining 4 or 5 blood samples at 6-hour intervals during a 24-hour period. In this study, 5 out of 7 autistic children showed irregular patterns of plasma 11-OHCS secretion. Despite the high occurrence rate of abnormal circadian rhythms, data presented for 6 autistic children showed sufficient reactivity to intravenous pyrogen in 4 of them. Although a majority of these autistic children were able to respond to a pyrogen stressor with an elevation of plasma 11-OHCS, the abnormal plasma 11-OHCS rhythmicity suggests a functional abnormality in the hypothalamic regulation of ACTH secretion (Yamazaki et al, 1975). Furthermore, a failure in the development of this rhythmic pattern could reflect a maturational delay of the CNS.

Campbell and associates (1978b) provided additional evidence of a neuroendocrine abnormality in a sample of 10 autistic children (ages 2.6 to 7.7 years). In response to an intravenous infusion of thyrotropin-releasing hormone (TRH), these children showed abnormalities in the kinetics of their thyroid stimulating hormone (TSH) and T_3 response, blunting of T_3, and exaggerated or subnormal TSH responses. These data suggest that impaired hypothalamic regulation of thyroid function occurs in at least some patients with infantile autism.

Neurostructural Abnormalities

Computerized axial tomography (CT) was used to detect the possible presence of subtle neurostructural abnormalities in a large sample of 45 autistic children (ages 2 years 7 months to 7 years 8 months) diagnosed according to DSM-III criteria (Campbell et al, 1982b). The autistic sample was relatively homogeneous as all of the children were within a narrow age range and without gross neurological abnormalities, seizure disorders or identifiable causes of the syndrome. Control CT scans were performed on a sample of 19 hospitalized children with normal intellectual function. These children received scans as part of a neurological workup but were determined to have "no neurological abnormalities due to brain pathology" and normal scans. The CT scans of the autistic children were performed with different generation scanners and ventricular size was determined by linear measurements and visual inspection. In this study, about 24% of the autistic sample (11 out of 45 autistic children) showed evidence of ventricular enlargement. However, no relationship could be determined between ventricular enlargement and any of a variety of clinical variables examined.

A pilot study was undertaken employing high resolution CT scanning with image analysis software and volumetric measurements (Rosenbloom et al, 1984). CT scans were performed on 13 autistic children (ages 3 to 8 years), selected according to DSM-III criteria, and 10 children of normal intellectual function (ages 3 to 10 years) who served as controls. The control subjects were scanned as part of a neurological workup and none had CT scan abnormalities. Although a few autistic patients showed ventricular and subarachnoid cisternal enlargement, no differences existed between the two groups on a variety of linear and volumetric measurements. With the exception of the left/right ventricular volume ratio, the autistic sample showed significantly greater variance for some of the measures. These data suggested that autistic patients may show greater uniformity than controls in having a smaller left ventricular to right ventricular volume ratio. This could indicate something unique about the relationship between hemispheres in autistic children. The large variance on a variety of measures in this small autistic sample suggests that subgroups may be resolved according to structural features.

Psychopharmacological Interventions and Their Rationale:
A Review of the Literature
Short-Term Studies

In view of impaired hypothalamic regulation of thyroid function in some autistic children (Campbell et al, 1978b), a clinical trial of daily, oral T_3 administration to 30 clinically-euthyroid, autistic patients (ages 2.3 to 7.2 years) was implemented (Campbell et al, 1978c). An earlier pilot study had suggested that T_3 administration to autistic children was beneficial for some patients (Campbell et al, 1973). The later study was placebo-controlled with a crossover design and patients were maintained on the optimal dosage (range 12.5 to 75 mcg/day, mean = 59.2 mcg/day) for 3 weeks, after a variable period of dosage regulation. When this sample was grouped according to IQ, the profoundly or severely retarded patients showed greater global improvement than the less retarded group while receiving T_3. Only 4 of the 30 children showed clear evidence of a beneficial response with greatest effect observed on "optimal" dosage of T_3. There was no characteristic that could select or identify the individual T_3 responders. The responders showed a reduction of stereotypies and improved behavioral performance at home. These positive changes on T_3 may be associated with a reduction of thyroxine (T_4) blood levels (Campbell et al, 1973, 1978c).

The hyperserotonemia in blood observed in some autistic patients has suggested treatment strategies designed to reduce serotonin levels. The rationale underlying these interventions is that behavioral symptoms are related to the elevated serotonin levels. The administration of L-dopa (2 to 4 g/day over 6 months) to 4 autistic patients (ages 3 to 16 years) resulted in significant reductions of serotonin in the 3 youngest children (Ritvo et al, 1971). Despite these reductions, no salutary effect of L-dopa was observed in this study. Campbell and associates (1976b) administered L-dopa (dosage range 900-2250 mg/day; mean daily dose = 1487 mg) to 12 autistic children (ages 3 to 6.9 years) and observed beneficial effects in 5 of these patients. However, therapeutic effects were not related to alterations of serotonin levels and included decreases in negativism and increases in play, energy and motor initiation in hypoactive children. None of these therapeutic changes reached statistical significance. Adverse effects of this intervention included worsening of preexisting stereotypies and emergence of stereotypies *de novo*.

The value of D-lysergic acid diethylamide (LSD) and methysergide, its methylated derivative, which are ligands that interact with and may block central serotonin receptors, in the treatment of infantile autism remains uncertain (Bender et al, 1963; Fish et al, 1969). Some patients displayed increased activity and alertness with decreased stereotypies (Bender et al, 1963). Methysergide caused less excitability than LSD in a pilot study involving 54 autistic children (ages 6 to 12 years) (Bender et al, 1963). In a study of 11 autistic children, methysergide resulted in a mixed reduction and worsening of symptoms (Fish et al, 1969). The 2 most retarded children in this sample of 11 patients showed greatest improvement with increased alertness and affective responsiveness.

The deterioration of one-half of a sample of 10 autistic children following administration of imipramine could have been due to the ability of this drug to facilitate serotonergic transmission (Campbell et al, 1971). This augmentation of central serotonin activity could also be responsible for the failure to demonstrate therapeutic efficacy of lithium when administered to autistic children (Campbell et al, 1972b).

Recent attention has focused upon the potential efficacy of the anorexogenic drug, fenfluramine, an agent which can deplete central stores of serotonin, in the treatment of infantile autism (Geller et al, 1982; Ritvo, et al, 1983). Fenfluramine reduces 5-HIAA in CSF suggesting that it decreases central turnover of serotonin. Geller and associates (1982) reported their preliminary results on fenfluramine administration to 3 autistic boys (ages 3 to 5.33 years). The dosage of fenfluramine was regulated to keep the blood serotonin concentration between 150 and 200 ng/ml, the normal range for children of this age. Alterations of blood serotonin levels were sensitive to dosage. All 3 patients improved behaviorally and 2 showed an increase in scores on serial IQ tests. These gains were maintained for at least 6 weeks after drug discontinuation. Ritvo et al (1983) issued a preliminary report of a multicenter study of 15 autistic patients, including 2 of Geller et al, ages 2.10 to 22 years. They were treated with 1.5 mg/kg of fenfluramine; 13 patients improved. The areas of improvement included decreased activity and increased attention, affectual response, language and speech, and relating to objects. Two older patients (ages 18 and 22 years) failed to show improvement possibly due to the long duration of illness. In these studies, no serious untoward effects were reported.

The existence of a hyperdopaminergic subgroup of autistic children is supported by neurochemical and pharmacological data. The excess dopaminergic activity appears to be related to lower IQ scores, hyperactivity and stereotypies in these children (Campbell et al, 1982a; Young et al, 1982). These children show elevations of HVA levels in CSF, suggesting increased dopamine turnover and release, and beneficial responses to low doses of haloperidol (0.5 to 3.0 mg/day), a potent antidopaminergic agent (Young et al, 1982; Campbell et al, 1982a; Anderson et al, 1984). Moreover, administration of dopamine agonists (L- and D-amphetamines, L-dopa) resulted in worsening of negativism, withdrawal, irritability, motor excitement and stereotypies, as well as emergence of stereotypies *de novo* in some children (Campbell et al, 1972a, 1976b). These data are consistent with hypotheses regarding hyperdopaminergic mechanisms in at least some autistic patients.

As reviewed by Campbell and associates (1977), a variety of different classes of neuroleptics has been studied in the treatment of autistic children. Most of these studies included heterogeneous diagnostic groups and failed to consider issues related to dosage regulation. Despite these limitations, those neuroleptics which are more purely antidopaminergic and have the least sedative properties appear to be most effective in reducing withdrawal, hyperactivity and stereotypies (Campbell et al, 1977, 1981, 1982a). In an extensive series of placebo-controlled, double-blind studies, using a crossover design, haloperidol, in a dosage range which does not cause sedation (e.g., 0.5 to 3.0 mg/day), promoted the facilitation and retention of learning in the laboratory and reduced a variety of behavioral symptoms (Campbell et al, 1978a, 1982a; Anderson et al, 1984). These symptoms included withdrawal, stereotypy, abnormal object relationships, fidgetiness, hyperactivity, negativism, and angry and labile affect.

Wolpert et al (1967) conducted an 8-week double-blind study comparing trifluoperazine with thiothixene in 16 children ages 8 to 15 years (mean 11 years, 4 months). The children were diagnosed childhood schizophrenia and had been hospitalized from 3 to 64 months (mean 23.2 months). As this paper states the study was designed to validate prior observations with thiothixene and cites Fish et al's work with thiothixene in autistic children and uses the Central Islip Nurses Rating Scale of Autistic Children, it is assumed they are autistic children. Mean daily dose of the 8 children on thiothixene was 13 to 20 mg/day (0.24 to 0.59 mg/kg). Four children improved, 3 showed no change and 1 worsened. The 8 children on trifluoperazine received 13 to 20 mg/day (0.35 to 0.61 mg/kg). Three children improved, 3 showed no change, and 2 worsened. No child in either group was rated as "much improved." Untoward effects were minimal.

Waizer et al (1972) reported a single-blind study of thiothixene in 18 children (17 boys and 1 girl) aged 5 to 13 years who appear to be autistic (they were diagnosed childhood schizophrenic based on the Nine Points of the British Working Party) (Creak, 1961). Following a 2-week placebo period, thiothixene was begun. The non-blind psychiatrist initially prescribed from 2 to 7 mg/day (mean 4.0 mg). This was titrated upward to a range of 10 to 24 mg/day (mean 16.9) by week 12. Children were rated on the Children's Psychiatric Rating Scale (CPRS) at weeks 1, 2, 4, 6, 8, 10 and 12 and on the Clinical Global Impressions Rating Scale (CGI) at week 12. All children improved on the CGI: 4 were "very much improved," 11 were "much improved," and 3 were "minimally improved." On the CPRS, there was significant improvement in motor activity, stereotyped behavior, coordination, sleeping, affect, exploratory behavior, concentration, eating habits, and range of communication. Untoward effects were mild and few in number.

Engelhardt and associates (1973) conducted a double-blind study comparing the efficacy of fluphenazine and haloperidol in 30 outpatient autistic children (26 males and 4 females) ages 6 to 12 years. Following 1 to 2 weeks on placebo, active medication was titrated upward to a possible maximum of 16 mg/day. Maximum improvement was reached by 6 weeks and maintained thereafter. Evaluations after 12 weeks showed the following: The fluphenazine group (N = 15) had optimal doses of 12.5 mg/day and the haloperidol group (N = 15) of 11.9 mg/day. All children had some improvement on the CGI. Ninety-three percent (14) of children on fluphenazine and 87% (13) of children on haloperidol showed "much" or "very much" improvement. Nine items on the CPRS-1 showed significant improvement over baseline in both groups. They were psychomotor activity, stereotyped behavior, responsiveness, relations with adults and with children, frustration tolerance, concentration, eating habits, and sleeping. Untoward effects were mild and relatively infrequent. The most common were extrapyramidal symptoms, increased salivation and drowsiness.

LeVann (1969) in the study described above included among his 100 subjects 25 mentally retarded children and adolescents ages 7-22 years (mean 11.9) and 7 non-retarded children ages 9-11 years (mean 10.0) all of whom were diagnosed juvenile autism. Dose ranges for haloperidol, the areas of significant improvement, and untoward effects were as described in the section on schizophrenic disorder.

Four of the 10 patients treated by Simeon et al (1973) as described above were diagnosed as infantile autism. In these 4 children, the maximum daily dosage of thiothixene ranged from 15 to 60 mg (average 28.75 mg) and optimal dosage from 10 to 15 mg/day (average 13.0 mg/day). On Clinical Global Improvement ratings compared to baseline placebo, one child showed marked improvement, one moderate improvement, and 2 slight improvement. As the authors did not analyze the data by diagnostic category, the areas of improvement and untoward effects are as described in the section on schizophrenic disorder.

The possible therapeutic synergism between haloperidol and behavior therapy in reduction of behavioral symptoms and facilitation of language acquisition was examined in a descriptively homogeneous sample of 40 autistic children (ages 2.6 to 7.2 years) (Campbell et al, 1978a). All children were randomly assigned to one of four treatment groups. Half of this total sample received a response-contingent reinforcement for imitative speech; whereas, the other half received similar training but rewards delivered on a time (noncontingent-reinforcement) rather than a response-contingent basis. Also, half of the children received active medication and half placebo. The behavioral protocols were implemented after the optimal dosage was identified for each individual during a variable period of dosage regulation. The optimal dosage range in this study was 0.5 mg to 4.0 mg/day. Subdividing the children according to age (i.e., above and below the mean age of 4.5 years) revealed that the older group of children responded to optimal dosage of haloperidol with a reduction of withdrawal and stereotypies. The group of autistic children receiving the combination of haloperidol-contingent reinforcement treatment mastered the greatest number of words per total number of training sessions. In terms of a rank ordering, the performance of this group was superior to the group receiving placebo-contingent reinforcement followed by the haloperidol-noncontingent reinforcement group (Campbell et al, 1978a). A mechanism for the observed synergism considered by these authors was that reduction of stereotypies and withdrawal contributes to improved learning ability.

In addition to its synergistic interaction with behavior therapy to facilitate language acquisition, haloperidol (optimal dosage range 0.5 to 3.0 mg/day) was shown to improve discrimination learning performance in the laboratory in a study involving 33 autistic children (ages 2.3 to 7.9 years) (Campbell et al, 1982a). In the laboratory, there was no reduction in duration of stereotypic behaviors between haloperidol and placebo groups. These data suggest that improved discrimination learning performance on haloperidol might be due to its positive effect on attentional or other learning mechanisms rather than to its reduction of behaviors which interfere with learning (Campbell et al, 1982a). These data also emphasize the importance of ecological environment to the appearance or emergence of certain target behaviors. As in the earlier study (Campbell et al, 1978a), haloperidol caused a reduction of a variety of behavioral symptoms (including withdrawal, stereotypy, abnormal object relationships, fidgetiness and hyperactivity) when assessed in a playroom environment with a semistructured interview. Thus, the failure to detect a reduction in duration of stereotypic behaviors in the laboratory could be a function of this ecological environment.

The ability of haloperidol (0.5 to 3.0 mg/day) to decrease behavioral symptoms was extended to a different series of 40 autistic children (2.33 to 6.92 years) (Anderson et al, 1984). In this study, the children served as their own controls in an A-B-A design which permitted a comparison of treatment effects across groups and within groups. Global clinical improvement and significant reductions of withdrawal, stereotypies, abnormal object relationships, fidgetiness, hyperactivity, negativism, and angry and labile affect were obtained with haloperidol in this group of mildly to profoundly retarded autistic children. Therefore, the behavioral efficacy of low-dose haloperidol in this population appears to be established.

The interaction between haloperidol and Gesell language developmental quotients (DQ) on discrimination learning performance was examined in a subset of 32 of the above 40 children (Anderson et al, 1984). When children were classified according to high and low language DQ scores, the salutary effect of haloperidol on discrimination learning performance became more pronounced. Children with lower language DQ scores receiving haloperidol performed as well or better on a discrimination learning task than children with higher language DQ scores receiving placebo. The authors again noted that facilitation of learning by haloperidol in the laboratory was independent of a reduction of stereotypies or hyperactivity in the laboratory environment. They speculated that haloperidol may improve learning by a positive effect on attentional mechanisms (Anderson et al, 1984).

Long-Term Studies

As reviewed, on several short-term, controlled studies involving large samples of autistic children, therapeutic efficacy of haloperidol (0.5 to 4.0 mg/day) in the reduction of behavioral symptoms and facilitation of learning in the laboratory has been shown (Campbell et al, 1978a, 1982a; Anderson et al, 1984). These results prompted the design of a study to assess long-term efficacy of haloperidol and relationship of long-term drug administration to emergence or alterations of abnormal movements in these children (Campbell et al, 1983b). Autistic children are known to display a high incidence of abnormal movements (e.g., stereotypies, grimacing and mannerisms) independent of and prior to any drug administration (Campbell et al, 1983a, b). The difficulty in differentiating between re-emergence of pre-existing stereotypies and tardive or withdrawal dyskinesias following drug discontinuation in this population highlights the importance of a long-term study with baseline assessments (Campbell et al, 1983b). Thirty-six of 40 autistic children (ages 2 years 10 months to 7 years 10 months), who were felt to have benefited from short-term administration of optimal doses of haloperidol (0.5 to 3.0 mg/day) by professional staff and parents, were enrolled in this long-term (6-month to 2½-year follow-up), double-blind study. Children were randomly assigned to either 6 months of continuous daily administration of their optimal haloperidol dose or 6 months of receiving optimal doses of drug for 5 days of the week alternating with for 2 placebo days. After 6 months, both continuous and discontinuous medication groups entered a 4-week placebo phase prior to reentry into the cycle of 6 months of drug administration. Behavioral efficacy and abnormal movements were assessed at fixed intervals during each phase of the study with multiple independent raters. During 6 months of active drug administration, haloperidol remained effective in reducing behavioral symptoms. Furthermore, clinical and behavioral deterioration occurred 1 week after drug discontinuation as reflected in worsening of stereotypies, fidgetiness, hyperactivity, withdrawal and object relations and Clinical Global Impressions (CGI). To date, 6 of the 36 children (16.5%) have developed movements *de novo* and 2 children (5.6%) showed alteration in topography or intensity of pre-existing movements. Therefore, in this study, 22% of the sample showed a relationship of abnormal movements to long-term neuroleptic administration. These abnormal movements were reversible and ceased, at various times, in all 8 patients although in two of the patients, they ceased after haloperidol was reinstituted. This study showed that with adequate baseline assessments neuroleptic-induced dyskinesias can be distinguished from pre-existing abnormal movements.

Psychopharmacological Treatment of Infantile Autism
Neuroleptics

Neuroleptics appear to be the most useful pharmacological agents as a part of a comprehensive treatment program in decreasing or controlling some of the symptoms of autistic children. Although significant improvements are frequent, some autistic children improve only minimally. In our clinical experience, the hypoactive autistic child does not respond well to neuroleptics although there are exceptions.

Based on both the literature and our extensive clinical and research experience, we feel, at present, haloperidol is the drug of choice for autistic children. Principles of administration and untoward effects are identical to those described in administering neuroleptics to children with schizophrenic disorder. Dose ranges are as in Table I.

Fenfluramine

While preliminary findings using this anorexic agent with antiserotonergic properties have been very promising, this has been in a total of only 15 patients. Further critical assessment of efficacy and safety in larger numbers of autistic patients is necessary before treatment with fenfluramine can be generally recommended.

TABLE I. Representative Major Tranquilizers and Dosages in Children and Adolescents

Class of Neuroleptic	Generic Name	Trade Name	Usual Oral Dose Range in mg/day*	Minimum Age at Which Use is Recommended
Phenothiazines (a) aliphatic	chlorproma-zine	Thorazine	10-200 (2.0 mg/kg/day maximum for children up to age 12)	2 years
(b) piperidine	thioridazine	Mellaril	10-200 (3.0 mg/kg/day maximum for children up to age 12)	2 years
(c) piperazine	trifluoperazine	Stelazine	1-15	6 years
Butyrophenones	haloperidol	Haldol	0.5-16.0 (0.15 mg/kg/day maximum for children up to age 12)	3 years
Thioxanthenes	thiothixene	Navane	6-30	12 years
Dibenzoxazepines	loxapine	Loxitane	20-100	16 years
Dihydroindolones	molindone	Moban	1-40	12 years

*Severely disturbed psychotic children and adolescents may require higher doses.

CONCLUSION

Major Affective Disorders (Major Depressive Disorder and Bipolar Disorder) with psychotic features and Schizophrenic Disorder are rare in childhood and uncommon in early adolescence. Consequently these conditions have been studied much more frequently in older adolescents and adults. On the other hand, Infantile Autism, another rare condition, which manifests itself in earliest childhood, has been much better studied in young children than has its progression into adolescence and adulthood. Only in the past 5 to 10 years has major progress been made in careful diagnosis and have well designed studies been conducted to elucidate these children's and adolescents' responses to psychopharmacological agents. These data have been summarized and evaluated critically. Further precision in diagnosis and larger clinical samples will be necessary before more definitive statements can be made.

REFERENCES

Akiskal, H.S., Rosenthal, R.H., Rosenthal, T.L., Kashgarian, M., Khani, M.K. and Puzantian, V.R.: Differentiation of primary affective illness from situational, symptomatic, and secondary depressions, *Arch. Gen. Psychiat.* 36:635-643, 1979.

Anderson, L.T., Campbell, M., Grega, D.M., Perry, R., Small, A.M. and Green, W.H.: Haloperidol in infantile autism: Effects on learning and behavioral symptoms, *Am. J. Psychiat.* 141(10):1195-1202, 1984.

Anthony, J. and Scott, P.: Manic-depressive psychosis in childhood, *J. Child Psychol. Psychiat.* 1:53-72, 1960.

Baron, M., Risch, N. and Mendlewicz, J.: Age at onset in bipolar-related major affective illness: clinical and genetic implications, *J. Psychiat. Res.* 17(1):5-18, 1983.

Bender, L., Faretra, G. and Cobrinik, L.: LSD and UML treatment of hospitalized disturbed children in Recent Advances in Biological Psychiatry Vol. 5 (J. Wortis, ed.), Plenum Press, New York, pp. 84-92, 1963.

Berg, I., Hullin, R., Allsopp, M., O'Brien, P. and MacDonald, R.: Bipolar manic-depressive psychosis in early adolescence, a case report, *Br. J. Psychiat.* 125:416-417, 1974.

Bowden, C.L. and Sarabia, F.: Diagnosing manic-depressive illness in adolescents, *Comprehensive Psychiatry* 21(4):263-269, 1980.

Campbell, M. and Green, W.H.: Pervasive developmental disorders of childhood. In: Comprehensive Textbook of Psychiatry IV, fourth edition, (H.I. Kaplan and B.J. Sadock, eds.), William & Wilkins, Baltimore, Md., 1672-1683, 1985.

Campbell, M., Fish, B., Shapiro, T. and Floyd, A., Jr.: Imipramine in preschool autistic and schizophrenic children, *J. Aut. Child. Schizo.* 1:267-282, 1971.

Campbell, M., Fish, B., David, R., Shapiro, T., Collins, P. and Koh, C.: Response to triiodothyronine and dextroamphetamine: A study of preschool schizophrenic children, *J. Aut. Child. Schizo.* 2:343-358, 1972a.

Campbell, M., Fish, B., Korein, J., Shapiro, T., Collins, P. and Koh, C.: Lithium and chlorpromazine: A controlled cross-over study of hyperactive severely disturbed young children, *J. Aut. Child. Schizo.* 2:234-263, 1972b.

Campbell, M., Fish, B., David, R., Shapiro, T., Collins, P. and Koh, C.: Liothyronine

treatment in psychotic and nonpsychotic children under 6 years, *Arch. Gen. Psychiat.* 29:602-608, 1973.

Campbell, M., Friedman, E., DeVito, E., Greenspan, L. and Collins, P.J.: Blood serotonin in psychotic and brain damaged children, *J. Aut. Child. Schizo.* 4:33-41, 1974.

Campbell, M., Friedman, E., Green, W.H., Collins, P.J., Small, A.M. and Breuer, H.: Blood serotonin in schizophrenic children: A preliminary study, *Int. Pharmacopsychiat.* 10:213-221, 1975.

Campbell, M., Friedman, E., Green, W.H., Small, A.M. and Burdock, E.I.: Blood platelet monoamine oxidase activity in schizophrenic children and their families: A preliminary study, *Neuropsychobiology* 2:239-246, 1976a.

Campbell, M., Small, A.M., Collins, P.J., Friedman, E., David, R. and Genieser, N.B.: Levodopa and levoamphetamine: A crossover study in schizophrenic children, *Curr. Ther. Res.* 18:70-86, 1976b.

Campbell, M., Geller, B., and Cohen, I.L.: Current status of drug research and treatment with autistic children, *J. Pediat. Psych.* 2:153-161, 1977.

Campbell, M., Anderson, L.T., Meier, M., Cohen, I.L., Small, A.M., Samit, C. and Sachar, E.J.: A comparison of haloperidol and behavior therapy and their interaction in autistic children, *J. Amer. Acad. Child Psychiat.* 17:640-655, 1978a.

Campbell, M., Hollander, C.S., Ferris, S. and Greene, L.W.: Response to TRH stimulation in young psychotic children: A pilot study, *Psychoneuroendocrinology* 3:195-201, 1978b.

Campbell, M., Small, A.M., Hollander, C.S., Korein, J., Cohen, I.L., Kalmijn, M. and Ferris, S.A.: A controlled crossover study of triiodothyronine in young psychotic children, *J. Aut. Child. Schizo.* 8:371-381, 1978c.

Campbell, M., Cohen, I.L. and Anderson, L.T.: Pharmacotherapy for autistic children: A summary of research, *Can. J. Psychiat.* 26:265-273, 1981.

Campbell, M., Anderson, L.T., Small, A.M., Perry, R., Green, W.H. and Caplan, R.: The effects of haloperidol on learning and behavior in autistic children, *J. Aut. Devel. Disorders* 12:167-175, 1982a.

Campbell, M., Rosenbloom, S., Perry, R., George, A.E., Kricheff, I.I., Anderson, L., Small, A.M. and Jennings, S.J.: Computerized axial tomography in young autistic children. *Am. J. Psychiat.* 139:510-512, 1982b.

Campbell, M., Grega, D.M., Green, W.II. and Bennett, W.G.: Neuroleptic-induced dyskinesias in children, *Clin. Neuropharm.* 6:207-222, 1983a.

Campbell, M., Perry, R., Bennett, W.G., Small, A.M., Green, W.H., Grega, D., Schwartz, V. and Anderson, L.: Long-term therapeutic efficacy and drug-related abnormal movements: A prospective study of haloperidol in autistic children, *Psychopharm. Bull.* 19(1):80-83, 1983b.

Campbell, M., Perry, R. and Green, W.H.: The use of lithium in children and adolescents, *Psychosomatics* 25(2):95-106, 1984a.

Campbell, M., Small, A.M., Green, W.H., Jennings, S.J., Perry, R., Bennett, W.G. and Anderson, L.: A comparison of haloperidol and lithium in hospitalized aggressive conduct disorder children, *Arch. Gen. Psychiat.* 41:650-656, 1984b.

Carlson, G.A.: Lithium carbonate use in adolescents: Clinical indications and management in Adolescent Psychiatry Vol. VII (S.C. Feinstein and P.L. Giovacchini, eds.) The University of Chicago Press, Chicago, pp. 410-418, 1979.

Carlson, G.A. and Strober, M.: Manic-depressive illness in early adolescence, *J. Amer. Acad. Child Psychiat.* 17:138-153, 1978.

Carroll, B.J., Feinberg, M., Greden, J.F., Tarika, J., Albala, A.A., Haskett, R.F., James, N.M., Kronfol, Z., Lohr, N., Steiner, M., DeVigne, J.P. and Young, E.: A specific laboratory test for the diagnosis of melancholia: Standardization, validation, and clinical utility, *Arch. Gen. Psychiat.* 38:15-22, 1981.

Chambers, W.J., Puig-Antich, J., Tabrizi, M.A. and Davies, M.: Psychotic symptoms in prepubertal major depressive disorder, *Arch. Gen. Psychiat.* 39:921-927, 1982.

Cohen, D.J., Caparulo, B.K., Shaywitz, B.A. and Bowers, M.B., Jr.: Dopamine and serotonin metabolism in neuropsychiatrically disturbed children: CSF homovanillic acid and 5-hydroxyindoleacetic acid, *Arch. Gen. Psychiat.* 34:545-550, 1977.

Coleman, M., Campbell, M., Freedman, L.S., Roffman, M., Ebstein, R.P. and Goldstein, M.: Serum dopamine-β-hydroxylase levels in Down's syndrome, *Clin. Genetics* 5:312-315, 1974.

Creak, M. (Chairman): Schizophrenic syndrome in childhood, *Developm. Med. Child. Neurol.* 3:501-504, 1961.

Cytryn, L., McKnew, D.H., Jr., Logue, M. and Desai, R.B.: Biochemical correlates of affective disorders in children, *Arch. Gen. Psychiat.* 31:659-661, 1974.

Deutsch, S.I. and Davis, K.L.: Schizophrenia: A review of diagnostic and biological issues. II. Biological issues, *Hosp. Comm. Psychiat.* 34:423-437, 1983.

Diagnostic and Statistical Manual (DSM), Mental Disorders. American Psychiatric Association Mental Hospital Service, Washington, D.C., 1952.

Diagnostic and Statistical Manual of Mental Disorders, Second Edition (DSM-II), American Psychiatric Association, Washington, D.C., 1968.

Diagnostic and Statistical Manual of Mental Disorders, Third Edition (DSM-III), American Psychiatric Association, Washington, D.C., 1980.

Endicott, J. and Spitzer, R.L.: A diagnostic interview: The schedule for affective disorders and schizophrenia, *Arch. Gen. Psychiat.* 35:837-844, 1978.

Engelhardt, D.M., Polizos, P., Waizer, J. and Hoffman, S.P.: A double-blind comparison of fluphenazine and haloperidol in outpatient schizophrenic children, *J. Aut. Child Schizo.* 3:128-137, 1973.

Faretra, G., Dooher, L. and Dowling, J.: Comparison of haloperidol and fluphenazine in disturbed children, *Amer. J. Psychiat.* 126:1670-1673, 1970.

Feighner, J.P., Robins, E., Guze, S.B., Woodruff, R.A. and Winokur, G., Diagnostic criteria for use in psychiatric research, *Arch. Gen. Psychiat.* 26:56-63, 1972.

Fish, B., Campbell, M., Shapiro, T. and Floyd, A., Jr.: Schizophrenic children treated with methysergide (Sansert), *Dis. Nerv. Syst.* 30:534-540, 1969.

Geller, E., Ritvo, E.R., Freeman, B.J. and Yuwiler, A.: Preliminary observations on the effect of fenfluramine on blood serotonin and symptoms in three autistic boys, *New Eng. J. Med.* 307:165-169, 1982.

Gil-Ad, I., Dickerman, Z., Weizman, R., Weizman, A., Tyano, S. and Laron, Z.: Abnormal growth hormone response to LRH and TRH in adolescent schizophrenic boys, *Amer. J. Psychiat.* 138:357-360, 1981.

Greden, J.F., Gardner, R., King, D., Grunhaus, L., Carroll, B.J. and Kronfol, Z.: Dexamethasone suppression tests in antidepressant treatment of melancholia. The process of normalization and testretest reproducibility, *Arch. Gen. Psychiat.* 40:493-500, 1983.

Green, W.H., Campbell, M., Hardesty, A.S., Grega, D.M., Padron-Gayol, M., Shell, J. and Erlenmeyer-Kimling, L.: A comparison of schizophrenic and autistic children, *J. Amer. Acad. Child Psychiat.* 23(4):399-409, 1984.

Hayes, T.A., Logan Panitch, M. and Barker, E.: Imipramine dosage in children: A comment on Imipramine and electrocardiographic abnormalities in hyperactive children, *Amer. J. Psychiat.*, 132:546-547, 1975.

Horowitz, H.A.: Lithium and the treatment of adolescent manic-depressive illness, *Dis. Nerv. Syst.* 38:480-483, 1977.

Hsu, L.K.G., Molcan, K., Cashman, M.A., Lee, S., Lohr, J. and Hindmarsh, D.: The dexamethasone suppression test in adolescent depression, *J. Amer. Acad. Child Psychiat.* 22:470-473, 1983.

Kallen, B. and Tandberg, A.: Lithium and pregnancy, *Acta Psychiatrica Scandinavica* 68(1):134-139, 1983.

Kelly, J.T., Koch, M. and Buegel, D.: Lithium carbonate in juvenile manic-depressive illness, *Dis. Nerv. Syst.* 37:90-92, 1976.

Kolvin, I.: Psychoses in childhood—a comparative study in Infantile Autism: Concepts, Characteristics and Treatment (M.

Rutter, ed.), Churchill Livingstone, Edinburgh, pp. 7-26, 1971.

LeVann, L.J.: Haloperidol in the treatment of behavioral disorders in children and adolescents, *Can. Psychiat. Assn. J.* 14:217-220, 1969.

Maher, K.R., Harper, J.F., Macleay, A. and King, M.G.: Peculiarities in the endocrine response to insulin stress in early infantile autism, *J. Nerv. Ment. Dis.* 161:180-184, 1975.

McKnew, D.H., Jr., and Cytryn, L.: Urinary metabolites in chronically depressed children, *J. Amer. Acad. Child Psychiat.* 18:608-615, 1979.

McKnew, D.H., Cytryn, L., Buchsbaum, M.S., Hamovit, J., Lamour, M., Rapoport, J.L., and Gershon, E.S.: Lithium in children of lithium-responding parents, *Psychiat. Res.* 4:174-180, 1981.

Meyers, B., Tune, L.E. and Coyle, J.T.: Clinical response and serum neuroleptic levels in childhood schizophrenia, *Amer. J. Psychiat.* 137:483-484, 1980.

Pallmeyer, T. and Petti, T.A.: Aggression as a side effect in the treatment of depressed children with imipramine, *Amer. J. Psychiat.* 136:1472, 1979.

Perry, R., Campbell, M., Grega, D.M. and Anderson, L.: Saliva lithium levels in children: Their use in monitoring serum lithium levels and lithium side effects, *J. Clin. Psychopharm.* 4(4):199-202, 1984.

Petti, T.A. and Wells, K.: Crisis treatment of a preadolescent who accidentally killed his twin, *Amer. J. Psychother.* 34 (3):434-443, 1980.

Physicians' Desk Reference (PDR) 38th Edition, Medical Economics Co., Oradell, N.J., 1984.

Pool, D., Bloom, W., Mielke, D.H., Roniger, J.J. and Gallant, D.M.: A controlled evaluation of loxitane in seventy-five adolescent schizophrenic patients, *Curr. Ther. Res.* 19(1):99-104, 1976.

Pope, H.G. and Lipinski, J.F.: Diagnosis in schizophrenia and manic-depressive illness, *Arch. Gen. Psychiat.* 35:811-828, 1978.

Poznanski, E.O., Carroll, B.J., Banegas, M.C., Cook, S.C. and Grossman, J.A.: The dexamethasone suppression test in prepubertal depressed children, *Amer. J. Psychiat.* 139:321-324, 1982.

Preskorn, S.H., Weller, E.B., Weller, R.A. and Glotzbach, E.: Plasma levels of imipramine and adverse effects in children, *Amer. J. Psychiat.* 140:1332-1335, 1983.

Puig-Antich, J.: Psychopharmacology update in childhood disorders (Course 32) presented at the 136th Annual Meeting of the American Psychiatric Association, April 30-May 6, 1983, New York, NY., 1983.

Puig-Antich, J., Blau, S., Marx, N., Greenhill, L.L. and Chambers, W.: Prepubertal major depressive disorder, *J. Amer. Acad. Child Psychiat.* 17:695-707, 1978.

Puig-Antich, J., Chambers, W., Halpern, F., Hanlon, C. and Sachar, E.J.: Cortisol hypersecretion in prepubertal depressive illness: A preliminary report, *Psychoneuroendocrinology* 4:191-197, 1979a.

Puig-Antich, J., Perel, J.M., Lupatkin, W., Chambers, W.J., Shea, C., Tabrizi, M.A. and Stiller, R.L.: Plasma levels of imipramine (IMI) and desmethylimipramine (DMI) and clinical response in prepubertal major depressive disorder: A preliminary report, *J. Amer. Acad. Child Psychiat.* 18:616-627, 1979b.

Puig-Antich, J., Tabrizi, M.A., Davies, M., Goetz, R., Chambers, W.J., Halpern, F. and Sachar, E.J.: Prepubertal endogenous major depressives hyposecrete growth hormone in response to insulin-induced hypoglycemia, *Biological Psychiat.* 16(9):801-818, 1981.

Puig-Antich, J., Goetz, R., Davies, M., Fein, M., Hanlon, C., Chambers, W.J., Tabrizi, M.A., Sachar, E.J. and Weitzman, E.D.: Growth hormone secretion in prepubertal major depressive children: II. Sleep related plasma concentrations during a depressive episode, *Arch. Gen. Psychiat.* 41:463-466, 1984a.

Puig-Antich, J., Goetz, R., Davies, M., Tabrizi, M.A., Novacenko, H., Hanlon, C., Sachar, E.J. and Weitzman, E.D.: Growth hormone secretion in prepubertal major depressive children: IV. Sleep related plasma concentrations in a drug-free fully recovered clinical state, *Arch. Gen. Psychiat.* 41:479-483, 1984b.

Puig-Antich, J., Novacenko, H., Davies, M., Tabrizi, M.A., Ambrosini, P., Goetz, R., Bianca, J., Goetz, D. and Sachar, E.J.: Growth hormone secretion in prepubertal major depressive children: III. Response to insulin-induced hypoglycemia after recovery from a depressive episode in a drug-free state, *Arch. Gen. Psychiat.* 41:471-475, 1984c.

Puig-Antich, J., Perel, J., Lupatkin, W., Chambers, W.J., Tabrizi, M.A., King, J., Davies, M. and Stiller, R.: Imipramine effectiveness in prepubertal major depressive disorders: I. Relationship of plasma levels to clinical response of the depressive syndrome. *Arch. Gen. Psychiat.* In press.

Redmond, D.E., Jr. and Huang, Y.H.: New evidence for a locus coeruleus-norepinephrine connection with anxiety, *Life Sciences* 25:2149-2162, 1979.

Rieder, R.O., Mann, L.S., Weinberger, D.R., van Kammen, D.P. and Post, R.M.: Computed tomographic scans in patients with schizophrenia, schizoaffective, and bipolar affective disorder, *Arch. Gen. Psychiat.* 40:735-739, 1983.

Ritvo, E.R., Yuwiler, A., Geller, E., Kales, A., Rashkis, S., Schicor, A., Plotkin, S., Axelrod, R. and Howard, C.: Effects of L-dopa on autism, *J. Aut. Child Schizo.* 1:190-205, 1971.

Ritvo, E.R., Freeman, B.J., Geller, E. and Yuwiler, A.: Effect of fenfluramine in 15 autistic patients, New research (NR90) presented at the 136th Annual Meeting of the American Psychiatric Association, April 30-May 6, 1983, New York, NY., 1983.

Rivera-Calimlim, L., Nasrallah, H., Strauss, J. and Lasagna, L.: Clinical response and plasma levels: Effect of dose, dosage schedules, and drug interactions on plasma chlorpromazine levels, *Amer. J. Psychiat.* 133:646-652, 1976.

Robbins, D.R., Alessi, N.E., Yanchyshyn, G.W. and Colfer, M.V.: The dexamethasone suppression test in psychiatrically hospitalized adolescents, *J. Amer. Acad. Child Psychiat.* 22:467-469, 1983.

Rogeness, G.A. and Macedo, C.A.: Therapeutic response of a schizophrenic boy to a methylphenidate-chlorpromazine combination, *Amer. J. Psychiat.* 140:932-933, 1983.

Rosenbloom, S., Campbell, M., George, A.E., Kricheff, I.I., Taleporos, E., Anderson, L., Reuben, R.N. and Korein, J.: High resolution CT scanning in infantile autism: A quantitative approach. *J. Amer. Acad. Child Psychiat.* 23(1):72-77, 1984.

Rutter, M.: Psychotic disorders in early childhood. In: Recent Developments in Schizophrenia (A. Coppen and A. Walk, eds.), *Brit. J. Psychiat.* Special Publication No. 1 Royal Medico-Psychological Association, Headly Brothers, Ltd., Ashford, Kent, pp. 133-158, 1967.

Saraf, K.R., Klein, D.F. and Gittelman-Klein, R.: Imipramine side effects in children, *Psychopharmacologia* (Berlin) 37:265-274, 1974.

Simeon, J., Saletu, B., Saletu, M., Itil, T.M. and DaSilva, J.: Thiothixene in childhood psychoses. Paper presented at the Third International Symposium on Phenothiazines, June 25-28, 1973, Rockville, Md.

Spitzer, R.L., Endicott, J. and Robbins, E.: Research diagnostic criteria: Rationale and reliability, *Arch. Gen. Psychiat.* 35:773-782, 1978.

Sternberg, D.E., van Kammen, D.P., Lerner, P., Ballenger, J.C., Marder, S.R., Post, R.M. and Bunney, W.E., Jr.: CSF dopamine-β-hydroxylase in schizophrenia. Low activity associated with good prognosis and good response to neuroleptic treatment, *Arch. Gen. Psychiat.* 40:743-747, 1983.

Strober, M. and Carlson, G.: Bipolar illness in adolescents with major depression, *Arch. Gen. Psychiat.* 39:549-555, 1982.

Träskman, L., Äsberg, M., Bertilsson, L. and Sjöstrand, L.: Monoamine metabolites in CSF and suicidal behavior, *Arch. Gen. Psychiat.* 38:631-636, 1981.

Waizer, J., Polizos, P., Hoffman, S.P., Engelhardt, D.M. and Margolis, R.A.: A single-blind evaluation of thiothixene with outpatient schizophrenic children, *J. Aut. Child Schizo.* 2:378-386, 1972.

Weizman, R., Weizman, A., Gil-Ad, I., Tyano, S. and Laron, Z.: Abnormal growth hormone responses to TRH in chronic adolescent schizophrenic patients, *Brit. J. Psychiat.* 141:582-585, 1982.

White, J.H. and O'Shanick, G.: Juvenile manic-depressive illness, *Amer. J. Psychiat.* 134:1035-1036, 1977.

Winokur, G., Behar, D., van Valkenburg, C. and Lowry, M.: Is a familial definition of depression both feasible and valid, *J. Nerv. Ment. Dis.* 166:764-767, 1978.

Wolpert, A., Hagamen, M.B. and Merlis, S.: A comparative study of thiothixene and trifluoperazine in childhood schizophrenia, *Curr. Ther. Res.* 9:482-485, 1967.

Yamazaki, K., Saito, Y., Okada, F., Fujieda, T. and Yamashita, I.: An application of neuroendocrinological studies in autistic children and Heller's syndrome, *J. Aut. Child. Schizo.* 5:323-332, 1975.

Young, J.G., Kavanagh, M.E., Anderson, G.M., Shaywitz, B.A. and Cohen, D.J.: Clinical neurochemistry of autism and associated disorders, *J. Aut. Developm. Dis.* 12:147-165, 1982.

CHAPTER 11

Vasopressin Effects on Learning in 6-OH Dopamine Treated Rats and Minimal Brain Dysfunction Children

Robert H. Belmaker
Rahel Hamburger-Bar
Jacques Eisenberg
Shella Chazan
Yehuda Shapira
Lawrence Greenberg
Elsa Shapiro
Batsheva Mandel

SUMMARY

The cognitive deficits of attention deficit disorder in childhood are poorly responsive to presently available medication. Vasopressin derivatives have been reported to enhance learning and memory in animals and in normal humans, in controlled studies. We studied vasopressin effects on learning in rats treated at day 5 of life with intracisternal 6-OH dopamine. Such dopamine-depleted rats have lasting cognitive deficits and have been proposed as an animal model of human attention deficit disorder. In an automated shuttle box design, vasopressin significantly ameliorated the learning deficits of such rats. Moreover, caudate vasopressin levels correlated significantly with performance in the shuttle box learning, both in 6-OH dopamine pretreated rats and in controls. Vasopressin treatment three times weekly for 6 weeks appeared to be more effective in enhancing learning and retarding extinction than vasopressin treatment only at the beginning of learning and the beginning of extinction. In 17 children with attention and learning disorders, postulated to result from central dopamine deficiency, vasopressin derivative was given daily for 10 days and compared with 10 days of placebo treatment in a randomized crossover double-blind design. Story memory plus position learning were significantly improved by vasopressin derivative compared to placebo. In 15 other children with attention and learning disorders, a single dose of vasopressin derivative was compared with placebo in a double-blind, randomized crossover design. No benefit was found. These parallel animal and human studies suggest that chronic but not acute vasopressin treatment may benefit childhood learning disorders. Such benefit is not dependent on intact brain dopaminergic mechanisms but may work independently in a manner that can complement current inadequate treatments with drugs such as methylphenidate.

Minimal brain dysfunction (MBD) (Wender, 1971) or, in more recent terminology, attention deficit disorder (ADD) (American Psychiatric Association DSM III, 1980), is a common behavioral disorder of childhood. Methylphenidate is an effective and widespread treatment of hyperactivity in human ADD (Barkley, 1977). The usefulness of methylphenidate in ADD is most marked on the symptoms of overactivity and attention (Rapoport and Zametkin, 1980). Learning disorders in ADD are much less markedly affected by methylphenidate (Riddle and Rapoport, 1976) and methylphenidate is not usually used in cognitive deficits of ADD individuals beyond childhood. New treatments for the cognitive deficits are critically needed.

Vasopressin and its derivatives have been reported to improve learning and memory in various animal models (Rigter and Crabbe, 1979). Conditioned avoidance in a shuttle box (Bohus et al., 1973), in a pole jumping paradigm (De Wied, 1971), a sexually-rewarded T-maze task (Bohus, 1977), and a food-rewarded task (Hostetter et al., 1977) have all been reported to be improved when preceded by administration of vasopressin or its derivatives. A single injection of vasopressin has been reported to retard extinction of learning in rats for several weeks (De Wied and Bohus, 1979). The effect of vasopressin derivatives on rat models of MBD or in children with learning and attention disorders has not previously been studied. This paper summarizes a parallel series of studies of a vasopressin derivative in a rat model of MBD and in children with cognitive deficits of MBD. DDAVP (1-desamino-8-D-arginine vasopressin) was chosen as it is already available and known to be safe for use in children with diabetes insipidus (Becker and Foley, 1978) or enuresis nocturna (Birkasova et al., 1978) and because it is the only vasopressin derivative reported to improve memory and learning in normal humans in a double-blind controlled design (Weingartner et al., 1981).

ANIMAL STUDIES

A rat model of ADD was first described by Shaywitz et al. (1976) and has been replicated in our laboratory (Hamburger-Bar et al., 1983). The animal model, produced by 6-OH dopamine (6-OH DA) injection at day 5 of life intracisternally (i.c.) after pretreatment i.p. with imipramine, shares key characteristics with the human disorder: 1) 6-OH DA treated pups are hyperactive between 15-23 days of age but later this activity declines to control levels, much as ADD humans with hyperactivity are overactive in childhood, but lose this aspect of the disorder in adolescence (Cantwell, 1975); 2) 6-OH DA treated pups show learning disorders which persist beyond 23 days of age, much as children with ADD usually have cognitive deficits that persist beyond childhood; and 3) hyperactivity in 6-OH DA treated pups is reversible with methylphenidate (Shaywitz et al., 1976).

In our studies male rat pups 5 days old were injected i.p. with imipramine (300 µg/rat in 25 µl) followed after one hour by i.c. 6-OH DA (100 µg/rat in 25 µl of 0.4% ascorbic acid in sterile saline) or with vehicle only.

The data of Fig. 1 and Fig. 2 confirm the reports of Shaywitz et al. (1976) that rat pups treated i.c. with 6-OH DA at day 5 of life are hyperactive between 15-23 days of life. Shaywitz et al. (1976) reported on learning deficits at age 27 days of life in these rats; we reported that such deficits remain at 2 months of age and are still present at 4 months of age (Hamburger-Bar et al., 1983). Such data are consistent with human reports of cognitive deficits in adult MBD (Wender, 1971).

DDAVP at doses of 10 µ/rat does not affect activity behavior (Fig. 1). This finding suggests that increased alertness, vigilance or motor agility is not a likely explanation of DDAVP effects on learning behavior. Such data clearly distinguishes DDAVP from stimulants such as methylphenidate, and encourages the possibility that DDAVP will work via different mechanisms and, hence, synergize with methylphenidate in the treatment of human ADD.

Kovacs et al. (1979) suggested that vasopressin effects on animal learning are mediated via catecholamines and dependent on intact catecholaminergic pathways. Shaywitz et al. (1978) have suggested that childhood MBD may involve a deficiency of brain DA. It, therefore, seemed important to study the interactions of catecholamines and vasopressin effects on learning. It is, of course, not possible to easily extrapolate effects in MBD model rats to children with MBD, but a finding that 6-OH DA treated rats are resistant to ameliorative effects of vasopressin on learning might dampen enthusiasm for a human trial of vasopressin in MBD. We, therefore, decided to study the effect of DDAVP on learning in 6-OH DA pretreated rats. The study was divided into two parts. In the first part, we studied the effect of lysine vasopressin (LVP)

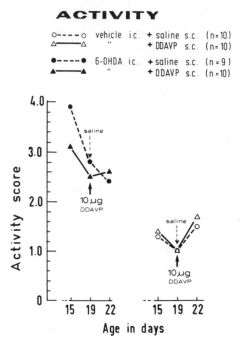

FIG. 11-1. The effect of a single high dose injection of DDAVP on activity of rats pretreated at day 5 of life with 6-OH DA or saline i.c.

All behavioral tests were performed in the second half of the dark period of the dark-light cycle (dark from 05.00 till 17.00). Activity was studied between two and three weeks of age. Each pup was placed in a plastic cage placed on the floor. Recording of activity began after 20 minutes of habituation and lasted for 30 minutes. Each minute the cages were scanned. Activity score was rated as follows: Walking or running about the cage received a rating of 5, climbing or rearing received a rating of 3, a rating of 1 was given to sniffing, grooming or scratching and a rating of 0 for standing or sitting motionless. The mean of 30 ratings per rat over 30 minutes was used for data analyses. DDAVP was administered s.c. one hour before the tests.

and of DDAVP on learning of 6-OH DA treated rats in a conditioned avoidance paradigm. In the second part of the study, levels of vasopressin in different brain areas were measured in 6-OH DA or control animals that were treated with DDAVP or saline and tested for active avoidance performance, one month before their sacrifice.

Figure 3 illustrates the learning curves in 6-OH DA treated rats treated later with saline, DDAVP or LVP and studied repeatedly in the automated two-way shuttle box. LVP-treated animals show significantly enhanced learning on the first, second, and fourth day of training and significantly less extinction on day 7. DDAVP-treated animals show similar improvement in both acquisition and extinction.

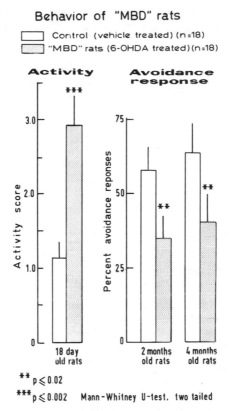

FIG. 11-2. Activity and shuttle box avoidance learning in rats pretreated with 6-OH DA at day 5 of life.

Learning was tested in a two-way shuttle box (Columbus "Reflex 6" instrument) at the age of 2 and 4 months of life. After adaptation of 5 minutes in the shuttle box a sound as conditioned stimulus (CS) was presented for maximally 10 seconds, followed by the CS with an electric shock of 0.5 mA through the grid floor to the rat's feet for a maximum of another 10 seconds. There was then an intertrial interval of 30-50 seconds. A session consisted of 15 trials. CAR was recorded if the rat crossed from one side of the box to the other within 10 seconds after the CS was presented.

A parallel group of rats was studied after treatment i.c. with vehicle rather than 6-OH DA on the fifth day of life. As expected, such normal animals performed significantly better with saline treatment than 6-OH DA treated animals with saline treatment on day 1 of testing (%CAR $\bar{x}$ = 24 vs. $\bar{x}$ = 12, p < .005 Mann Whitney U). LVP significantly enhanced learning in these normal rats on day 4 and retarded extinction as expected from the reports of De Wied (1971). The effects of LVP and DDAVP in these normal animals were less than in 6-OH DA pretreated

CONDITIONED AVOIDANCE OF 6-OHDA TREATED MALE RATS ONE HOUR AFTER S.C. ADMINISTRATION OF:

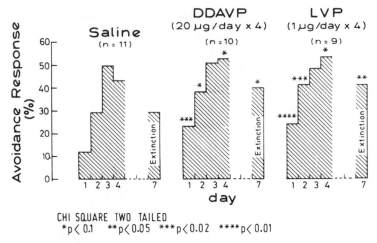

CHI SQUARE TWO TAILED
*p< 0.1   **p< 0.05   ***p< 0.02   ****p< 0.01

FIG. 11-3 The effect of vasopression derivatives on conditioned avoidance of 6-OH DA treated rats.

Learning was tested in a two-way shuttle box (Columbus "Reflex-6" instrument) at the age of 2 months of life. After adaptation of 5 minutes in the shuttle box a sound as conditioned stimulus (CS) was presented for maximally 10 seconds, followed by the CS with an electric shock of 0.5 mA through the grid floor to the rat's feet for a maximum of another 10 seconds. There was then an intertrial interval of 50-70 seconds. A session consisted of 15 trials. DDAVP (20 μ/rat), LVP (1 μ/rat) or saline were administered s.c. (0.5 ml/rat) one hour before each learning session. Doses were chosen based on the approximately 20:1 ratio for behavioral activity of DDAVP and LVP reported by Walter et al. (1978). Treatments were given for 4 consecutive days on days 1, 2, 3 and 4 of testing in the shuttle box. Extinction was studied 3 days after the last treatment (day 7). CAR was recorded if the rat crossed from one side of the box to the other within 10 seconds after the CS was presented.

animals (Fig. 3) although these differences did not reach statistical significance. Thus 6-OH DA pretreatment does not prevent the effect of vasopressin to improve learning but, if anything, perhaps enhances it. Such results encourage the possibility that vasopressin may enhance learning in MBD children with a postulated DA deficiency (Shaywitz et al., 1978).

We have reported (Hamburger-Bar et al., in press (b)) the vasopressin levels in various brain areas of these rats treated and studied for four days in shuttle box learning as described above and sacrificed one month later. In general, vasopressin levels found in the various regions in this study are similar to levels reported by other groups (Kasting and Martin,

1983). 6-OH DA treatment does not change vasopressin levels in any brain area studied except pituitary. DDAVP treatment does not change vasopressin levels in any brain area except pituitary. 6-OH DA treatment significantly reduces pituitary vasopressin content and DDAVP treatment significantly enhances pituitary vasopressin content in animals whose pituitary vasopressin is reduced by 6-OH DA pretreatment. Most importantly, caudate vasopressin levels correlated significantly with conditioned avoidance response learning averaged over four daily sessions (Fig. 4). Correlations for each individual day of learning revealed no pattern for caudate vasopressin to correlate specifically with early or late learning. Moreover, the correlation of caudate vasopressin levels is present in control rats ($r = .69$, $N = 8$), 6-OH DA treated rats ($r = .64$, $N = 8$) and 6-OH DA plus DDAVP treated rats ($r = .60$, $N = 9$). Since no significant mean differences in caudate vasopressin levels are present in these three groups, they were pooled; and a correlation of .59 ($N = 25$) between conditioned avoidance response and caudate vasopressin was found. In pituitary, hypothalamus and hippocampus correlations of vasopressin levels with learning behavior were not significant ($r = .20$, $N = 25$ for hypothamalus, and $r = .08$, $N = 23$ for hippocampus. The latter negative finding, surprising in view of the importance of the hippocampus for memory, is illustrated in Fig. 5.

Thus, injection of 6-OH DA on the fifth day of life leads to a persistent learning deficit and persistent reduction in brain DA levels. However, the results are that such DA-depleted animals are at least as sensitive to the learning ameliorative effects of vasopressin derivatives as are control animals. This suggests that DA, at least in the caudate, is not an obligatory mediator of vasopressin effects. Conversely, these DA-depleted animals have clear learning deficits despite normal caudate vasopressin levels. This suggests that the mechanism of the learning deficit in 6-OH DA treated animals is not mediated via a reduction in vasopressin. Such results imply that, as in many biological systems, there are several independent pathways through which learning can be affected, positively or negatively. The marked correlation of caudate vasopressin levels with performance in the shuttle box is present both in animals with high or low caudate DA and with resultant high or low mean performance levels in the shuttle box. The persistence of this correlation despite manipulations of the DA system is further evidence of the independence of DA effects and vasopressin effects on learning. The significant reduction in pituitary vasopressin content after 6-OH DA treatment may be due to dopaminergic control of posterior pituitary vasopressin-containing neurons (Kimura et al., 1981).

Correlation of caudate vasopressin levels with learning ability in the shuttle box is especially impressive in view of its specificity to the caudate. No other brain region showed a similar consistent trend. Hippo-

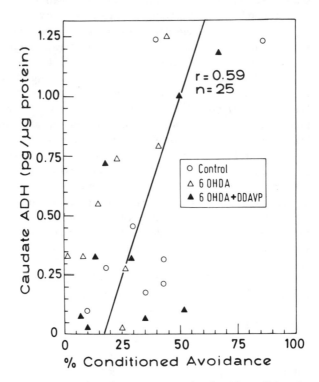

FIG. 11-4. Correlation of caudate vasopressin levels with conditioned avoidance performance. Animals as in Fig. 3, sacrificed one month after learning experiments.

Individual pituitaries are homogenized in 2.0 ml of a 0.1 n HCl solution in a glass teflon homogenizer. The homogenate is then transferred to plastic mini-vials and homogenized with a polytron homogenizer (setting number 5) for 5 seconds. A similar procedure is followed for individual caudate nuclei, hippocampi and hypothalami. After homogenization the samples are centrifuged at 1500 x g for 20 minutes. A sample is then taken for protein analysis using the method of Lowry.

The acidified brain extracts are purified using an ODS-silica column (Immunonuclear Corp., Stillwater, Minn.) using the following procedure: 1 ml of the acidified samples are passed through a commercially prepared ODS-silica column and washed with 20 ml of 4% acetic acid. Peptide is then eluted in 4 ml absolute methanol and dried down at 37°C with a stream of dry nitrogen. The precipitate is then redissolved in 1 ml 1% BSA-borate buffer, vortexed and placed at 37°C for 10 minutes. A sample is then taken for assay using a radioimmunoassay for vasopressin (Immunonuclear Corp., Stillwater, Minn.).

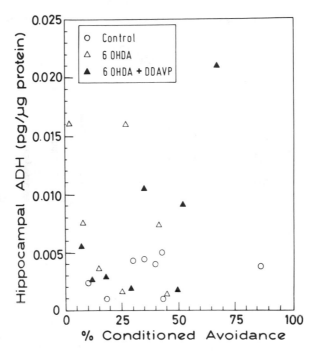

FIG. 11-5. Absence of correlation between hippocampal vasopressin levels and % conditioned avoidance. Methods as for Fig. 4.

campal vasopressin levels were so low, however (Fig. 5), and at the limit of sensitivity of the RIA, that possible correlations might have been obscured. It is speculatively possible that individuals with low caudate ADH might benefit most from exogenous vasopressin administration. A study of such individual differences in the animal model is under way in our laboratory, as a basis for a planned human study of CSF vasopressin in severe learning disorders. It is possible that low CSF vasopressin individuals may be most likely to respond to vasopressin treatment of learning disorder (see below).

De Wied (1971) reported that a single injection of vasopressin retarded extinction of active avoidance learning in rats. Although several authors have used multiple doses of vasopressin in animal learning experiments (De Wied et al., 1974; Bohus et al., 1973; Hamburger-Bar et al., in press (a), (b)), systematic comparisons of varying durations of administration of vasopressin have not been performed. We, therefore, decided to compare the effects of single dose vasopressin vs. repeated doses, both on acquisition of learning and on extinction. Fig. 6 illustrates the results of acute or chronic vasopressin treatment in 6-OH DA pre-

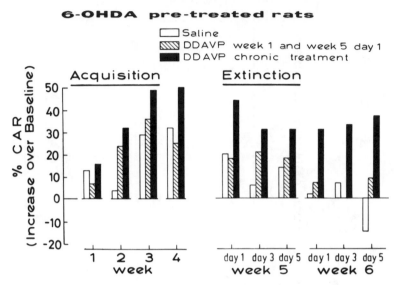

FIG. 11-6. The effect of acute vs. chronic DDAVP treatment on conditioned avoidance learning of rats pretreated with 6-OH DA at day 5 of life.

Conditioned avoidance was measured as in the legend to Fig. 3. Sessions of 10 trials were conducted three times weekly for 4 weeks with shock reinforcement and then 3 times weekly for week 5 and week 6 with no shock reinforcement. Saline was given 1 hour before each session in one group (N = 8); DDAVP 20 µg/rat was given once before each of the three sessions of week 1 and once before the first session of week 5 for another group ("acute" DDAVP, N = 9); and DDAVP 20 µg/rat was given 1 hour before each of the 18 sessions in a third group ("chronic" DDAVP, N = 7). Results are expressed as increases over baseline performance in the week preceding onset of treatment. The chronic DDAVP group is significantly better than the acute DDAVP group in week 3 and 4 of acquisition and throughout extinction.

treated rats. Acute vasopressin treatment is not significantly different from saline treatment on acquisition, except for week 2 (p < .001); whereas, the vasopressin chronically treated animals perform better than saline treated animals by the 2nd, 3rd and 4th weeks of learning. Chronic vasopressin significantly prevents extinction through the end of week 6 and is significantly more effective than a single vasopressin injection or controls.

These results, illustrated in Fig. 6, find clear effects of chronic vasopressin treatment on retarding extinction and on acquisition. In extinction, a single dose of vasopressin had no significant lasting effects compared with saline treated animals. Chronic vasopressin, by contrast, maintained conditioned avoidance response behavior at almost peak levels for almost 60 trials after the end of reinforcement. The learning and extinction curves of Fig. 6 suggest that continued vasopressin treatment is desirable for maintenance of the effects achievable by vasopressin on memory and learning (Hamburger-Bar et al., submitted).

In animal studies, using active avoidance tests, long-lasting positive results after single treatments were reported only for selected highly-responsive pretreated animals (De Wied, 1971, 1976; Walter et al., 1978). In our study such a selection was not applied. It should be noted also that in animal studies, using passive avoidance tests and acute vasopressin treatments, enhanced learning/memory could be obtained only after prior experience with learning situations (Rigter, 1982).

These animal results favoring chronic over acute vasopressin treatment could be specific to 6-OH DA pretreated rats (MBD model rats). They encourage, in any case, the use of chronic treatment in the design of clinical studies of vasopressin in MBD children.

HUMAN STUDIES

Human studies of vasopressin in memory disorders of aging (Tinklenberg et al., 1982) or post-traumatic amnesia (Oliveros et al., 1978; Jenkins et al., 1979) have been inconclusive. A study in six normal volunteers by Weingartner et al. (1981) using 30-60 µg of DDAVP three times daily for 2-3 weeks in an own-control design showed small, but statistically significant improvement in serial learning, recall of semantically-related words, and prompted free recall. Beckwith et al. (1982) also studied normal volunteers using 60 µg DDAVP single dose in 18 subjects, saline control in 21 subjects and no treatment in 15 subjects. DDAVP significantly enhanced learning in a concept shift task but had no effect on simple visual memory. Although the above studies achieved results that were too small to be of probable clinical siginificance, Swaab and Boer (1982) have proposed that the developing organism's brain may be more sensitive to vasopressin effects. Anderson et al. (1979) reported that 2 of 3 children with Lesh-Nyhan disease who were unable to learn a passive avoidance task were able to do so after treatment with DDAVP.

DDAVP is a synthetic vasopressin derivative with a plasma half-life of 75 minutes compared to the plasma half-life of 14 minutes for LVP (Edwards et al., 1973). DDAVP has powerful antidiuretic endocrine activity and has been in use for years (Becker and Foley, 1978). It has very little pressor activity compared with AVP and blood pressure changes are not reported (Beckwith et al., 1982; Kaye et al., 1982; Laczi et al., 1982). Although some animal studies suggest that DDAVP has less effect on memory than AVP (Walter et al., 1978), the human studies of Weingartner et al. (1981), Beckwith et al. (1982) and Anderson et al. (1979) all used DDAVP with positive results. Since DDAVP is clinically available and used widely in children for diabetes insipidus (Becker and Foley, 1978) and enuresis nocturna (Birkasova et al., 1978), we planned a study of DDAVP in children with learning disorders (Eisenberg et al., in press).

Sixteen boys and one girl participated in the study, age range 7-14. Seven children were referred by the psychological service of a regular school and diagnosed as suffering from ADD and/or learning problems at school. All were of normal intelligence. Three children came from a special education school, were suffering from severe learning disabilities and had a low average intelligence. A third group (7 children) came from a special education school which is part of a total care program for children with emotional and behavior disorders. The group was heterogeneous in regard to intelligence level. None of the children suffered from psychosis, seizure disorders or other physical illness. Informed consent was obtained from the parents of each child.

A controlled, double-blind crossover design was used. A psychometric pretest preceded medication. Following ten days of DDAVP ($20\mu g$ intranasally) or placebo, children were retested with the same test form two hours after the last dose of drug or placebo. After a 3-week washout period, the children were given the alternative test form, the appropriate crossover medication as before and retested with the same alternative test forms. No side effects were observed.

Results are shown in Fig. 7. The improvement in total score of position learning and story memory was greater in DDAVP-treated children (13.6 ± 11 units) than in placebo-treated children (7.4 ± 12 units), $p < .05$ one-tailed (Mann Whitney $U = 94$, $N = 17$) or $p = .035$ one-tailed (Wilcoxon matched pairs signed ranks $T = 35$, $N = 16$ because of one tie).

These present results represent the first study of vasopressin derivatives in childhood disorders of learning. The design was vigorously double-blind with balanced crossover. The intranasal drops containing DDAVP or vehicle only were identical in taste and impossible to distinguish; moreover, DDAVP treatment has very few side effects compared with most psychotropic drugs and the blind appeared to be exceptionally good. Preservation of the double-blind is important in interpreting the results which are quantitatively small and which could easily be due to expectation effects if the double-blind were not excellent. Moreover, the study used a carefully randomized balanced crossover design. This is critical in such studies because of order effects and practice effects that vary widely from test to test and setting to setting. Laczi et al. (1982), for instance, gave all subjects placebo first for 7 days and then DDAVP for 7 days. The greater improvement he reported for vasopressin could be due to greater cooperation by the subjects in the second half of the study.

The dosage used in the present study was identical to the starting dosage used for diabetes insipidus in children or enuresis nocturna in children (Becker and Foley, 1978; Birkasova et al., 1978). Ethical guide-

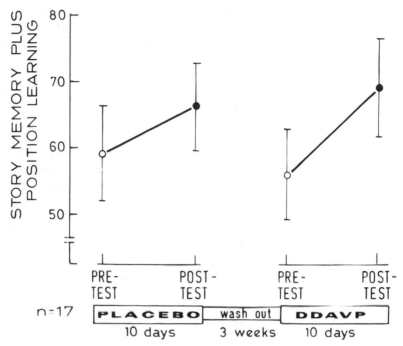

FIG. 11-7. The effect of 10 days of DDAVP or placebo treatment on the sum of story memory and position learning tests.

Of the 17 children who participated, 9 began with placebo and 8 with active DDAVP. The same pre-test and post-test was used for the first period for all children; an alternative form for the second period pre-test and post-test was used for all children. Story memory scores were added to position learning after weighting to give the two tests equal weight. The increase on DDAVP was significantly greater than the increase with placebo (Eisenberg et al., submitted (a)).

lines for research in children (Belmaker et al., in press) dictated this dosage which was lower than that used by Beckwith et al. (1982) or Weingartner et al. (1981) in adults and much lower than the dosage which might be predicted to be therapeutic from animal studies. The positive results are encouraging of the possibility of pharmacological treatment of these disorders with vasopressin derivatives even if the present results are not quantitatively of clinical significance. In the total absence of side effects, further studies may be carried out using higher dose DDAVP or using DGAVP, a vasopressin derivative active on CNS processes but devoid of effects on the kidney (Greven and De Wied, 1981). The time-dose-response relationship of vasopressin's learning effects in animals is unusual, and these are clearly long-lasting effects not dependent on the drug's plasma half-life (De Wied, 1971).

The clinical population studied in this trial was heterogeneous. Thirteen of the 17 children met DSM III criteria for ADD, 6 with hyperactivity and 7 without. The mean improvement score of ADD diagnosed children with DDAVP (14.6 ± 11) vs. placebo (7.3 ± 11) was similar to that of the total group. Seven of the children were inpatients at a unit for disturbed but not psychotic children. The mean improvement score of inpatient children with DDAVP (10.7 ± 8) vs. placebo (8.0 ± 11) was smaller than that of the total group. Dividing the children according to baseline performance, there was a nonsignificant trend for more impaired children to benefit less from DDAVP compared to placebo than children with less baseline impairment. While animal experiments suggest that vasopressin improves learning independently of the animal's state, both in normal animals, in hypophysectomized animals (Bohus et al., 1973), in CO_2-treated amnesic animals (Rigter and Crabbe, 1979), and ECS-treated amnesic animals (Pfeifer and Bookin, 1978), we reported that 6-OH DA treated animals (ADD model animals) (Hamburger et al., 1983) seemed more sensitive to vasopressin's ameliorative effects. It is possible that some diagnostic groups may be identified with learning disorders specifically responsive to vasopressin. Alternatively, vasopressin may be diagnostically nonspecific, like methylphenidate effects on hyperactivity; and the decision to prescribe it may depend on clinical judgement of need rather than diagnosis.

Since 20 µg of DDAVP is a small dose compared to the 60-180 µg daily reported to improve memory in normal adults by Weingartner et al. (1981), we hypothesized that a higher dose might result in greater improvement. On the other hand, De Wied's studies (1979) have suggested that a single dose of vasopressin may have lasting effects on the brain. Such lasting effects could be clinically important as a tactic for achieving clinical benefit with DDAVP without possible kidney side effects from continual dosing. We, therefore, planned an experiment to test single dose effect of DDAVP in children with attention and learning disorders (Eisenberg et al., submitted).

Methods were similar to those in the chronic DDAVP study, but an entirely non-overlapping patient population was used. Fifteen children were studies between the ages of 7 and 13. Five met RDC criteria for ADD with hyperactivity, 7 met RDC criteria for ADD without hyperactivity and 3 met RDC criteria for developmental reading disorder. All the children were free of drugs, seizure disorders or other medical problems. Informed signed consent was obtained from parents of each child.

Prior to the learning session, each child was administered 60 µg DDAVP (0.6 cc) intranasally or placebo identical in taste, in a random, double-blind crossover design. Blood pressure was measured at the beginning and end of the session. The child was administered several tests of attention, learning, retrieval and recognition. Three weeks later each

TABLE 1. Effect on psychometric tests of a single dose of 60 μg DDAVP in 15 children

Test (N = 15)	Placebo x̄ ± SD	DDAVP x̄ ± SD
Digit Span	4 ± 1	4 ± 1 NS
Word List	4.1 ± 2.8	4.8 ± 2.7 NS
Position Learning Test	33 ± 13	37 ± 10 NS
Story Memory	9.5 ± 7.7	9.4 ± 5.4 NS

subject was administered the alternate drug and an alternate form of test in the same manner as before.

Table 1 illustrates the results of DDAVP or placebo treatment on the psychometric tests administered. There was no significant drug effect on any of the measures. There were no side effects reported during the sessions, nor any change in blood pressure. Thus single intranasal dose of 60 μg of DDAVP had no measurable effect on psychometric measures in this group of children. This contrasts with the effect of 10 days of 20 μg of DDAVP intranasally in a diagnostically similar group (of different individuals) studies by the same investigators (Eisenberg et al., in press). These results may indicate that chronic treatment is required in humans for vasopressin effects on learning in MBD children.

The present series of studies illustrates the utility of parallel animal and clinical research. The effect of vasopressin to improve learning in rats treated at day 5 of life with 6-OH DA encouraged us to study vasopressin effects in MBD children. The improvement in learning of MBD children induced by DDAVP strengthens the validity of the rat MBD model that predicted this effect. Further animal studies may clarify dosage schedules and specific vasopressin derivatives to maximize clinical potential in further clinical studies.

REFERENCES

American Psychiatric Association: DSM-III: Diagnostic and Statistical Manual of Mental Disorders. 3rd ed. APA, Washington, D.C., 1980.

Anderson, L.T., David, R., Bonnet, K. and Dancis, J.: Avoidance learning in Lesh Nyhan disease: Effect of 1-desamino-8-arginine vasopressin. *Life Sci.* 24:905-910, 1979.

Barkley, R.A.: A review of stimulant drug research with hyperactive children. *J. Child Psychol. Psychiat.* 18:137-165, 1977.

Becker, D. and Foley, T.P.: DDAVP in treatment of central diabetes insipidus. *J. Pediat.* 92:1011-1018, 1978.

Beckwith, B.E., Petros, T., Kanaan-Beckwith, S., Couk, D.I., Haug, R.J. and Ryan, C.: Vasopressin analog (DDAVP) facilitates concept learning in human males. *Peptides* 3:627-630, 1982.

Belmaker, R.H., Klein, E. and Dick, E: Ethics and psychopharmacologic research. In: Impact on Clinical Psychiatry, (D.W. Morgan, ed), Ishiyaku EuroAmerica. (In press).

Birkasova, M., Birkas, O., Flynn, M.J. and Cort, J.H.: Desmopressin in management of nocturnal enuresis in children. *Pediatrics* 62:970-974, 1978.

Bohus, B., Gispen, W.H. and De Wied, D.: Effect of lysine vasopressin and ACTH 4-10 on conditioned avoidance behavior of hypophysectomized rats. *Neuroendocrinology* 11:137-143, 1973.

Cantwell, D.P.: The Hyperactive child: Diagnosis, Management and Current Research, Spectrum Press, New York, 1975.

De Wied, D.: Long term effect of vasopressin on the maintenance of a conditioned avoidance response in rats. *Nature* 232:58-60, 1971.

De Wied, D., Bohus, B. and Van Wimersma Greidanus, T.J.B.: The hypothalamoneurohypophyseal system and the prevention of conditioned avoidance behavior in rats. *Prog. Brain Res.* 41:417-428, 1974.

De Wied, D. and Bohus, B.: Modulation of memory processes by neuropeptides of hypothalamic-neurohypophyseal origin. In: Brain Mechanisms in Memory and Learning, (M.A. Brazier, ed.), Raven Press, New York, 1979.

Edwards, C.R.W., Kitan, M.J., Chard, T. and Besser, G.M.: Vasopressin analog DDAVP in diabetes insipidus. *Brit. Med. J.* 3:374-378, 1973.

Eisenberg, J., Chazan-Gologorsky, S., Hattab, J. and Belmaker, R.H.: A controlled trial of vasopressin treatment of childhood learning disorders. *Biol. Psychiat.* (In press).

Eisenberg, J., Belmaker, R.H. and Shapira, Y.: Single-dose administration of vasopressin in children with learning and attention disorders. (Submitted).

Greven, H.M. and De Wied, D.: Neuropeptides and behavior. In: Perspectives in Peptide Chemistry, (A. Eberle, R. Geiger and T. Wieland, eds.), Karger Press, Basel, pp. 356-371, 1981.

Hamburger-Bar, R., Gak, S. and Belmaker, R.H.: The effect of a vasopressin derivative on conditioned avoidance learning in a rat model of minimal brain dysfunction. In: Advances in Neuropsychopharmacology (G.D. Burrows, ed.), John Libbey, London, 1983.

Hamburger-Bar, R. and Belmaker, R.H.: (a) Dose-response relationships of vasopressin effects on conditioned avoidance learning in a rat model of minimal brain dysfunction. In: Symposium on Neuronal Communications, (B.J. Meyer and S. Kramer, eds.), A.A. Balkema, Cape Town. (In press).

Hamburger-Bar, R., Ebstein, R.P. and Belmaker, R.H.: (b) Vasopressin effect on learning in 6-OH DA pretreated rats: Correlation with caudate vasopressin levels. *Biol. Psychiat.* (In press).

Hamburger-Bar, R., Klein, A. and Belmaker, R.H.: The effect of chronic vs. acute injection of vasopressin on animal learning and memory. (Submitted).

Hostetter, G., Jubb, S.L. and Kozlowski, G.P.: Vasopressin affects the behavior of rats in a positively rewarded discrimination task. *Life Sci.* 21:1323-1328, 1977.

Jenkins, J.S., Mather, H.M., Coughlan, A.K. and Jenkins, D.G.: Desmopressin in post traumatic amnesia. *Lancet* 1245-1246, 1979.

Kasting, N.W. and Martin, J.B.: Changes in immunoreactive vasopressin concentrations in brain regions of the rat in response to endotoxin. *Brain Res.* 253:127, 1983.

Kaye, W.H., Weingartner, H., Gold, P., Ebert, M.H., Gillin, J.C., Sitaram, N. and Samllberg, S.: Cognitive effects of cholinergic and vasopressin-like agents in patients with primary degenerative dementia. In: Alzheimer's Disease—A Report of Progress, (S. Corkin, K.L. Davis, J.H. Growdon, E. Usdin and R.J. Wurtmann, eds.), Raven Press, New York, 1982.

Kimura, T., Share, L., Wang, B.C. and Crofton, J.T.: Central effects of dopamine and bromocriptine on vasopressin release and blood pressure. *Neuroendocrinology* 33:347, 1981.

Kovacs, G.L., Bohus, B. and Versteeg, D.H.G.: The interaction of posterior pituitary neuropeptides with monoaminergic neurotransmission: significance in learning and memory processes. *Prog. Brain Res.* 53:123, 1980.

Laczi, F., Valkusz, S., Laszio, F.A. Wagner, A., Jardanhazy, T., Szasz, A., Szilard, J. and Telegdy, G.: Effect of LVP and DDAVP on memory in healthy individuals and diabetes insipidus patients. *Psychoneuroendocrinology* 7:185-193, 1982.

Oliveros, J.C., Jandali, M.K., Timsit, B.M., Remy, R., Benghezal, A., Audibert, A. and Moeglen, J.M.: Vasopressin in amnesia. *Lancet* 8054, 1978.

Pfeifer, W.D. and Bookin, H.B.: Vasopressin antagonizes retrograde amnesia in rats following electro-convulsive shock. *Pharmacol. Biochem. Behav.* 9:261-263, 1978.

Rapoport, J.L. and Zametkin, A.: Attention deficit disorder. *Psych. Clin. North America* 3:425-441, 1980.

Riddle, K. and Rapoport, J.: A two-year follow-up of 72 hyperactive boys. *J. Nerv. Ment. Dis.* 162:126-134, 1976.

Rigter, H. and Crabbe, J.C.: Modulation of memory by pituitary hormones and related peptides. *Vit. Hormones* 37:153-241, 1979.

Rigter, H.: Vasopressin and memory: The influence of prior experience with the training situation. *Behav. Neural. Biol.* 34:337-351, 1982.

Shaywitz, B.A., Klopper, J.H., Yager, R.D. and Gordon, J.W.: Paradoxical response to amphetamine in developing rats treated with 6-hydroxydopamine. *Nature* 261:153-155, 1976.

Shaywitz, B.A., Klopper, J.H. and Gordon, J.W.: Methylphenidate in 6-hydroxydopamine treated developing rat pups: effects on activity and maze performance. *Arch. Neurol.* 35:463-479, 1978.

Swaab, D.F. and Boer, G.J.: Neuropeptides and brain development. Current perils and future potentials. *J. Dev. Physiol.* 5:67-75, 1983.

Tinklenberg, J.R., Pigache, R., Pfefferbaum, A., Berger, P.A.: Vasopressin peptides and dementia. In: Alzheimer's Disease: A Report of Progress, (S. Corkin, K.L. Davis, J.H. Growdon, E. Usdin and R.J. Wurtmann, eds.), Raven Press, New York, pp. 463-467, 1982.

Walter, R., Van Ree, J.M. and De Wied, D.: Modification of conditioned behavior of rats by neurohypophyseal hormones and analogues. *Proc. Natl. Acad. Sci.* 75:2493-2496, 1978.

Weingartner, H., Gold, P., Ballenger, J.C., Smallberg, S., Summers, K., Rubinow, D.R., Post, R.M. and Goodwin, F.W.: Effect of vasopressin on human memory functions. *Science* 211:601-603, 1981.

Wender, P.M.: Minimal brain dysfunction in children. J. Wiley and Sons, New York, pp. 12-30, 1971.

CHAPTER 12

Update on Pharmacology: Clinical Use and Side Effects of Lithium

Robert J. Pary, M.D.
Kenneth E. Goolsby, M.D.
Angel Rodriguez, M.D.

INTRODUCTION

Lithium is the third element on the periodic table, and its salt has been prescribed as a medical treatment for over a century. Its use in psychiatry is credited to Cade (1949) when he discovered that lithium had a anti-manic effect.

The magnitude of that discovery is such that by 1982, over 9500 medically-related articles on lithium have been published (Jefferson, Griest, Ackerman, 1983). There have been many excellent reviews, but of special note is a project of Jefferson, Greist, and Ackerman of Madison, Wisconsin. They have developed the Lithium Information Center and use three computer programs: lithium library, lithium index, and lithium consultation. Direct on-line access to the computer programs is available for a nominal fee to institutions and individuals.

The lithium index, which is frequently updated, was extremely helpful in the preparation of this chapter. The book version of the index is the *Lithium Encyclopedia for Clinical Practice* (Jefferson, Greist and Ackerman, 1983).

Unless stated overwise, lithium will refer to one of the lithium salts; the anion will be any of those mentioned in the section on Preparations.

PHARMACOLOGY
Absorption

Generally, lithium salts are thought to be completely absorbed from the gut, although Caldwell (1971) found only 75% absorption with some sustained-release preparations. Thronhill (1981) calculated the absorption half-life as 0.78 ± 0.05 hr. (standard preparation) and 3.73 ± 0.37 hr. (sustained-release). Thornhill also found peak plasma values at 6 hr. (standard preparation) and 12 hr. (sustained-release). These values are considerably delayed compared with the 1.5-2 hr. (standard) and 4-4.5 hr. (sustained-release) that are conventionally given for peak plasma values (Jefferson, Greist, and Ackerman, 1983). The reasons for the discrepancy are not clear.

Distribution

The volume of distribution approximates the total body water volume. Lithium crosses the blood brain barrier, placenta, and appears in maternal milk (Thornhill, 1981). It is not protein bound.

Spirtes (1976) examined five rhesus monkeys who were on chronic oral dosages yielding plasma lithium concentrations of 1.0/mEq/l and examined one manic-depressive patient at 12 hr. post-mortem. Average brain concentrations were approximately half of the plasma ones. Increased brain concentrations were in the thalamus and caudate nucleus while lower brain levels were found in the temporal lobe (0.4 mEq/kg). Of the non-brain areas, concentrations greater than plasma concentrations were found in bile, erythrocytes, skin, bone, and thyroid. Liver and fat had the lowest values. Of potential clinical significance, is that saliva concentrations are higher than plasma and gave similar and consistent kinetics (Groth, Prellivitz, and Jahnchen, 1974).

Elimination

Despite the finding of greater concentrations in the bile than plasma, fecal excretion appears clinically insignificant. Lithium is excreted through the kidneys and competes with sodium for reabsorption in the proximal tubules of the kidney (Schou 1968). Hence in states of relative sodium deficiency (e.g. sodium-depleting diuretics) proportionally more lithium will be reabsorbed leading to high plasma concentrations. The converse is true with sodium excess.

Using a two compartment kinetic model, Groth (1974) found the plasma elimination half-life to be 14-24 hrs. However, Goodnick, Fieve and Meltzer (1981) showed that elimination half-life is significantly longer (2.43 days ± 0.91) in eleven patients who had been on lithium for more than a year than in thirteen patients who had no previous lithium treatment (1.2 days ± 0.38).

Mechanism of Action

Lithium's mechanism of action may likely remain unknown until either etiologies or effective animal models for affective illnesses become well established. Numerous physiological actions have been reported with lithium; yet the significance for the clinician remains unclear. Bloom et al (1983) was pessimistic that any of the preclinical studies in animals of amines or neuropeptides, etc. would have much clinical relevance in the absence of a good animal model of affective illness.

With that caveat, the following is a brief discussion of lithium's various actions.

NEUROTRANSMITTERS

Dopamine

Bunney and Garland (1983) reviewed the effects of lithium in preventing haloperidol-induced behavioral supersensitivity. Most studies found that lithium did prevent the supersensitivity although a few did not (Bloom 1983, Reches 1982). The implication is that lithium might prevent haloperidol-induced supersensitivity in man. Dopamine supersensitivity is postulated as an etiology for tardive dyskinesia. However, as mentioned later, lithium as a treatment for tardive dyskinesia has not been encouraging so far.

Norepinephrine

A proposed mode of action of antidepressant drugs is through down-regulation of beta-adrenergic receptors (Sulser, 1979). Early reports of decreases in cortical beta-receptor binding (Treiser and Kellar, 1979) have not been supported by later investigations (Pandey and Davis, 1981) (Kafka, 1982).

Bunney and Garland (1983) reviewed the effectiveness of lithium in blocking alpha- and beta-receptor sub and supersensitivity. Lithium appears to be ineffective in blocking the subsensitivity of beta receptors (Rosenblatt 1979). Pert el al (1978) demonstrated blockade of alpha- and beta-supersensitivity while Mailman (1980) could not find blockade of 6-OHDA-induced beta supersensitivity.

Adenylate Cyclase

Perhaps of more immediate clinical relevance than the work on dopamine or norepinephrine has been the work on adenylate cyclase.

Lithium has been found to inhibit adenylate cyclase, the enzyme converting ATP to cAMP, the "second messenger" Pandey and Davis, 1979). Adenylate cyclase inhibition appears to be the mechanism for several of lithium-induced side effects such as hypothyroidism, diabetes insipidus, hyperglycemia in diabetic patients on lithium, and psoriasis.

Circadian Rhythms

Jefferson et al (1983) summarized the evidence that lithium's effect may act through altering the phase of the circadian rhythm. Compared to placebo, lithium causes small though significant delays (14.2 minutes) in the sleep-wake circadian rhythm of 23 volunteers (Kripke 1979). The significance is that depression may be related to an alteration of circadian cycles and thus lithium may normalize the cycle.

Preparations

Schou (1981) listed 52 available lithium preparations worldwide. Of these, Jefferson et al (1983) condensed the list to 21 preparations which have been referenced in the literature. The anions available are carbonate, acetate, citrate, gluconate in the standard release form and carbonate, citrate and sulfate in the slow release form. The theoretical advantage of the slow released compounds is to minimize side effects due to high serum-level peaks and to increase patients' compliance from a Q.I.D. or T.I.D. schedule to B.I.D. It should be noted that the standard release lithium citrate (available in the U.S.) and lithium gluconate are liquid preparations.

Pre-Lithium Workup

A pre-lithium workup usually includes serum creatinine, BUN, electrolytes, thyroid function tests, EKG, CBC, serum glucose. This establishes baseline data since lithium is known to affect several organ systems (Bernstein 1983).

Dosages

With the narrow therapeutic index, in almost all cases one must use serum levels to guide lithium prescribing. There have been two strategies; one is to pick some starting dose. For example, in manic adults under 50 years, 600 mg T.I.D. adjusted according to steady state serum level (drawn 12 hrs. after the last dose) and/or clinical status. The dosage would be given to achieve a serum level of 0.8 mEq/l to 1.5 mEq/l (Jefferson, 1983). An alternative strategy is to give a single 600 mg dose and draw a serum lithium level 24 hours later (Cooper and Simpson 1976). That level is used to predict the dosage schedule needed to achieve a steady state level from 0.6 mEq/l to 1.2 mEq/l. One drawback to the second method is that the patient must be lithium free prior to the test dose. Despite the predictive dosages, one still needs to monitor clinically and to obtain periodic steady state serum levels.

A variation of the second method involves giving the patient 600, 900, 1200, or 1500 mg. of lithium carbonate, depending upon age and weight on the evening of first day (Perry 1982). Serum lithium levels are drawn after 12 and 36 hrs., using a lithium kinetics computer program in basic. The program states half-life and number of days to achieve a particular steady level expected from various dosing schedules. One drawback is that the program is based on a one-compartment pharmacokinetic model.

Naiman (1981) offers caution in using a lithium dosage guide in ordinary practice. He emphasizes the potential difficulty of getting serum levels at appropriate times and obtaining patient compliance.

Monitoring

Two basic procedures are used to quantitate lithium in biological fluids, flame emission and atomic absorption. Cooper (1981) found that the techniques can be used interchangeably. Although flame emission has a lower limit of detection, Cooper does not believe this is a practical concern because even atomic absorption's lowest detectable limit is over 100 times greater than is needed to assay 1.0 mmol/l.

Unless toxicity is suspected, there are two crucial factors in monitoring: (1) blood is drawn 12 hrs. after the last dose; and (2) steady state, five times the elimination of half-life, has been achieved within 4-5 days for patients with no previous lithium treatment and probably within 8-12 days for elderly patients or patients who have been on lithium for over a year.

Jefferson (1983) warns that the therapeutic serum lithium level has not been fully resolved. Guidelines do exist, 0.8 to 1.5 mEq/l for acute mania and 0.6 to 1.0 mEq/l for maintenance, although the ideal is to treat maintenance with the lowest effective level. A serum level never replaces the clinical assessment for toxicity (See below).

Treatment

Lithium has been considered a potential treatment in many psychiatric illnesses, and these will be reviewed in the following summary. However, lithium is currently indicated by the FDA only for the treatment of manic episodes of manic-depressive illness and for maintenance therapy in manic-depressive patients with a history of mania.

AFFECTIVE DISORDERS ASSOCIATED WITH PHYSICAL CONDITIONS (including organic brain syndrome)

Numerous case reports have shown lithium to exert a beneficial effect in the treatment of affective disorders associated with physical conditions. These have included affective symptoms precipitated by such physical disorders as cerebrovascular accidents with subsequent surgery, hemodialysis, brain stem injury, and closed head injury (Rosenbaum 1975, Procci 1977, Oyewumi 1981, Cohn 1977). Some case reports have shown lithium alone to be ineffective in the treatment of affective symptoms possibly related to physical disorders, but effective in combination with carbamazepine (Forrest, 1982).

Lithium has also been reported effective in the treatment of affective disorders associated with OBS in several case reports (Young 1977, Mehta 1976). Williams (1979) evaluated the cognitive and affective responses to lithium in ten patients with chronic brain syndromes, six of whom were alcoholics. Six of the ten patients improved dramatically with both cognitive (improved memory and speech) and affective symptoms. Hale (1982) examined the usefulness of lithium in the treatment of five patients with OBS and some characteristics of affective instability. All patients showed improved symptoms of affective instability, and three patients showed improved cognitive function. However, a recent case report of a patient with Alzheimer's disease treated with lithium had improvement of affective symptoms but no improvement in cognitive function (Havens, 1982).

Aggressive Behavior

Lithium has been shown to have an anti-aggressive effect in animal (Sheard, 1978). In a single-blind, placebo-controlled evaluation of prison inmates, Sheard (1971) found an anti-aggressive effect of lithium with levels above 0.6 Meq/l. Tupin (1973) in an open study examined 27 male convicts for 3-18 months and found an anti-aggressive effect of lithium in most patients with levels averaging 0.82 Meq/l. However, this study included eight schizophrenic and four possible schizophrenic patients. Case reports and open trials with mentally retarded patients have shown lithium to decrease self-mutilation and aggression towards others with levels between 0.7-0.9 Meq/l (Cooper 1973, Dostal 1970). Worral (1975), in a double-blind, controlled study, found lithium to be effective in decreasing aggression in some mentally retarded patients. Of the eight patients studied, two had significant decrease in the number and intensity of aggressive episodes and one had slightly decreased aggression. Effective levels ranged from 0.7-0.93 Meq/l. Two patients, developed neurotoxicity at levels above 1.1 Meq/l. In another double-blind trial, Sheard (1976) found lithium to decrease the number of infractions in a group of male delinquents convicted of serious crimes. Levels ranged from 0.64-0.89 Meq/l. It is important to note that in several studies both the ward personnel and the patients reported the beneficial effects of lithium (Schou, 1980).

Alcoholism

Lithium has received much recent publicity as a possible treatment of alcoholism and accompanying affective disorders. McMillian (1981) summarized non-blind and uncontrolled studies using lithium as a treatment for alcoholism. He found an overall reduced morbidity for both alcoholic and affective components for long periods of time. However, he viewed these results with some skepticism because of difficulty in classification, selection, and criteria for improvement.

An uncontrolled study, not included in the above review, used strict diagnostic categories in a six-week trial and found lithium's effect of decreasing alcohol consumption to be independent from its effect on mood (Himmelhoch, 1980).

Kline (1974) evaluated the use of lithium in a double-blind study with a group of chronic alcoholics, some of which had depressed features. The first year drop-out rate was 59%. He found that the patients given lithium had fewer disabling drinking episodes than those given placebo, but depression was alleviated similarly in both groups (Kline, 1974). In another double-blind study, (Merry, 1976) found lithium to be superior to placebo in a depressed group of alcoholics, but no differences were noted in the non-depressed group. However, there was no significant difference in the alleviation of depression between the two groups. They had a 46% drop-out rate. Pond (1981), found no improvement in alcohol consumption or depression in a six-month, double-blind crossover study with lithium. The drop out rate was 60%.

Anorexia Nervosa

Several case reports have suggested a beneficial effect of lithium in the treatment of anorexia nervosa. These patients had weight gains of approximately 30% and sustained an improved mood over one to four years (Jefferson, 1983).

The only double-blind, controlled study to date was performed by Gross (1981). He found significant improvement of weight gain by lithium over placebo when used in combination with behavior modification. Lithium levels ranged from 0.9-1.4 Meq/l.

Attention Deficit Disorder

A case report found lithium to augment the response of pemoline in a patient with attention deficit disorder (Brown, 1983). However, several double-blind studies comparing lithium with dextrophetamine, antipsychotics or placebo in hyperactive children showed only partial effectiveness (Jefferson, 1983). Reasons for the conflicting reports may, in part, be related to diagnostic difficulties with attention deficit disorder and other childhood disorders with hyperactivity. The FDA advises not using lithium in children under 12 years of age.

Depression, Acute

Ramsey (1980) reviewed twelve controlled studies comparing placebo or antidepressants with lithium in depressed patients. As Ramsey indicates, there are already several treatments (e.g. tricyclics, MAOIs, and ECT) that have demonstrated efficacy in the treatment of depression. Thus, while nine of the controlled studies demonstrated an antidepressant effect for lithium, the fundamental question is whether there is a subgroup of depressed patients in which lithium is the treatment of choice? That cannot be definitively answered. Use of lithium for depression appears to be linked to either treatment of refractory depression (see below) or else in bipolar patients who have manic episodes precipitated by tricyclic antidepressants. Ramsey (1980) outlined features that predicted response to lithium in recurrent unipolar patients who don't seem to respond well to tricyclic antidepressants. The lithium-responsive subgroup has a "tinge" of bipolarity either in their history (mood liability or mild hypomania) or in their families. For a further discussion of lithium in acute depression see depression, refractory.

Depression, Prophylaxis

There have been many studies suggesting lithium's efficacy in the prophylaxis of depression in some patients. Baastrup (1967) found lithium to be equally effective in the prophylaxis of both bipolar and depression. Schou (1979) reviewed the studies comparing lithium with placebo and antidepressants in the prophylaxis of depression. He concluded that lithium produced about a 20% relapse rate versus 70% with placebo, and this was true for both unipolar and bipolar patients. In direct comparison studies, he found lithium to be more effective than antidepressants in the prophylaxis of bipolar depression, and lithium equal or slightly superior in unipolar depression. Davis (1976), in another review, concluded lithium to be equally effective in the prophylaxis of unipolar and bipolar depression. However, Priens (1979) suggested that lithium's efficacy in the prophylaxis of depression has not been established.

In a double-blind study with bipolar II patients, Dunner (1976) found no statistical differences in the number of depressive relapses with lithium or placebo for a 15-month period. However, Dunner (1982) did find a prophylactic effect when the bipolar II patients were evaluated after 33 months of lithium treatment. Fieve (1976) in a double-blind study, concluded lithium to be effective in the prophylaxis of bipolar I, bipolar II, and unipolar patients. Kane (1982) also found lithium in a double-blind study to be effective in the prophylaxis of unipolar and bipolar II patients. However, Peselow (1982) found a limited prophylactic effect of lithium in unipolar, bipolar II and cyclothymic patients.

Depression, Refractory

Many studies have suggested a possible antidepressant effect of lithium in selected patients (See Acute Depression). Recent evidence has suggested that lithium may also be effective in the treatment of refractory depression. However, conclusive reviews, such as Ramsey (1980) evaluating the efficacy of lithium in the treatment of acute depression, are not available for the use of lithium in refractory depression. Therefore, the case reports and open studies will be summarized. Any conclusions must be regarded only as tentative.

Kline (1978) reported on three depressed patients unresponsive to treatment with antidepressants. After lithium therapy was initiated, all three patients showed an improvement in depression within 2-7 days. The two lithium levels reported were 0.6 and 0.45 Meq/l. It was implied that the patients were taking no medications with the lithium. De Montigny (1981) examined eight patients with major unipolar depression refractory to treatment for at least three weeks with tricyclic antidepressants. Lithium was added to the antidepressant, and all eight patients had relief of their depression within 48 hours. Levels ranged from 0.5-1.0 Meq/l. Nelson (1982) reported that the addition of lithium to the regimen of three patients previously unresponsive to phenelzine resulted in an improvement of depression in five days. Lithium levels were not listed. Price (1983) examined the effect of lithium augmentation in six patients with delusional depression previously unresponsive to combined neuroleptic-tricyclic treatment. Five of the six patients showed improvement with lithium, but over a more variable length of time (48 hours to three weeks). DeMontigny (1983) evaluated the addition of lithium to the treatment of depressed patients previously unresponsive to tricyclic antidepressants. They found a 50% improvement in 48 hours in 30 of 42 observations. The same authors studied the effect of lithium addition in patients with depression refractory to pre-treatment with either amitriptyline or placebo. All the amitriptyline pre-treated patients showed at least 50% improvement in 48 hours; however, only one of the placebo pre-treated patients showed a marked response. Also, they studied the effect of lithium withdrawal in nine antidepressant-resistant patients who had responded to lithium. Only five of the nine patients relapsed within five days after lithium discontinuation. Effective levels in all of these studies were 0.4-1.2 Meq/l (1983).

Heninger (1983) recently performed a double-blind, placebo-controlled study with lithium in depressed patients refractory to antidepressants. In comparison with placebo, lithium augmentation produced a small but significant improvement in two days, a more variable course during the next four days, and a significant and clinically-meaningful improvement in the 7th through the 12th day. Individually, one-third of the patients responded within six days, and the remainder responded during the next six day period. Lithium levels ranged from 0.5-1.1 Meq/l.

Mania, Acute

Lithium has been considered a potentially effective treatment for mania since Cade's report in 1949. There have since been a multitude of studies demonstrating lithium's effectiveness in the treatment of acute mania. In a review of the open and single-blind studies, Goodwin (1979) found an 81% rate of improvement with lithium in the treatment of mania. He also found a 76% lithium response rate when evaluating placebo-controlled studies.

In a review of the double-blind studies comparing lithium with neuroleptics, Kocsis (1981) concluded that lithium was an effective treatment and should be tried alone in most acutely manic patients. Combining the results of uncontrolled and controlled studies, Kocsis (1980) concluded that approximately 75-80% of typical manic patients of mild to moderate severity will improve within two weeks of lithium therapy. Since some patients required levels greater than 1.5 Meq/l, he suggested that plasma levels be gradually increased until remission of symptoms or signs of toxicity occurs, but this should be carefully monitored in a hospital setting. In a review of the double-blind studies comparing lithium with antipsychotics, Goodwin (1979) concluded that lithium was associated with marked improvement in at least 70% of the patients. The authors suggested that lithium was superior to chlorpromazine in the treatment of most patients with acute mania, but considered chlorpromazine to be probably superior to lithium in the initial control of patients with increased psychomotor activity. Garfinkel (1980) also found higher potency neuroleptics to be preferable initially for the rapid control of highly agitated patients. Jefferson (1983) suggests using an antipsychotic drug alone with extremely violent patients and adding lithium gradually after the acute phase has passed. Then the antipsychotic drug should be gradually discontinued and, in most patients, treatment should be continued with lithium alone. However, it is important to note that the combination of lithium and neuroleptics has led to reports of neurotoxicity in some patients (Spring 1981, Charney 1979).

Although lithium is well accepted in the treatment of mania, some patients fail to respond with lithium alone. Several case reports have shown manic episodes refractory to treatment with lithium alone to be responsive to a combination of lithium and carbamazepine (Forrest 1982, Moss 1983, Lipinski 1982). Levels of carbamazepine ranged from (4.5-9.5mg/ml). Another case report showed L-tryptophan to be effective in combination with lithium in a patient refractory to lithium alone (Chouinard, 1979).

Mania, Prophylaxis

Lithium has for many years been considered an efficacious treatment in the prophylaxis of mania. Davis (1976) reviewed the double-blind, placebo-controlled studies evaluating lithium's prophylaxis in affective disorders. He found that lithium had a substantial prophylactic effect which was statistically significant and consistently demonstrated in all studies. Several of the studies found lithium to have a larger quantitative effect in the prevention of mania, while others showed similar effects against both mania and depressive phases.

Others have also evaluated the controlled studies and found lithium to be superior to placebo in the prophylaxis of mania (Prien 1979), Spring

1980). Effective serum levels are usually lower than for acute episodes, with a minimum between 0.6 and 0.8 Meq/l Jefferson (1983).

Obsessive-Compulsive Disorder

There have been few studies evaluating the efficacy of lithium in the treatment of obsessive-compulsive disorders. Reports of two patients showed lithium to relieve severe obsessions and compulsions. However, two placebo-controlled trials failed to show lithium to be of value in the treatment of obsessive-compulsives (Jefferson, 1983). Also, studies evaluating the response of lithium in the treatment of depressed patients with obsessional features have been mixed (Donnelly 1979, Kupfer, 1975).

Personality Disorder

The category "personality disorders" is quite broad; case reports have primarily examined borderline, cyclothymic, and dysthmic personality disorders (Jefferson 1983, Akiskal 1983). Bernstein (1983) reports on uncontrolled study of approximately 100 patients with borderline symptomatology that he has treated with lithium.

He observed that it may be difficult to differentiate borderline patients from those classified as schizoaffective and that severe borderline with suicide threats or attempts tended to do better when low-dose high potency neuroleptic was added.

Phobic Disorder

Little information is available regarding the efficacy of lithium in the treatment of patients with phobic disorders. The information available is in the form of case reports, and these results are contradictory. Lithium does not appear to be useful in primary phobic disorders (Jefferson, 1983).

Psychoses, Drug-Induced

Several studies have demonstrated lithium to be useful in steroid induced psychoses. Lithium in several case reports has been effective in the prophylaxis of prednisone-induced psychoses (Siegal 1978, Goggans, 1983). Other case reports have shown lithium to be effective in the prophylaxis of corticotropin-induced psychoses (Falk 1979, Kemp 1977). Effective levels ranged from 0.8-1.4 Meq/l.

Several case reports have also suggested a positive effect of lithium in the treatment of cocaine induced psychoses (Scott 1981, Flemenbaum, 1977). Others have suggested a prophylactic effect of lithium in bipolar patients with tricyclic antidepressant-induced mania (Jann 1982). Lithium has also been effective in case reports of levodopa-induced psychosis (Ryback 1971, Braden 1977), as well as phencyclidine-induced mania (Slavney, 1977).

Schizoaffective Disorder

Lithium has been shown to have mixed results in the treatment of schizoaffective patients. A major difficulty in determining the efficacy of lithium has been the imprecision of the diagnostic criteria in schizoaffective disorder (Watanabe, 1980).

One review of the uncontrolled studies found a positive response in 77% of schizoaffectives treated with lithium (Procci, 1976). Other reviews of case reports and uncontrolled studies have suggested benefits of lithium in schizoaffective patients especially in reducing affective symptoms (Delva, 1982). Double-blind studies comparing chlorpromazine with lithium have shown mixed results. Although the affective symptoms responded well to lithium, they also suggested a possible antipsychotic action of lithium in some patients. Delva (1982) also reviewed the controlled studies and concluded that in the clearly defined schizoaffectives, and in the less clearly defined marginal group, the favourable response to lithium is at least 75%. The usual effective levels ranged from 0.7-1.2Meq/l. In a review of the uncontrolled and controlled double-blind studies, Watanabe (1980) concluded that lithium benefits 60-70% of patients with schizoaffective psychosis, manic type, with the target symptoms of affect. Other studies have suggested that lithium is of more benefit in schizoaffective patients with periodicity or psychomotor acceleration (Miller 1979).

Several studies have shown lithium to be effective in combination with other medications. A recent double-blind study found lithium plus L-tryptophan resulted in a significantly greater improvement in schizoaffective patients than lithium and placebo; however, the L-tryptophan group received slightly larger doses of neuroleptics than the placebo group (Brewerton, 1983). Other reports have suggested a synergistic effect of lithium when added to neuroleptics in schizoaffective patients (Carman 1981 and Biederman 1979). However, Spring (1980) stated that there were no well-controlled studies which demonstrate the superiority of lithium plus neuroleptics and recommended treating acute schizoaffectives of the excited, manic type with neuroleptics alone.

There is some evidence to suggest a prophylactic effect of lithium in schizoaffective patients. Delva (1982) found that three of five studies examining this prophylactic effect showed lithium to have a significant benefit. However, additional studies are needed to examine this question.

Schizophrenia

There have been conflicting reports regarding the efficacy of lithium in the treatment of schizophrenia. This is, in part, related to the past diagnostic imprecision in the classifications of schizophrenia. Earlier studies probably included some schizoaffective patients.

Gershon (1960) reviewed articles prior to 1960 on 269 schizophrenics and concluded that 60% improved with lithium. However, in the majority of cases improvement was limited to decreased psychomotor activity and not to improvement of basic condition. Delva (1982) reviewed the uncontrolled and controlled studies of lithium treatment with schizophrenic patients and concluded that between 40-55% of schizophrenic patients without affective overlay or excitement respond to lithium. This is a lower response rate than seen with schizoaffective disorder. Effective levels range from 0.7-1.2 Meq/l. However, Watanabe (1980), in another review, concluded that the effects of lithium in the treatment of schizophrenia are still controversial and require further studies. Spring (1980) stated that no research or clinical data support the use of lithium with schizophrenic patients.

Delva (1982) evaluated the effects of lithium withdrawal in six schizophrenic patients stabilized on lithium and neuroleptics for at least two years with levels between 0.6-1.2 Meq/l. Two of the six patients relapsed in two weeks, and four had not relapsed after one year.

Tardive Dyskinesia

For a discussion of lithium preventing dopamine supersensitivity, refer to previous section on mechanism of action, neurotransmission.

Animal, studies have shown conflicting reports regarding the efficacy of lithium in the prevention of dopamine supersensitivity caused by neuroleptics (see section on Dopamine).

In open trials with human subjects, lithium has shown some effectiveness in decreasing the symptoms of tardive dyskinesia. In four open trials with a total of ten patients treated, three had dosage-related improvement, one had complete remission, and the other six had small but statistically significant improvement. In a fifth trial, lithium was combined with an antidepressant in agitated, depressed patients to treat tardive dyskinesia and major depression; and 11 of 19 patients showed marked improvement in both depression and tardive dyskinesia (Jefferson, 1983).

Controlled studies have shown less encouraging results. Gerlach (1975) and others compared the use of lithium with a placebo in a double-blind, cross-over trial in 15 patients with tardive dyskinesia. The patients had various psychiatric diagnoses. Each drug was tried for a period of three weeks, and previous drugs were also continued. There were marked individual differences, but symptoms were reduced by an average of 25% while taking lithium. Simpson (1976) evaluated lithium in a single-blind trial and a placebo-controlled, double-blind trial in elderly patients with tardive dyskinesia. Previous medications were continued during the single-blind trial, but were discontinued during the double-blind trial. The investigators found no statistically significant effect of lithium in either the single-blind or double-blind trial. Mackay (1980) performed a double-blind, placebo-crossover trial in 11 patients with tardive dyskinesia who continued to take background medications. There was no significant effect after five weeks of lithium treatment. Jus (1978) compared lithium, deanol, and placebo in a double-blind, cross-over trial. The patients continued to take neuroleptics. Neither drug produced statistically significant improvement, but some improved; and individual responses varied greatly.

SIDE EFFECTS AND TOXICITY

With the increased clinical use of lithium therapy over the last ten years comes a concomitant increase in the number and variety of reported side effects. Some side effects are innocuous and transient, even with the continuation of lithium treatment. Others are reversible with discontinuation of the drug. Finally, there are reports of potentially irreversible side effects.

Early side effects in the initiation of lithium therapy, as well as the ones occurring during maintenance therapy, are expressed against therapeutic serum lithium concentration (0.6-1.4 mEq/L). Toxicity is usually associated with high serum lithium concentration (above 2.0 mEq/L), this is not always the case (Jefferson 1983).

SIDE EFFECTS ACCORDING TO SYSTEMS
Dermatological

Acne may begin or worsen during lithium treatment (Deandra, 1982). Psoriasis has also been reported to be worsened by lithium therapy; and, unless lithium is discontinued, antipsoriatic treatment is generally ineffective. There have been 19 recent cases of papular and 2 cases of nonpapular rashes (Jefferson, 1983). Frenk (1981) describes verrucous hyperplasia after 5 years of lithium treatment.

Hair loss in both hypothyroid and euthyroid patients receiving lithium can occur (Heng 1982, Dawber 1982). Etiology is unclear. Initial treatment is to observe; some dermatological problems clear spontaneously. Topical steroid cream or antihistamines may be useful (Bernstein, 1983). If problem persists, consider discontinuing lithium. Reinstitution of lithium has not always led to resumption of problem (Bernstein, 1983).

Endocrinological
Thyroid

Lithium can cause hyperthyroidism, goiter and hypothyroidism (Mannisto, 1980). Approximately 5% of patients will develop goiter, and 3–4% will develop hypothyroidism. Lazarus reported up to 30% of patients had an elevated TSH level and up to 50% had an exaggerated response to thyrotropin releasing factor. Clinical hypothyroidism occurs in patients with a preliminary history of thyroid abnormalities and occurs much more frequently in women. Goiter, however, is seen slightly more in men than women (Jefferson, 1983). Generally, lithium-induced hypothyroidism is felt to be reversible after discontinuation of the drug; however, Perrid (1978) described two irreversible cases. If lithium is continued, supplemental use of exogenous thyroid extract can restore thyroid functions.

Hyperthyroidism and exophthalmus have also been occasionally reported (Rabin, 1981). The mechanism is unclear.

Parathyroid hormone and calcium metabolism

Frank (1982) found elevated levels of parathyroid hormone, serum calcium and magnesium with no clinical manifestations. However, a case of an acute hypoparathyroid and hypercalcemic state has been reported (Rothman, 1982).

Diabetes mellitus

Lithium may impair insulin release. High glucose and glucogen levels may stimulate a compensatory increase in insulin release resulting in normalization of glucose metabolism (Waziri 1978). However, for the insulin-dependent diabetic on lithium, insulin resistance can occur, and increased insulin may be required.

Gastrointestinal

Gastrointestinal complaints commonly appear. Anorexia, vomiting, loose stools, nausea and abdominal pains have been extensively reported, especially with higher doses of lithium; and if the drug is taken on an empty stomach (Lydiard, 1982). Vestergard, 1980, reported 20% of 237 patients receiving lithium for 5.2 years complaining of troublesome diarrhea.

Gastrointestinal effects are related to GI absorption. They can be treated with the passage of time, more frequent administration of smaller doses, ingestion of the drug with meals and the use of slow release preparations or the use of citrated form. Although generally benign, GI symptoms may also be an early warning of severe lithium intoxication, and one should assess for other signs of toxicity.

Cardiovascular

The most documented cardiovascular effect of lithium treatment is a benign change in ECG repolarization; at regular doses, a dependent "T" wave flattening or inversion developed within the first few weeks and disappeared spontaneously. Risch (1981) reported at toxic levels S-T segment depression and Q-T prolongation. Sinus node abnormalities, sinoatrial and atrioventricular blocks, atrial and venticular arrythmias, as well as cardiomyopathy have occasionally been described (Weintraub, 1983 and Albrecht, 1980).

Jefferson (1983) concluded that lithium had no clinically relevant effects on blood pressure.

Hematological

Jefferson concluded that the most consistent hematological effect is a reversible granulocytosis, representing an increase in total body granulocytosis in addition to a shift from bone marrow reserve. The leukocytosis primarily consists of an increase in mature neutrophils whose phagocytic ability remains intact, although Friedenberg (1980) reported reduced bactericidal activity.

Hussain (1973) reported fatal aplastic anemia; however, other medications were administered concurrently, and a definite casual relationship has not yet been determined.

Neurological

One of the most common early side effects of lithium therapy, and perhaps the most common neurological side effect, is tremor. Vestergaard (1980) reported 45% of 237 patients on long-term therapy with fine tremors. Distinction should be made between fine tremor and the coarse hand tremors that may be indicative of lithium intoxication. (See Below). Although fine tremors usually improve with time, treatment may be necessary. Jefferson (1983) advised to reduce the lithium level and caffeine intake. If still symptomatic, use a beta adrenergic blocker (e.g. propranolol). Other mild side effects are confusion, fatigue, muscle weakness, and lethargy. Treatment is through dose adjustment, either more frequent divided doses or a sustained release form (Jefferson, 1983).

Long-term memory impairment and a slowing of information processing have been described. However, Ananth (1981) found no differences between lithium-treated, tricylic-antidepressant treated and untreated psychiatric patients although lithium seems to enhance memory deficits of ECT (Bernstein, 1983).

Unilateral EEG spiking in patients on lithium for a least 5 years has been reported by Tyrer (1980). However, there was the suggestion of pre-existing EEG irregularities as a predisposing factor. This group also found that lithium increases slow wave (delta) sleep, decreases the duration of rapid eye movements (REM) sleep, and decreases REM latency but does not change total sleep time, differing from most REM suppressors by not being associated with REM rebound.

More severe neurological symptoms may be prodromal signs of impending lithium intoxication, usually initiated by dysarthia and ataxia. Coarse hand tremors, muscular fasiculations and twitching, slurred speech and extrapyramidal effects, and cogwheel rigidity have been reported (Vestergaard 1980, Ghadivian 1980).

Lithium intoxication is primarily a neurotoxicity. Besides the above neurotoxic signs, marked neuromuscular irritability, seizures, impaired consciousness, irreversible neurological damage, coma and death have been reported (Ghadivian 1980), as well as a severe peripheral neuropathy (Pamphlett 1982).

Schou (1980) advises that if the lithium level is less than 3mEq/l and clinical signs are mild, correction of fluid and electrolyte abnormalities are usually sufficient. If the lithium level is above 3 mEq/l or with signs of severe intoxicity, then hemodialyze the patient.

Renal

Renal biopsy studies of patients on lithium have found higher than expected incidence of nonspecific morphological damage characterized by intestinal fibrosis (Lippoman 1982). It is hard to suggest lithium as the sole factor. Similar abnormalities have been reported in the kidney of patients with affective disorders who have not received lithium, making patients with mood disorders probably a predisposed factor for the development of renal damage (Lydiard 1982). Despite renal anatomical abnormalities associated with long-term lithium use, glomeular filtration appears to be well preserved (Vestergaard 1982, Wallin 1980).

It is conceivable that toxic lithium levels are required to produce renal damage, but the possibility of irreversible renal damage must be considered and prevented. Some preventive measures have been recommended by Jefferson (1983): screen for pre-existing renal pathology or family history of nephropathy; assess urine concentration capacity such as urine osmolity after a 12-hour, overnight dehydration; measure or estimate 24-hour creatinine clearance; and rule out diabetes mellitus, hypertension, and other causes of nephropathy. Renal function should be reassessed and monitored during the course of lithium therapy on a regular basis. Unless otherwise indicated by the patients' clinical condition or history, testing should be restricted to measuring serum creatinine every six months. Patients should be treated only for appropriate indications and at the lowest effective dosage level.

Increased thirst was described in a recent study in 40% of 237 lithium treated patients (Vestergaard 1980). Frequent urination has also been reported with increased thirst. Although early in therapy the concentration capacity of the kidney may not be affected and the polyuria appears to be dosage dependent, with the long-term administration of lithium, the polyuria may range from mild and well tolerated to severe nephogenic diabetis insipidus, a condition which may be aggravated by the concurrent administration of antipsychotic medication (Plengk 1982).

The impaired concentration capacity is believed to be a result of reduced renal response to the antidiuretic hormone (ADH). Lithium is reported to interfere with the formation of cyclic adenosine monophosphate (cAMP) by ADH-sensitive renal adenylate cyclase and also with the utilization of cAMP by a protein urinase. Also, lithium impairs fluid reabsorption in the proximal tubule (Schou 1968). Mild nephrogenic diabetes insipidus can be treated by ensuring sufficient fluid intake. Severe, nephrogenic diabetes insipidus requires reduction or discontinuance of lithium. Alternate concurrent administration of a thiazide diuretic with a decrease in lithium dosage can be tried (Singer 1981).

Developmental and reproductive effects

Lithium has teratogenic effects in lower species and probably in man. The most sensitive developmental period appears to be the first trimester of gestation (Lydiard 1980). Due to the unanswered question in regard to dysgenesis, it seems prudent to avoid considering lithium during the first third to the first half of pregnancy (Jefferson 1983). Also since lithium is excreted in breast milk and the potential dangers to the infant are unknown, lactating mothers should avoid breast feeding.

Reports of impotence and loss of libido are rare, and their incidence is difficult to estimate (Jefferson 1983). It has been suggested that lithium decreases sperm viability (Levin, 1981). However there is no evidence that the male fertility is reduced or that the risk of fetal malformation is increased in fathers taking Li + at the time of conception. Adverse effects on sexual function in women have not been reported.

Others

Intermittent edema was reported in 10% of the 237 patients used in (Vestergaard's study (1980). The mechanism for this edema is unclear and is usually resolved spontaneously.

Weight gain is a common and troublesome complication more likely to occur in patients who have had weight problems prior to lithium treatment and usually due to increase in flesh rather than fluid retention (Vestergaard 1980). Also, there has been a correlation established between lithium response and weight gain, with responses gaining significantly more weight than intermediate responses and nonresponders gaining no weight. Paselow (1980) found 13 out of 21 patients taking lithium had increased their pre-lithium weight by more than 5%, and only 2 out of 21 on placebo increased their weight. The mechanism behind weight gain is not fully known. The insulin effects of Li + on carbohydrate metabolism and the probable effect on lipid metabolism would contribute to fat formation. Other contributing factors to weight gain include the concurrent administration of antipsychotic or antidepressant medications and lithium-induced polydipsia with an excessive intake of high-calorie beverages.

In the management of weight gain, instructions for a sensible reducing diet that does not limit severely Na+ fluid intake and for an increase in the level of activities for patients are needed.

Isolated case reports of altered taste (Bressler 1980) and sialorrhea have been described in recent literature (Donaldson 1982).

It is interesting to mention that in Vesterguard's study (1980), only 10% of the patients did not have any complaints. A marked variation in the severity and extent of side effects is expected from patients undergoing lithium treatment. Clinical judgment is the key to determining if lithium's therapeutic benefits is worth the cost of its side effects. Having this in mind, obtaining and documenting the necessary baseline through screening and periodic monitoring of the different values to determine changes should provide clear guidelines for the management of these side effects.

SUMMARY

a. In the United States, lithium is currently approved by FDA for mania and for prophylaxis against mania in patients with manic-depressive illness.

b. Prior to initiation of lithium, obtain creatinine, BUN, electrolytes, thyroid function tests, EKG, CBC, urinalysis and serum glucose.

c. Severely-agitated, manic patients will usually need a neuroleptic to initially control their symptoms because lithium has a seven- to ten-day latency. Unless the patient is schizoaffective, once mania remits, the neuroleptic can be discontinued.

d. Unless toxicity is suspected, lithium levels are drawn twelve hours after last dose once steady state is achieved. Steady state is usually reached after five times the elimination half-life. This is usually by five days in patients without previous treatment, but *may* be eight to fourteen days in elderly patients or in patients on lithium for at least a year, as suggested by Goodnick (1981).

e. Lithium is generally considered for prophylaxis after at least two distinct manic episodes, each lasting at least a month. Baastrup (1980) believes that the case for prophylaxis of mania is strengthened if the patient is at least 40 years old, has a bipolar course, and may face significant stress.

f. Lithium appears to be useful for endogenous depression. Bipolar patients probably respond better than unipolar. Recurrent unipolar patients are more likely to respond if there are: a) family history of bipolar illness, b) history of mild hypomania or cyclothymia, c) history of post-partum depression, d) hypersomnia or hyperphagia during depression, e) early age of onset (Ramsey, 1982).

g. Lithium may augment monoamine oxidase inhibitors or tricyclic antidepressants in unipolar depressives who had been previously refractory.

h. Schizophrenia and schizoaffective disorder may show improvement. It is unclear if thought disorder improves. Overall research is hampered by imprecise diagnostic criteria.

i. Steroid-induced psychoses respond to lithium.

j. Lithium may be of value in chronic assaultive behavior or poor impulse control. Lithium may enable the person to delay acting on impulse.

k. Other conditions such as tardive dyskinesia, anorexia nervosa, obsessive-compulsive disorder, phobic disorder, and attention deficit disorder need further study before recommending lithium.

l. Studies of lithium in the treatment of alcoholism are hampered by high drop rates. Results, as yet, are inconclusive.

m. With the reports of renal problems associated with lithium use, it seems prudent to get baseline renal studies and reassess regularly. Increased polyuria may suggest a need to reassess.

n. Lithium toxicity may need to be treated with hemodialysis if level goes above 3 mEq/l or if symptoms are severe. Otherwise, treatment is by fluid and electrolyte replacement.

o. Besides reports of renal problems, side effects have been noted in almost every organ system, although many appear to be mild.

REFERENCES

Akisal, H.S.: Dysthymic Disorder: Psychopathology of Proposed Diagnostic Subtypes, *Am. J. Psychiat.* 140:11-20, 1983.

Ananth, J., Gold, J., Ghadirian, A.M. and Engelsmann, F.: Long-Term Effects of Lithium Carbonate on Cognitive Functions, *J. Psych. Tr.*3:551-555, 1981.

Baastrup, P.C. and Schou, M.: Lithium As a Prophylactic Agent: Its Effect Against Recurrent Depressions and Manic-Depressive Psychosis, *Arch. Gen. Psychiatry* 16:162-172, 1967.

Baastrup, P.C.: Lithium in the Prophylactic Treatment of Recurrent Affective Disorders. In: Handbook of Lithium Therapy, (F.N. Johnson, ed.), Lancaster, MTP Press, 26-38, 1980.

Bernstein, J.G.: Lithium in Handbook of Drug Therapy in Psychiatry, John Wright Psg., Inc., Boston, 1983.

Biederman, J., Lerner, X. and Belmaker,

R.H.: Combination of Lithium Carbonate and Haloperiodol in Schizoaffective Disorder, *Arch. Gen. Psychiatry* 36:327-333, 1979.

Bloom, F.E., Baetge, G., Deyo S., Ettenberg, A., Kodal, L., Magistretti, P.J., Shoemaker, W.J. and Staunton, D.A.: Chemical and Physiological Aspects of the Actions of Lithium and Antidepressant Drugs, *Neuropharmacology* 22:359-365, 1983.

Braden, W.: Response to Lithium in a Case of L-Dopa-Induced Psychosis, *Am. J. Psychiatry* 134:808-809, 1977.

Bressler, B.: An Unusual Side Effect of Lithium: Case Report Psychosomatics, August, 1980, Vol. 21, No. 8, pp. 688-689, 1980.

Brewerton, T.D. and Reus. V.J.: Lithium Carbonate and L-Tryptophan in the Treatment of Bipolar and Schizoaffective

Disorders, *Am. J. Psychiatr.* 140:757-759, 1983.

Brown, R.P., Ingber, P.S. and Tross, S.: Pemoline and Lithium in a Patient with Attention Deficit Disorder, *J. Clin. Psychiatry* 44:146-148, 1983.

Brown, W.T.: The Pattern of Lithium-Side Effects and Toxic Reactions in the Course of Lithium Therapy. In: Handbook of Lithium Therapy, (F.N. Johnson, ed.), MTP Press, Lancaster, pp. 279-288, 1980.

Bucht, G., Wahlin, A., Wentzel, T. and Winblad, B.: Renal Function and Morphology in Long-term Lithium and Combined Lithium-Neuroleptic Treatment, *A.C.T.A. Med. Science* 208:381-385, 1980.

Bunney, W.E. and Garland, B.L.: Possible Receptor Effects of Chronic Lithium Administration, *Neuropharm.* 22:367-372, 1983.

Cade, J.F.J.: Lithium Salts in the Treatment of Psychotic Excitement, *Med. J. Aust.* 36:349-352, 1949.

Caldwell, H.C., Westlake, W.J. and Connor, S.M.: A Pharmacokinetic Analysis of Lithium Carbonate Absorption from Several Formulations in Man, *J. Clin. Pharmacol.* 11:349-56, 1971.

Carman, J.S., Bigelow, L.B. and Wyatt, R.J.: Lithium Combined with Neuroleptics in Chronic Schizophrenia and Schizoaffective Patients, *J. Clin. Psych.* 42:124-128, 1981.

Chouinard, G., Jones, B.D. and Young, S.N.: Potentiation of Lithium by Tryptophan in a Patient with Bipolar Illness, *Am. J. Psychiatr.* 136:719-720, 1979.

Cohn, C.K., Wright, J.R. and Devaul, R.A.: Post Head Trauma Syndrome in an Adolescent Treated with Lithium Carbonate-Case Report, *Dis. Ner. Syst.* 38:630-631, 1977.

Cooper, A.F. and Fowlie, H.C.: Control of Gross Self-Mutilation with Lithium Carbonate., *Br. J. Psychiatr.* 122:370-371, 1973.

Coppen, A. and Abou-Saleh, M.T.: Lithium in the Prophylaxis of Unipolar Depression: A Review, *J. Royal Society Med.* 76:297-301, 1983.

Cooper, T.B. and Simpson, G.M.: The 24-HR Lithium Level as a Prognosticator of

Dosage Requirements: A Two-Year Follow-up Study, *Am. J. Psychiatr.* 133:440-443, 1976.

Cooper, T.B. and Carroll, B.J.: Monitoring Lithium Dose Levels: Estimation of Lithium in Blood and Other Body Fluids. *J. Clin. Psychopharm.* 1:53-58, 1981.

Davis, J.M.: Overview: Maintenance Therapy in Psychiatry: II Affective Disorders, *Am. J. Psychiatr.* 133:1-13, 1976.

Dawber, R. and Mortimer, P.: Hair Loss During Lithium Treatment, *Br. J. Dermatol* 107:124-125, 1982.

Deandrea, D., Walker, N., Mehlmauer, M. and White, K.: Dermatological Reactions to Lithium: A Critical Review of the Literature, *J. Clin. Psychopharm.* 2:199-204, 1982.

Delva, N.J. and Letemendia, F.J.J.: Lithium Treatment in Schizophrenia and Schizoaffective Disorders, *Br. J. Psychiatr.* 141: 387-400, 1982.

Delva, N.J., Letemendia, F.J.J. and Prowse, A.W.: Lithium Withdrawal Trial in Chronic Schizophrenia, *Br. J. Psychiatr.* 141:401-406, 1982.

De Montigny, C., Grunberg, F., Mayer, A. and Deschenes, J.P.: Lithium Induces Rapid Relief of Depression in Tricyclic Antidepressant Drug Non-Responders, *Br. J. Psychiat.* 138:252-256, 1981.

De Montigny, C., Cournoyer, G., Morissette, R., Langlois, R. and Caille, G.: Lithium Carbonate Addition in Tricyclic Antidepressant-Resistant Unipolar Depression, *Arch. G. Psychiat.* 40:1327-1334, 1983.

Donaldson, S.R.: Sialorrhea As a Side Effect of Lithium: A Case Report, *Am. J. Psychiatry* 139:10, pp. 1350-1351, October, 1982.

Donnelly, E.F., Murphy, D.L. and Waldman, I.N.: Obsessionalism and Response to Lithium, *Br. Med. Journal* 1:1627-1628, 1979.

Dostal, T. and Zvolsky, P.: Antiaggressive Effect of Lithium Salts in Severe Mentally Retarded Adolescents, *Int. Pharmacopsychiat.* 5:203-207, 1970.

Dunner, D.L., Stallone, F. and Fieve, R.: Lithium Carbonate and Affective Disorders, *Arch. G. Psychiat.* 33:117-120, 1976.

Dunner, D.L. and Stalloe, F.: Prophylaxis with Lithium Carbonate: An Update, *Arch. Gen. Psychiatry* 39:1344-1345, 1982.

Falk, W.E., Mahnke, M.W. and Poskanzer, D.C.: Lithium Prophylaxis of Corticotropin-Induced Psychosis, *J.A.M.A.* 241: 1011-1012, 1979.

Fieve, R.R., Kumbaraci, T. and Dunner, D.: Lithium Prophylaxis of Depression Bipolar I, Bipolar II, and Unipolar Patients, *Am.J. Psychiat.* 133:925-929, 1976.

Flemenbaum, A.: Antagonism of Behavioral Effects of Cocaine by Lithium, *Pharmacol. Biochem. Behav.* 7:83-85, 1977.

Forrest, D.V.: Bipolar Illness After Right Hemispherectomy, *Arch. G. Psychiat.* 39: 817-819, 1982.

Franks, R.D., Dubovsky, S.L. and Lifshitz, M.: Long-term Lithium Carbonate Therapy Cause Hyperparathyroidism, *Arch. G. Psychiat.* 39:1074-1077, 1982.

Frenk, E.: Inflammatory Verrucous Hyperplasia of the Skin, and Unusual Side-Effect of Long-Term Lithium Therapy, *Arch. Dermatol Res.* 270-226, 1981.

Friedenberg, W.R. and Marx, J.J.: Effect of Lithium Carbonate on Lympocyte Granulocyte and Platelet Function, *Cancer* 45:91-97, 1980.

Garfinkel, P.E., Strancer, H.C. and Persad, E.: A Comparison of Haloperidol Lithium Carbonate, and their Combination in the Treatment of Mania, *J. Affective Dis.* 2:279-288, 1980.

Gerlach, J., Thorsen, K. and Munkvad, I.: Effect of Lithium on Neuroleptic-Induced Tardive Dyskinesia Compared with Placebo in a Double-Blind Cross-Over Trial, *Pharmakopsych.* 8:51-56, 1975.

Gershon, S. and Yuwiler, A.: Lithium Ion; A Specific Pharmacological Approach to the Treatment of Mania, *J. Neuropsychiat.* 1:229-241, 1960.

Ghadirian, A.M. and Lehmann, H.E.: Neurological Side Effects of Lithium: Organic Brain Syndrome, Seizures, Extrapyramidal Side Effects, and EEG, Changes, *Comp. Psychiat.* 21:327-335, 1980.

Goggans, F.C., Weisberg, L.J. and Koran, L.M.: Lithium Prophylaxis of Prednisone Psychosis: A Case Report, *J. Clin. Psychiat.* 44:111-112, 1983.

Goodnick, P.J., Fieve, R.R., Melzer, H.L. and Dunner, D.: Lithium Elimination, Half Life and Duration of Therapy, *Clin. Pharmacol Ther.* 29:47-50, 1981.

Goodwin F.K. and Zis, A.P.: Lithium in the Treatment of Mania: Comparisons with Neuroleptics, *Arch. G. Psychiat.* 36:840-844, 1979.

Gross, H.A., Ebert, M.H., Faden, V.B., Goldberg, S.C., Nee, L.E. and Kaye, W.H.: A Double Blind Controlled Trial of Lithium Carbonate in Primary Anorexia Nervosa, *J. Clin. Psychopharm.* 1:376-381, 1981.

Groth, U., Prellwitz, W. and Jahnchen, E.: Estimation of Pharmacokinetic Parameters of Lithium from Saliva and Urine, *Clin. Pharm. Ther.* 16:490-98, 1974.

Hale, M.S. and Donaldson, J.O.: Lithium Carbonate in the Treatment of O.B.S. *J. Nerv. and Ment. Dis.* 170:362-365, 1982.

Hansen, H.E.: Renal Toxicity of Lithium Drugs, (6):461-476, Dec. 22, 1981, (96 Ref.).

Havens, W.N., Cole, J.: Successful Treatment of Dementia With Lithium, *J. Clin. Psychopharm.* V2:71-72, 1982.

Heng, M.C.Y.: Cutaneous Manifestations of Lithium Toxicity, *Br. J. Dermatol* 106:107-109, 1982.

Heninger, G.R., Charney, D.S. and Sternberg, D.E.: Lithium Carbonate Augmentation of Antidepressant Treatment, *Arch. G. Psychiatr.* 40:1335-1342, 1983.

Himmelhoch, J.M., Hill, S., Steinberg, B. and May, S.: Lithium, Alcoholism, and Psychiatric Diagnosis Presented at the Annual Meeting of the APA, San Francisco, 1980.

Hussain, M.Z., Khan, A.G. and Chaudhry, Z.A.: Aplastic Anemia Associated with Lithium Therapy, *CAN Med. Assoc. J.* 108:724-728, 1973.

Jann, M.W., Bitar, A.M. and Rao, A.: Lithium Prophylaxis of Tricyclic-Antidepressant-Induced Mania in Bipolar Patients, *Am. J. Psychiatr.* 139:683-684, 1982.

Jefferson, J.W., Greist, J.H. and Ackerman, D.L.: Lithium Encyclopedia for Clinical Practice, *American Psychiatric Press, Inc.* Wash, D.C., 1983

Jus, A., Villeneuve, A. and Gautier, J.: Deanol, Lithium, and Placebo in Treatment of Tardive Dyskinesia-Double-Blind Cross Over Study *Neuropsychobiology* 4:140-149, 1978.

Kafka, M.S., Wirz-Justice, A., Naber, D., Marangos, P.J., O'donohue, T.L. and Wehr, T.A.: The Effect of Lithium on Circadian Neurotransmitter Receptor Rhythms, *Neuropsychobiology* 8:41-50, 1982.

Kane, J.M., Quitkin, F.M. and Rifkin. A., et al.: Lithium Carbonate and Imipramine in the Prophylaxis of Unipolar and Bipolar II Patients, *Arch. Gen. Psychiatry* 39:1065-1069.

Kemp, K., Lion, J.R. and Magram, G.: Lithium in the Treatment of a Manic Patient with Multiple Sclerosis, *Dis. Nerv. Syst.* 38:210-211, 1977.

Kline, N.S., Wren, J.C., Cooper, T.B. Varga, E. and Canal, O.: Evaluation of Lithium Therapy in Chronic and Periodic Alcoholism, *Am. J. Med. Sci.* 268:15-22, 1974.

Kline, N.A.: Lithium and Crisis Intervention: Dampening Affective Overload, *Psychosomatics* 19:401-405, 1978.

Kocsis, J.H.: Lithium in the Acute Treatment of Mania. In: Handbook of Lithium Therapy, (F.N. Johnson, ed.), MTP Press, Lancaster, pp. 9-16, 1980.

Kocsis, J.H.: Treatment of Mania, *Comp. Psychiatr.* 22:596-602, 1981.

Kripke, D.F., Judd, L.L., Hubbard, B., Janowsky, D.S. and Huey, L.Y.: The Effect of Lithium Carbonate on the Circadian Rhythm of Sleep in Normal Human Subjects, *Biological Psychiatr.* 14:545-548, 1979.

Kupfer, D.J., Pickar, D., Himmelhoch, J.M. and Detre, T.P.: Are There Two Types of Unipolar Depression, *Arch. G. Psychiatr.* 32:866-871, 1975.

Lazarus, J.H., John, R., Bennit, E.H., Chalmers, R.J. and Crockett, G.: Lithium Therapy and Thyroid Function: A Long Term Study, *Psychol. Med.* 11:85-92, 1981.

Levin, R.M., Amsterdam, J.D., Windkur, A. and Wein, A.J.: Effects of Psychotropic Drugs on Human Sperm Motility, *Fertil. Steril.* 36:503-506, 1981.

Lipinski, J.F. and Pope, H.G., Jr.: Possible Synergistic Action Between Carbamazepine and Lithium Carbonate in the Treatment of Three Acutely Manic Patients, *Am. J. Psychiatr.* 139:948-949, 1982.

Lippmann, S.: Is Lithium Bad for the Kidneys?, *J. Clin. Psychiatry* 43(6):220-224, June, 1982.

Lydiard, R.B. and Gelenberg, A.J.: Hazards and Adverse Effects of Lithium, *Ann. Rev. Med.* 33:327-44, 1982.

Mackay, A.V.P., Sheppard, G.P., Saha, B.K., Motley, B. Johnson, A.L. and Marsen, C.D.: Failure of Lithium Treatment in Established Tardive Dyskinesia, *Psychol. Med.* 10:583-587, 1980.

Mannisto, P.T.: Endocrine Side Effects of Lithium. In: Handbook of Lithium Therapy (F.N. Johnson, ed.), MTP Press, Lancaster, pp. 310-322, 1980.

Mailman, R.B., Kilts, C.B., Mueller, R.A., Harden, T.K. and Breese, G.R.: Lithium (Li) Administration Does Not Reverse G-Hydroxydopamine (G-OHDA)-Induced Supersensitivity, *Science* 39:1007, 1980.

McMillan, T.M.: Lithium and the Treatment of Alcoholism: A Critical Review, *Br. J. Addict.* 76:245-258, 1981.

Mehta, D.B.: Lithium and Affective Disorders Associated with O.B. Impairment, *Am. J. Psychiatr.* 133:236, 1976.

Mendels, J.: Role of Lithium as an Antidepressant, *Mod. Probl. Pharmacopsychiatr.* 18:138-144, 1982.

Merry, J., Reynolds, C.M., Bailey, J. and Coppen, A.: Prophylactic Treatment of Alcoholism by Lithium Carbonate (A Controlled Study) *Lancet* 2:481-482, 1976.

Miller, F.T. and Libman, H.: Lithium Carbonate in the Treatment of Schizophrenia and Schizo-Affective Disorder: Review and Hypothesis, *Society of Biol. Psychiatr.* 14:705-710, 1979.

Moss, G.R. and James, C.R.: Carbamazepine and Lithium Carbonate Synergism in Mania, *Arch. G. Psychiatr.* 40:588-589, 1983.

Naiman, I.F., Muniz, C.E., Stewart, R.B. and Yost, R.L.: Practicality of a Lithium Dosing Guide, *Am. J. Psychiatr.* 138:1369-1371, 1981.

Nelson, J.C. and Byck, R.: Rapid Response to Lithium in Phenelzine Non-Responders, Br. J. Psychiatr. 141:85-86, 1982.

Oyewumi, L.H. and Lapierre, Y.D.: Efficacy of Lithium in Treating Mood Disorder Occurring After Brain-Stem Injury, Am. J. Psychiatr. 138:110-111, 1981.

Pamphlett, R.S. and Mackenzie, R.A.: Severe Peripheral Neuropathy Due to Lithium Intoxication, Letters Journal of Neurology, Neurosugery, and Psychiatry 45:656-661, 1982.

Pandey, G.N. and Davis, J.M.: Cyclic-AMP and Adenylate Cyclase in Illness in Neuropharmacology of Cyclic Neucleotides, G.C. Palmer Urban and Scharzenberg, Baltimore, pp. 112-151, 1979.

Pandey, G. and Davis, J.M.: Treatment with Antidepressants, Sensitivity of B-Adrenergic Receptors and Affective Illness in Neuroreceptors Basic and Clinical Aspects (E USD,N, W.E. Bunney, J.M. Davis, eds.), Wiley, N.Y. pp. 99-120, 1981.

Perrid, H., Madsen, S.P. and Hansen, J.E.M.: Side Effects of Drugs: Irreversible Myxoedema after Lithium Carbonate, Br. Med. J. 1:1108-1109, 1978.

Perry, P.J., Alexander, B., Dunner, F.J., Schoenwald, R.D., Pfdhl, B. and Miller, D.: Pharmacokinetic Protocol for Predicting Serum Lithium Levels, J. Clin. Psychopharm. 2:114-118, 1982.

Pert, A., Rosenblatt, J.E., Sivit, C., Pert, C.B. and Bunney, W.E., Jr.: Long-Term Treatment with Lithium Prevents Development of Dopamine Receptor Supersensitivity, Science 201:171-173, 1977.

Peselow, E.D., Dunner, D.L., Fieve, R.R. and Lautin, A.: Lithium Carbonate Weight Gain, J. Affective Disord. 2:303-310, 1980.

Peselow, E.D., Dunner, D.L. and Fieve, R.R.: Lithium Prophylaxis of Depression in Unipolar, Bipolar II, and Cyclothymic Patients, Am. J. Psychiat. 139:747-752, 1982.

Peselow, E.D., Gulbenkian, G., Dunner, D.L., Fieve, R.R. and Deutsch, S.I.: Relationship Between Plasma Lithium Levels and Prophylaxis Against Depression in Bipolar I, Bipolar II, and Cyclothymic Patients, Comp. Psychiat. 23:176-182, 1982.

Plenge, P., Mellerup, E.T., Bolwig, T.G., Brun, C., Hetmar, O., Ladefoger, J. and Rafaelsen, O.J.: Lithium Treatment: Does The Kidney Prefer One Daily Dose Instead of Two?, Acta. Psychiat. Scand. 6:121-128, 1983.

Pond, S.M., Becker, C.E., Vandervoort, R., Phillips, M., Bowler, R.M. and Peck, C.C.: An Evaluation of the Effects of Lithium in the Treatment of Chronic Alcoholism I: Clinical Results, Alcoholism Clin. Exp. Res. 5:247-251, 1981.

Price, L.H., Conwell, Y. and Nelson, J.C.: Lithium Augmentation of Combined Neuroleptic-Tricyclic Treatment in Delusional Depression, Am. J. Psychiat. 140:318-322, 1983.

Prien, R.J.: Lithium in the Prophylactic Treatment of Affective Disorders, Arch. G. Psychiat. 36:847-848, 1979.

Procci, W.R.: Mania During Maintenance Hemodialysis Successfully Treated with Oral Lithium Carbonate, J. Nerv. Ment. Dis. 164:355-358, 1977.

Procci, W.R.: Schizoaffective Psychosis: Fact or Fiction?, Arch. G. Psychiat. 33:1167-1178, 1976.

Rabin, P.L. and Evan, D.C.: Exophalmos and Elevated Thyroxine Levels in Association with Lithium Therapy, J. Clin. Psych. 398-400, 1981.

Ramsey, T.A. and Mendels, J.: Lithium in the Acute Treatment of Depression. In: Handbook of Lithium Therapy, (F.N. Johnson, ed.), MTP Press, Lancaster, pp. 17-25, 1980.

Reches, A., Wagner, H.R., Jackson, V. and Fahn, S.: Chronic Lithium Administration Has No Effect on Haloperidol-Induced Supersensitivity of Pre- and Postsynaptic Dopamine Receptors in Rat Brain, Brain Research 172-177, 1982.

Rosenbaum, A.M. and Barry, M.J.: Positive Therapeutic Response to Lithium in Hypomania 2° to OBS, Am. J. Psychiat. 132:1072-1073, 1975.

Rosenblatt, J.E., Pert, C.B., Tallman, J.F., Pert, A. and Bunney, W.E., Jr.: The Effect of Imipramine and Lithium on Alpha and Beta Receptor Binding in Brain Research, 160:186-191, 1979.

Rothman, M.D.: Acute Hyperparathyroidism in a Patient After Initiation of Lithium Therapy, *Am. J. Psychiatry* 139(3): 362-363, March, 1982.

Ryback, R.S. and Schwab, R.S.: Manic Response to Levodopa Therapy: Report of a Case, *N.E.J.M.* 825:788-789, 1971.

Schou, M.: Lithium in Psychiatry: A Review Proceedings of the Sixth Annual Meeting of the American College of Neuropsychopharmacology in Psychopharmacology—A Review of Progress 1957-1967 (D.H. Efron, ed.), PHS. No. 1836, U.S. Gov. Printing Off., Wash., D.C, 1968.

Schou, M.: Lithium as a Prophylactic Agent in Unipolar Affective Illness, *Arch. G. Psychiat.* 36:849-851, 1979.

Schou, M.: a) Lithium Preparations Currently Available. In: Handbook of Lithium Therapy, (F.N. Johnson, ed.), MTP Press, Lancaster, Eng., pp. 237-242, 1980.

Schou, M.: b) The Psychiatric Uses of Lithium Outside Manic-Depressive Illness. In: Handbook of Lithium Therapy, (F.N. Johnson, ed.), MTP Press, Lancaster, pp. 68-72, 1980.

Scott, M.E. and Mullaly, R.W: Lithium Therapy for Cocaine-Induced Psychosis: A Clinical Perspective, *Southern Med. Journal* 74:1475-1477, 1981.

Sheard, M.H.: Effect of Lithium on Human Aggression, *Nature* 230:113-114, 1971.

Sheard, M.H., Marini, J.L., Bridges, C.I. and Wagner, E.: The Effect of Lithium on Impulsive Aggressive Behavior in Man, *Am. J. Psychiat.* 133:1409-1413, 1976.

Sheard, M.H.: The Effect of Lithium and Other Ions on Aggressive Behavior Psychopharmacology and Aggression (L. Valzelli, ed.), *Mod. Probl. Pharmacopsychiat.* Kargen Basel, 13:53-68, 1978.

Shopsin, B., Gershon, S. and Thompson, H.: Psychoactive Drugs in Mania: A Controlled Comparison of Lithium Carbonate, Chlorpromazine and Haloperidol, *Arch. G. Psychiat.* 32:34-42, 1975.

Shopsin, B. and Waters, B.: The Pharmacotherapy of Major Depressive Syndrome, *Psychosomatics* 21:542-556, 1980.

Shopsin, B., Johnson, G. and Gershon, S.: Neurotoxicity with Lithium: Differential Drug Responsiveness, *Int. Pharmacopsychiat.* 5:170-182, 1970.

Siegal, F.P.: Lithium for Steroid-Induced Psychosis, N.E.J.M., 299:155-156, 1978.

Simpson, G.M., Branchey, M.H., Lee, J.H., Voitashevsky, A. and Zovbok, B.: Lithium in Tardive Dyskinesia, *Pharmakopsych.* 9:76-80, 1976.

Singer, I.: Lithium and the Kidney-Nephrology Forum, *Kidney Int.* 19:374-387, 1981.

Slavney, P.R., Rich, G.B. and Pearlson, G.D.: Phencyclide Abuse and Symptomatic Mania, *Biol. Psychiat.* 12:697-700, 1977.

Spirtes, M.A.: Lithium Levels in Monkeys and Human Brain After Chronic Therapeutic Oral Dosage, *Pharmacol. Biochem. Beh.* 5:143-147, 1976.

Spring, G.K.: The Relative Efficacies of Lithium and Alternative Modes of Treatment. In Handbook of Lithium Therapy, (F.N. Johnson, ed.), Lancaster, MTP Press 80-91, 1980.

Spring, G. and Frankel, M.: New Data on Lithium and Haloperiodol Incompatibility, *Am. J. Psychiat.* 138:818-821, 1981.

Staunton, D.A., Magistretti, P.J., Shoemaker, W.J. and Bloom, F.E.: Effect of Chronic Lithium Treatment on Dopamine Receptors in the Rat Corpus Striatum, I. Locomotor Activity and Behavior Supersensitivity, *Brain Research* 232:391-400, 1982.

Sulser, F.: New Perspectives on the Mode of Action of Antidepressant Drugs, *Tr. Pharmacol. S.C.* 1:92-94, 1979.

Tanimoto, K., Maeda, K. and Chihara, K.: Antagonizing Effect of Lithium on the Developing of Dopamine Supersensitivity in the Tuberoinfundibular System, *Brain Research* 245:163-166, 1982.

Thornhill, D.P.: The Biological Disposition and Kinetics of Lithium, *Biopharm. and Drug Disposition* 2:305-322, 1981.

Treiser, S. and Kellar, K.J.: Lithium Effects on Adrenergic Receptor Supersensitivity in Rat Brain, *Evr. J. Pharmacol.* 58:85-86, 1979.

Tupin, J.P., Smith, D.B. and Clanon, T.L.: The Long-Term Use of Lithium in Aggressive Prisoners, *Comp. Psychiat.* 14: 311-317, 1973.

Tyrer, S., Shopsin, B.: Neural and Neuro-muscular Side Effects of Lithium. In: Handbook of Lithium Therapy, (F.N. Johnson, ed.), MTP Press Lancaster, England, pp. 289-309, 1980.

Vestergaard, P. and Amdisen, A.: Lithium Treatment and Kidney Function: A Follow-up Study of 237 Patients in Longterm Treatment, Acta. Psychiat. Scand. 63:333-345, 1981.

Vestergaard, P., Amdisen, A. and Schou, M.: Clinically Significant Side Effects of Lithium Treatment: A Survey of 237 Patients in Long-Term Treatment, Acta. Psychiat. Scand. 62:193-200, 1980.

Vestergaard, P., Schou, M. and Thomsen, K.: Monitoring of Patients in Prophylactic Lithium Treatment: An Assessment Based on Recent Kidney Studies, Br. J. Psychiat. 140:185-187, 1982.

Wallin, L., Alling, L. and Aurell, M.: Impairment of Renal Function in Patients on Long-term Lithium Treatment, Clin. Nephrol. 18:23-28, 1982.

Watanabe, S. and Ishino, H.: Special Cases of Affective Disorder and Their Treatment with Lithium. In: Handbook of Lithium Therapy, (F.N. Johnson, ed.), Lancaster, MTP Press 39-46, 1980.

Waziri, R. and Nelson, J.: Lithium in Diabetes Mellitus: A Paradoxical Response, J. Clin. Psychiat. 39:623-625, 1978.

Weintraub, M., Hes, J.P., Rotmensch, H.H., Soferman, G. and Liron, M.: Extreme Sinus Bradicardia Associated with Lithium Therapy, Isr. J. Med. Sci. 19:353-355, 1983.

Williams, K.H. and Goldstein, G.: Cognitive and Affective Responses to Lithium in Patients with OBS, Am. J. Psychiat. 136:800-803, 1979.

Worrall, E.P., Moody, J.P. and Naylor, G.J.: Lithium in Non Manic-Depressives: Antiaggressive Effect and Red Blood Cell Lithium Values, Br. J. Psychiat. 126:464-468, 1975.

Young, L.D., Taylor, I. and Holmstrom, V.: Lithium Treatment of Patients with Affective Illness Associated with OBS, Am. J. Psych. 134:1405-1407, 1977.

CHAPTER 13

Psychopharmacology of Cocaine: Behavior, Neurophysiology, Neurochemistry and Proposed Treatment

Karl Verebey, Ph.D.
Mark S. Gold, M.D.

INTRODUCTION

The aim of this review is the examination of our current knowledge of the psychopharmacology of cocaine. The behavioral effects will be correlated with neurophysiological and neurochemical events.

As with any other drugs of dependence, cocaine effects are variable depending on many factors. Such variables are the purity of the preparation, the route of administration, the chronicity of use, the personality and mental health of the user, the past and present use of other drugs or alcohol, the environment in which the drug is used and the other drugs which are knowingly or unknowingly taken along with the drug of interest. Thus the same set of observations described by a particular user will not occur exactly in each individual even with the identical dose of cocaine. But the general trend which was described by many users, by many observers over many years will describe adequately the typical effects of cocaine. By attempting to look at what cocaine does behaviorally and physiologically, how cocaine does it and what are the physiological roles of the substances cocaine effects we may be able to understand better "the drug" called the "Champagne of Drugs" and may arrive at a rational treatment proposal of the cocaine "addict."

THE BEHAVIORAL EFFECTS OF COCAINE

Cocaine effects at low to average doses as described by many investigators, textbooks and subjects, provide a generally enjoyable state referred to as euphoria (Jaffe, 1965). The users experience an increase in self confidence and self image. But what is considered by low to average doses? It is difficult to say definitely due to adulterants in street preparations. In general 10 mg cocaine is referred to constitute a "line" by users (Wesson and Smith, 1978). The name line is derived from the ⅛" by 1" arrangement of the white powder on a piece of glass or mirror, prepared for intranasal administration (or snorting). This being the most common method of cocaine administration by recreational users.

Before getting into the behavioral effects of cocaine another question must be answered: How pure are the street preparations and about what percent of cocaine can be expected in street cocaine? Pure cocaine is generally not available in street preparations. The most common substances mixed into cocaine are: mannitol, lactose, glucose, inositol to produce increased weight and lidocaine, procaine, tetracaine, amphetamines, PCP, heroin, quinine and taste and additional CNS stimulant effects (Bastos and Hoffman, 1976). The concentration of cocaine in street preparations ranges from 10 to 50% most being between 15 to 20% (Gupta et al., 1974). Both the cocaine concentration and obviously the adulterants in the various preparations affect the observed responses. The effects listed in Table 1 describe typical reactions to a single 25 mg intranasal dose of pure pharmaceutical cocaine hydrochloride (Byck and Van Dyke, 1977). Within minutes the effects of cocaine are felt. Euphoria and seldom dysphoria are observed. Whether an individual likes or dislikes cocaine may depend on his or her adrenergic or thyroxin dependent regulation of his normal state of excitation. Certain individuals in their normal state are more subdued than others. On the other hand there

TABLE 1. Cocaine effects. Low to average doses (25-150 mg)
($\approx$ 20-30 mg/line)

Generally enjoyable effects with great increase in self-image. A rapid onset of "high" with the following components:
  1. Euphoria, seldom dysphoria
  2. Increased sense of energy
  3. Enhanced mental acuity, alertness
  4. Increased sensory awareness (sexual, auditory, tactile, visual)
  5. Decreased appetite (anorexia)
  6. Decreased need of sleep
  7. Allows postponement of fatigue
  8. Increased self-confidence-egocentricity
  9. Delusions–dependence
  10. Physical symptoms of a generalized sympathetic discharge

---

are hyperexcited individuals as well in the population. In fact, all people fit somewhere in between the two extremes based on their steady state level of stimulation which may be regulated by adrenalin and/or thyroxine among other internal regulators. Cocaine is often misclassified into the sympathomimetic amines' class due to its similarity to amphetamines in its behavioral effects. Although cocaine is a local anesthetic it is a powerful stimulant of the central nervous system (CNS) (Stripling and Ellingwood, 1976). It is quite logical therefore that an individual with average or especially low level of excitation would enjoy the cocaine related effects and would be euphoric from the alertness, energy and overall stimulation cocaine provides. On the other hand individuals who are in their normal state are already hyperexcited and hypomanic may feel uncomfortable and dysphoric and may even develop paranoid psychosis from the cocaine related major sympathetic discharge. Similarly, psychosis was often observed in predisposed individuals after the administration of even low doses of amphetamines (Gold and Bowers, 1978). These effects may be diagnostic in patients with psychotic tendencies who do not appear overly psychotic in their daily routine. Such amphetamine sensitive individuals may have problems with cocaine as well. In another psychological disorder, depression, cocaine was found to worsen symptomatology (Post, 1976). Thus biologically depressed individuals are likely to experience exaggerated affect after cocaine use, manifested by dysphoria. This is a paradoxical situation since in some individuals cocaine (as amphetamines) can act like antidepressants, but in biological depression cocaine worsens depressive symptoms.

The feeling of well being in cocaine users may result from a generalized sympathetic discharge. One of the major effects of E is shifting the blood supply from the skin and the viscera into skeletal musculature (Vander, 1981). By the same adrenergic mechanism, there is increased levels of oxygen and by glycolysis higher concentrations of sugar in blood (Caldwell, 1976). In essence the cocaine stimulated reactions in the body are mimicking a natural physiological response; the generalized adrenergic discharge, stimulates the energy producing mechanisms to prepare the CNS and skeletal muscles for "fight or flight." This is a physiological purpose to prepare against impending threat. Being an important survival mechanism may be the reason for the lack of severe withdrawal symptoms after acute cocaine use. The organism quickly adjusts by having large reservoirs and using various backup systems by resynthesis of neurotransmitters, hormones and regeneration of the bioelectric mechanisms of CNS neurons. After depleting the reservoirs, these backup regenerating systems may not be as effective after chronic cocaine use thus physical withdrawal signs can be observed.

Are the feelings of increased mental acuity and alertness real or

illusional? The answer is a conditional yes, based on the electrical recordings from the CNS. EEG and ECG recordings show a general desynchronization of the brain waves after cocaine administration (Wallach
and Gershon, 1971). Desynchronization, especially in the reticular formation are convincing evidence for the cocaine related induction of alertness, since this brain location thought to be involved in the regulation
of conscious awareness and attention on one hand and sleep on the
other. While synchronization of neuronal, firing in the reticular formation, represent relaxation and sleep, desynchronization, as observed
after cocaine use, is a sign of arousal of the CNS (Wallach and Gershon,
1971). There is no evidence, however, that individuals gain deeper su-
pernatural ability and greater knowledge. They may feel omnipotent but
it is only illusional, their abilities are not above their natural level when
examined realistically. The confidence is greater, inhibitions absent and
it is often misinterpreted for greater knowledge and physical ability.

Cocaine is reported to produce increase in sensory awareness and
perception (auditory, visual and tactile). This is best explored by looking
at cocaine's effect on subjective reports of increased sexual stimulation.
There is considerable anatomical, neurological and biochemical evidence
that the amygdala is the major CNS center and dopamine (DA) the
neurotransmitter which is primarily involved in sexual excitation (Gatz,
1966). Cocaine is thought to effect this system specifically. So extreme
is cocaine's effect in this respect that following intravenous (IV) or in-
trapulmonary (freebase; FB) administration it alone can replace the sex
partner of either sex. Furthermore, when administered IV or FB, cocaine
can produce spontaneous ejaculation without direct genital stimulation
(Dimijian, 1974). Tolerance to the sexual stimulating effect of cocaine
rapidly develops and subsequently impotence and sexual frigidity are
seen in chronic cocaine users (Siegel, 1982). Direct application of cocaine
to the genitals lengthens sexual intercourse due to decreased sensation.
This effect is due to the local anesthetic property of cocaine.

Cocaine and the sympathomimetic amines, especially the amphetamines decrease appetite. Cocaine is thought to act through DA inac-
tivating the feeding center located in the lateral hypothalamus (Gropetti
and DiGuilio, 1976).

Decreased need of sleep may result from the cocaine induced release
and blockade of reuptake of DA and NE, which are stimulant neurotransmitters. Simultaneously, cocaine also depletes serotonin which
among its other functions is known as the "sleep transmitter" and it
antagonizes the stimulating effects of NE and DA. In cocaine naive individuals the negative balancing effects of serotonin may cause less
stimulation initially. In chronic cocaine use less and less serotonin is
available for release because cocaine interferes with its synthesis. Thus
the excitatory effects of NE and DA become even greater, since NE and

DA synthesis are stimulated by cocaine. This mechanism may be responsible for the observed "reverse tolerance" (Post and Rose, 1976; Stripling and Ellingwood, 1977). That is, greater excitation is achieved by subsequent doses than by the initial dose of cocaine.

The generalized energy mobilization and alert reaction produces a tremendous increase in self-confidence, self-image and egocentricity. The drug has the potential to produce megalomania and feelings of omnipotence in most individuals. The cocaine induced feelings of increased physical power and mental sharpness provides confidence which is best demonstrated by the professional defensive end who tries to pick up ("press") the offensive player or the high pressure sales man who feels that he could "sell the world" when using cocaine. The cocaine related increased energy, loquaciousness and self-confidence seems to help other professions as well. Entertainers and musicians and other modern day celebrities (e.g. physicians) also like cocaine, which provides them with bubbling energy and confidence and a "star-like" image. Their problems with cocaine dependence surfaces only after prolonged use. There is a price which has to be paid for all the CNS stimulation and self-confidence building. Due to the short time action of cocaine the undesirable side effects start to surface. These range from depression, fatigue, paranoia to outright acute toxic psychosis depending on the size of the dose and the route of administration. Looking at the neurochemical mechanisms, of cocaine action, it becomes clear that there is a limit to increasing CNS activity. After chronic excitation, rest, resynthesis of the transmitters and energy mechanisms must be accomplished for normal mental and physical functioning.

A commonly cited effect of cocaine is production of psychological dependence (Altshuler and Burch, 1976). Cocaine is deceptively addictive. Most recreational and moderate users would testify that they can take or leave cocaine. This in fact is not true. Given free access to cocaine a large percentage if not all cocaine users would soon find that all their lives revolve around cocaine: acquiring or using it. This delusion causing property of cocaine is most dangerous. There is a controversy polarizing medical and lay public opinion—one claiming that cocaine is safe, the other that it is dangerous. This diagonally different thinking is partly created by cocaine's delusional effects. Elite recreational users convincingly and eloquently misled psychiatrists and scientific investigators for years by "selling" the idea that while they use cocaine everything is under control with their lives and cocaine habits. The truth in most cases was that the control over cocaine's dependence was not self-regulated but it depended either on cocaine supply or price.

More rigorous inquiry into large numbers of cocaine users history, collected over the 800-Cocaine hotline, noted that even when the users still insisted that everything was alright in their lives, everything was slowly falling apart. The classic "cocaine delusion" was not recognized in the past as the source of general confusion over the dangers or safety of cocaine use. Clearly, one cannot accept the judgement of a cocaine user at full value about cocaine use because his or her reality is clouded by the cocaine related delusion.

One of the most convincing experiments demonstrating the dangers of cocaine came from self-administering monkey studies (Deneau et al., 1969). The self-administering monkeys demonstrated various behaviors which are similar to that seen in human abuse and toxicity. Such symptoms were: hyperactivity, paranoid psychosis, self-mutilation, convulsions, cardiovascular collapse and respiratory failure among others. The most striking phenomenon was that no other drug but cocaine was self administered until death. Other stimulants such as amphetamines, sympathomimetics, caffeine and nicotine were also self-administered but in binges. None were self-administered till self-destruction by death. In order to prolong the cocaine self-administration experiments beyond 30 days the intake of cocaine had to be restricted by the computer to one dose per hour no matter how often the lever was pushed.

Interestingly cocaine use is still not considered dangerous by the lay public and even by many psychiatrists and physicians. But if the extreme human users are reviewed (Gay et al., 1982), users for whom money was no object to purchase unlimited supply of cocaine, the observed behavior problem is very similar to the ones described in the monkey experiments. Intake constantly increases and the subjects are approaching or succeeding self-destruction. Thus, apparently the current safety of cocaine is strictly economical: high price and limited availability. Although more recently the price of cocaine is decreasing and is more available to a wider segment of the population than in the past. If cocaine would be legalized, based on the behavioral observations, there would be a great increase in the numbers and severity of cocaine related complications, accidents, overdoses and toxicity.

Another issue which has currently divided opinions is the presence or absence of physical dependence following chronic use of cocaine. Most text books of pharmacology claim that no physical dependence occurs because no signs and symptoms of withdrawal were seen following discontinuation of cocaine (Eddy et al., 1965). It is clear that no severe withdrawal symptoms such as seen in opiate withdrawal are present. But there is a group of milder symptoms of physical dependence which were observed and reported (Resnick and Schuyten-Resnick, 1976). The data on cocaine withdrawal signs in Table 2 are highly subjective. Half of the subjects responded that they "crashed" or were physically dependent after cocaine use. The specific psychological and physical withdrawal signs were: paranoia, depression, fatigue, craving, agitation, sweating and chills, insomnia and nausea/vomiting. There are

TABLE 2. Percent of subjects who experience "crashing" and "crash effects" most frequently reported

Do you "crash" after cocaine?		What effects do you get when you crash?	
		Effects	Number of subjects reporting
Yes	48%	Fear/paranoia	29
No	47%	Depression	28
No response	5%	Tired	27
		Want more	26
		Nervous	24
		Sweating/chills	13
		Insomnia	8
		Nausea/vomiting	8

Resnick R.B., Schuyten-Resnick, E. (1976).

two cautions which should be exercised when evaluating this data. First, similarly as in opiate dependence the severity of withdrawal symptoms and the percentage of subjects reporting physical dependence would depend on the size of cocaine dose and the length of time used. In this study, we have no information on these parameters could be obtained. Without controlled administration of cocaine no one can be certain how much drug was used by the subjects. Neither the subjects nor the investigators can be certain that the street preparation actually contained cocaine. Furthermore each subject had probably different sources of cocaine and different level of dependence. However, even with these deficiencies, the data appears significant, indicating that physical dependence develops after chronic administration of cocaine. Many of the signs indicate that the sympathetic nervous system is effected, and treatment should aim to reestablish the neurochemical balance to alleviate the various withdrawal symptoms listed in Table 2. It may be hypothesized that given a week of unlimited supply of pure pharmaceutical cocaine to the subjects interviewed (Table 2), the statistics of their responses would change significantly toward "yes" on the question of "crashing" and to the more serious complaints in the column of specific adverse effects.

When cocaine is administered in high to toxic doses either acutely or chronically, the effects change, compared to the ones described for the low to average doses. Table 3 lists the most commonly reported psychological effects, physical symptoms and toxic overdose effects after the administration of greater than 200 mg of cocaine (Gay and Inaba, 1976). Often such large doses are not only snorted but injected (IV) or administered by freebase smoking. The concensus is that the cocaine related "high" is significantly intensified but the behavorial complications listed in Table 3 are part of the severe price the cocaine addict must pay for taking such large doses. The psychological effects ranged from initial agitation and restlessness to intense anxiety. Hallucination, delusion and paranoid ideation are also observed after IV infusion of large doses of cocaine (Gay and Inaba, 1976). Most of these effects can be explained by the release and inhibition of reuptake of NE, DA, and depletion of serotonin by cocaine. Agitation, restlessness and anxiety are effects of NE hyperactivity, while paranoia, delusion and hallucination are part of DA hyperactivity especially in the hypothalamus and the amygdala. Insomnia is a dual effect of the increased NE, DA and decreased serotonin concentrations. Thus the upset of neurochemical balance by cocaine triggers CNS hyperactivity and crisis. Verbalization of impending doom by the subject should be taken seriously and emergency medical care provided immediately to prevent overdose death. The list in Table 3, second column describes the physical symptoms which precede the toxic effects described in the third column. These are rapid heart and breathing rates and pupillary mydriasis, etc. The physical symptoms are the familiar list of autonomic effects of E seen after generalized sympathetic discharge which as mentioned earlier, prepares the organism for "fight and flight" responses.

Symptoms of toxic overdose are listed in Table 3. Hyperexcitation on the CNS leads to convulsions. The very high fever can also be life threatening. This effect of cocaine is thought to be caused by resetting the medullary CNS thermostat (Ritchie et al., 1965). Treatment of this condition should be attended by providing ice baths or alcohol rubs to reduce body temperature. The fast heart rate along with high blood pressure often lead to a chain of events: ventricular fibrillation, circulatory failure, and respiratory failure. If the peripheral autonomic toxicity

TABLE 3. Cocaine effects. High to toxic doses >200 mg.

Generally intensification of the "High" but the price for that is bizarre often violent, paranoid psychotic symptomatology.

Psychological effects	Physical symptoms	Toxic overdose
1. Agitation, restlessness	1. Very rapid heart rate	1. Convulsions
2. Intense anxiety	2. Fast breathing rate	2. Tremors/muscular twitching incoordination
3. Hallucination	3. Pupillary mydriasis	3. Very high fever
4. Delusion	4. Increased sweating	4. Ventricular fibrillation
5. Insomnia	5. Paleness of the skin	5. Circulatory failure
6. Paranoia-suspiciousness	6. Hyperactive reflexes	6. Respiratory failure
7. Verbalization of impending doom	7. High body temperature	7. Paralysis of medullary centers
		8. Exitus

did not kill the subject, cocaine in high doses paralyzes the medullary cardio respiratory centers, causing death (Gay, 1982).

MEDICAL TREATMENT OF COCAINE TOXICITY

Depending on the severity of the cocaine toxicity syndrome two different approaches are suggested by Gay, 1982 and Rappolt et al., 1979 (Table 4). For the acute less severe type of cocaine toxicity diazepam is recommended. It is an excellent minor tranquilizer with anticonvulsant activity and a large therapeutic index. Its sedative effects are especially soothing for the hyper excited cocaine user. Muscle tension and spasms are visibly resolved 20 to 30 minutes after drug administration. The oral route is preferable because the needle may present threat to the paranoid subject. In more serious cocaine toxicity cases, seen mostly in chronic users, propranalol, a B-adrenergic blocking agent is recommended. A subject designated for such treatment would have symptoms of hyperkinesia with increased heart rate, blood pressure and respiratory rate. His limbs would show muscle jerks and tremor and his behavior would be characterized by having distorted perception. He would often be violent and delusional. The B-adrenergic blockade manifested by rapid decline in adrenergic tone would occur 3 to 5 minutes after IV propranolol or 15 to 30 minutes after oral doses.

Certain antipsychotic medications are actually contraindicated (Rappolt et al., 1979). Chlorpromazine and haloperidol are known to lower seizure threshold. The CNS of the cocaine user is already hyperstimulated and predisoposed to convulsions. The tricyclic antidepressants are not recommended during severe cocaine toxicity because they may trig-

TABLE 4. Medical treatment of acute cocaine toxicity

Acute	Chronic
(Single overdose)	(3-14 days use)
Diazepam	**Propranolol**
15-20 mg/6 to 8 hours	Intravenously—give in slow increments from 1 to 6 mg
Oral route preferable	
For night 20 mg	Orally 40-80 mg/4 to 6 hours for up to 1 week
Ideal for sedative and anticonvulsant activity	(A pulse of 90 or less is the goal)
	Acidify urine (NH$_4$ Cl) 75 mg/kg/dose 4 times/day
	Diazepam at bedtime
Contra-indicated	**Recommended supportive therapy**
CPZ and Haloperidol avoided because it lowers seizure threshold	Properly balanced diet
	Vitamin supplement
Tricyclic antidepressants avoided due to life threatening cardiac arrhythmias	Restful setting
	Psychological counseling

ger life threatening cardiac arrhythmias. While MAO inhibitors block cocaine degradation and prolong its effects, an action not needed in severe toxicity.

These procedures treat medical emergencies, leaving the common cocaine user and experienced user without effective treatment. Because the majority of the cocaine abusing population are slowly destroying their lives by their cocaine obsession, without major medical crisis, the only available treatment for moderate and novice cocaine abusers is behavior modification. Because of this open territory, it is worthwhile to investigate the literature carefully to explore how cocaine's pharmacological effects are produced and what neurophysiological and neurochemical systems are affected? The answers may provide clues for the reestablishment of the neurochemical equilibrium, upset by cocaine. Thus withdrawing subjects could be treated pharmacologically to prevent withdrawal symptoms and subsequent return to cocaine use.

THE LOCAL ANESTHETIC EFFECTS OF COCAINE

Cocaine was the first local anesthetic agent introduced into medical practice by Koller in 1884 (Stripling and Ellingwood, 1976). Now cocaine is often classified with the sympathomimetic agents because of its great similarity in its behavioral actions to amphetamines. The only legitimate medical use of cocaine today is in otolaryngal surgery because of its vasoconstrictive activity. While providing anesthesia it prevents bleeding into the otolaryngal pharynx (Barash, 1977). The mechanism of local anesthetic action is reasonably well understood (Figure 1) (Ritchie et al.,

COCAINE'S DIFFERENTIAL BLOCK OF NERVE CONDUCTION

Recording from a mixed nerve fiber of myelinated and non-myelinated fibers.

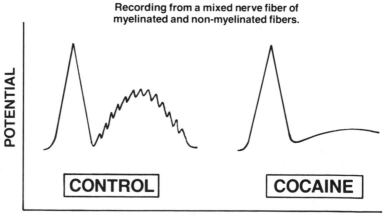

POTENTIAL

CONTROL

COCAINE

TIME (m sec)

1965). Although most behavioral actions of cocaine are explained by its sympathomimetic effects it is possible that its local anesthetic property is also involved in its overall activity. The figure shows that single action potentials in myelinated fibers are transmitted but the multipotentials of unmyelinated sensory fibers are completely blocked. Thus the sensation of pain is blocked because the sensory transmission from the site of injury is inhibited. It is possible that cocaine does block transmission of small nonmyelinated fibers in the CNS as well. The mechanism of inhibition presented in Figure 1 is referred to as "differential block." This means that local anesthetics at usual doses only block small unmyelinated neuronal fibers while the myelinated motor fibers are uneffected.

NEUROPHYSIOLOGICAL EFFECTS OF COCAINE

Many investigators and reports describe the effects of cocaine on the brain's electrical activity (Altshuler, et al., 1976; Eidelberg et al., 1963; Rothbeller, 1957; Stripling and Ellingwood, 1976; Matsuzaki, 1976; Matsuzaki, 1977; Matsuzaki, 1978). An electrocorticogram of a monkey is presented in Figure 2 which is from the work of Matsuzaki et al (1978). The tracings demonstrate electrical activity before and after chronic cocaine treatment for 6 months. The figure shows great increase in the amplitude of electrical activity in all areas of the CNS after chronic cocaine administration. Electrical energy output is seen after chronic cocaine administration, compared to the pre-drug condition. Chronic cocaine user's EEG tracings also have similar high amplitude nervous activity which is likely to drain the CNS of stored bioelectric resources. This information suggests that the CNS energy generating system need to be replenished.

Cocaine's pharmacological effects are typically associated with "behavioral arousal." This event is manifested in EEG tracings by desynchronization of cortical activity especially in anatomical locations of the reticular formation and rhythmical slow activity in the hypocampus (Rothbeller, 1957; Stripling and Ellingwood, 1976). A typical and most prominent effect of cocaine is its generation of "spindle activity," (Figure 3). Recording directly from the amygdala in the absence of drugs, no spindle activity is observed while after cocaine use there is frequent occurrence of spindles. Interestingly a local anesthetic, lidocaine, produces similar spindle activity in the mygdala while amphetamine does not (Stripling and Ellingwood). This CNS effect of cocaine is possibly related to cocaine's local anesthetic property.

Various cocaine related behavior such as violence and increased sex drive may be mediated through the amygdala. Surgical removal of the amygdala causes violent reaction in cats, while producing tame and 1970; Gropetti et al, 1973; Prioux-Gruyonneau et al, 1975). Nevertheless, it is possible to construct a model describing a theoretical mechanism of

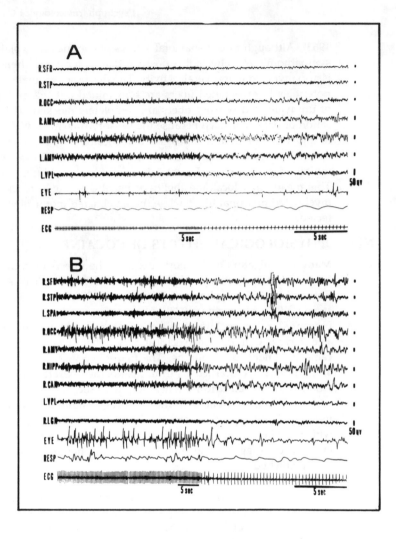

5.0 MG/KG COCAINE
HYDROCHLORIDE (I.V.)

	PRE-INJECTION	INJECTION + 15 SECONDS	INJECTION + 100 SECONDS	INJECTION + 180 SECONDS	
L. OLFACTORY BULB					$100\mu V$
R. OLFACTORY BULB					$100\mu V$
L. AMYGDALA					$100\mu V$
R. AMYGDALA					$100\mu V$
L. OLFACTORY TUBERCLE					$100\mu V$
L. N. ACCUMBENS					$100\mu V$

1 SECOND

docile effects in monkeys and rats. Interestingly, the same procedure increases sexual drive in all three species (Gatz, 1966). The antipsychotic agent chlorpromazine may also act through the amygdala. It causes excitation in cats while sedation in monkeys, rats and humans. Thus the cocaine related spindle activity in the amygdala may be the neurophysiological parallel of cocaine's behavioral effects. Spindles recorded from the olfactory bulb are correlated with stimulation of the reticular formation. This stimulatory effect seems responsible for the behavioral arousal seen after cocaine use.

COCAINE'S EFFECTS AT NEURONAL JUNCTIONS

Studies on the effect of cocaine on neurotransmitters in the brain and in the periphery are numerous and often the results are contradictory (Carmichael and Israel, 1973; Ross and Renji, 1967; Rudzik and Johnson, cocaine action (Figure 4). Cocaine seems to stimulate release of NE, DA and serotonin. There is also indication for the blocking of the reuptake of these neurotransmitters and inhibiting the intraneuronal enzyme MAO. These effects would create the observed increase in sympathetic activity. Some studies found that even after tremendous increase in behavioral effects and electrical CNS activity there is no significant change in the concentration of NE and DA (Gropetti et al, 1973; Prioux-Gruyonneau et al, 1975). This can only be logically accepted if, in addition to the above effects, the synthesis of the neurotransmitters is stimulated and rapidly replaced. This appears to be true for NE and DA, however

COCAINE'S LOCAL ANESTHETIC AND SYMPATHOMIMETIC EFFECTS

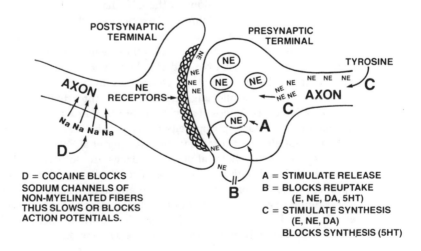

D = COCAINE BLOCKS SODIUM CHANNELS OF NON-MYELINATED FIBERS THUS SLOWS OR BLOCKS ACTION POTENTIALS.

A = STIMULATE RELEASE
B = BLOCKS REUPTAKE (E, NE, DA, 5HT)
C = STIMULATE SYNTHESIS (E, NE, DA) BLOCKS SYNTHESIS (5HT)

not for serotonin. Following release, cocaine inhibits its synthesis (Knapp and Mandell, 1972). The result is depletion of serotonin while NE and DA activities are high.

Before we accept this logical picture of cocaine's neurochemical mechanism of action, is there any experimental evidence for the involvement of the various neurotransmitters in cocaine's effects? There is evidence to support the fact that cocaine acts through DA, NE and E through pharmacological techniques which eliminate a group or selected neurotransmitters. Reserpine is known to deplete monoamines while -methylparatyrosine inhibits their synthesis. When given to animals both agents antagonized cocaine related locomotor hyperactivity and stereotyped behavior (Sayers and Handley, 1973). These studies imply that if the neurotransmitters are not present in the CNS in sufficient concentration cocaine cannot exhibit its usual behavioral effects. This further suggests that cocaine's effects are not direct but at least partly neurotransmitter mediated.

Serotonin in homeostasis seems to be the balancing neurohormone opposing the excitatory effects of NE and DA. This is partly supported by the experiment using parachlorphenylalanine which is known to deplete serotonin by blocking its synthesis. When cocaine was administered to parachlorphenylalanine treated animals an increase of the locomotor activity was seen (Scheel-Kruger et al, 1976). This study indicates that in the absence of serotonin an even greater excitatory effect of cocaine can be seen. Thus serotonin appears to be a physiological balancing neurotransmitter, opposing NE and DA in certain of their actions.

Acetylcholine is the major parasympathetic neurotransmitter in the periphery opposing or balancing at many sites NE, the sympathetic neurotransmitter. Such functions in the CNS have not been identified. However, there are reports stating that excess acetylcholine did decrease the cocaine induced psychomotor effects (Scheel-Kruger et al, 1976; Hatch and Fischer, 1972). Thus acetylcholine seems to antagonize the excitation caused by excess NE and DA. However, the tremendous increase in neuro-electrical activity by chronic cocaine use tend to decrease Ach levels and this would augment the stimulant activity of cocaine through NE and DA. These observations are further supported by the fact that atropine and scopolamine, which are Ach antagonists, increase the behavioral effects of cocaine (Scheel-Kruger et al, 1976).

The specific neurochemical effects of drugs are not easily followed in a dynamic *invivo* setting. In the case of cocaine it seems that a logical hypothesis may be constructed. Cocaine apparently achieves its excitatory stimulating effects by increasing adrenergic tone through NE and DA release and increased synthesis while decreasing the activity of the neurotransmitters which normally oppose excitation such as serotonin and Ach. The upset in the CNS chemical equilibrium may result in the reported physical signs after discontinuation of chronic cocaine use.

CORRELATION OF THE NEUROTRANSMITTERS WITH BEHAVIORAL EFFECTS

We discussed earlier the effects of cocaine on behavior. Also, we looked at how cocaine affects the various neurotransmitters. Now, lets look at how the various neurotransmitters affect behavior (Table 5). The list includes DA, NE, E, Ach and 5-HT (serotonin). The table differentiates the observed effects at physiological concentrations (normal), excess and deficiency levels. DA at normal concentration affects normal locomotor activity, decrease appetite and increase sexual drive. In excess in animals locomotor hyperactivity and stereotyped behavior is observed while in human subjects the familiar schizophrenic symptomatology of hallucination, suspiciousness and paranoia are seen (Hartman, 1976). DA deficiency is commonly observed in Parkinson's Disease manifested by depression, extrapyramidal muscle tremors and decreased sexual drive (Scheel-Kruger et al, 1976). NE physiologically is responsible for providing alertness, energy and increased assertiveness (Fernstrom, 1981). Excess NE activity results in agitation, restlessness, aggression and anx-

TABLE 5. Behavioral and physiological effects correlated with neurotransmitters

DA	NE	E	ACH	5-HT
NORMAL				
Locomotor hyperactivity Anorexia Sexual stimulation	Increased energy Increased assertiveness (Euphoria)	Increased energy Mobilization	Increased mental acuity Muscular coordination	Sleep Tranquilization Antidepressant Activity
EXCESS				
Stereotyped activity Hallucinations Suspiciousness Paranoia	agitation Restlessness Anxiety Aggression	Cardio-respiratory Over stimulation Leading to failure	Muscle tremor & incoordination Memory problems	Euphoria Mood elevating
DEFICIENCY				
Extra Pyramidal symptoms (Parkinsonism) Depression	Depression Lethargy	Lethargy	Mental confusion Hallucination	Insomnia Depression Agitation

iety commonly seen after chronic large doses of cocaine. While a deficiency state produces lethargy and depression. The physiological function of E is the hormonal regulation of the sympathetic side of the autonomic nervous system (Fernstrom, 1981). Its effects are increased energy by enzymatic stimulation (glycolysis and lypolysis) and energy mobilization by shifting the blood supply into skeletal muscles. Excess amounts of E create overstimulation of the heart and lungs leading to vertricular fibrillation and death, often seen in acute toxic cocaine emergencies. E deficiency if it occurs would manifest in lethargy since the parasympathetic side of the autonomic nervous system would be in control.

This leads us to Ach which is the neurotransmitter of the parasympathetic nervous system (Fernstrom, 1981). With the exception at some organ systems the sympathetic and parasympathetic nervous system regulate autonomic activity, trying to keep a physiologic balance between the two opposing systems, stimulation by E and inhibition by Ach. Ach appears to have CNS functions as well but while mood and memory maintainance is proposed the exact mechanism(s) is unknown. For purposes of this analysis Ach increases mental acuity and provides an equilibrium for skeletal muscle coordination. Excess Ach causes muscle fasciculation and skeletal muscle incoordination. Ach deficiency is often seen in toxicity cases caused by anticholinergic drugs such as atropine and scopolamine (Innes and Nickerson, 1965). The effects are mental confusion and hallucination. The great demand on the electrical activity of the CNS induced by cocaine may deplete among others Ach and confusion and hallucination seen in heavy cocaine users may result from Ach deficiency.

5-HT in physiologic levels has regulatory activity of sleep. It is also a tranquilizer and anti-depressant. Excess levels of 5-HT are correlated with elevated mood, and euphoria, while deficiency with insomnia, depression and agitation (Fernstrom, 1981).

This table is by no means complete. There are other neurotransmitters and putative neurotransmitters with various physiological and/or behavioral effects. Examples of neurochemicals not discussed are: GABA, glutamine, other amino acids, ACTH, cortisol, MSH, melatonin, LH, FSH, Prolactin, GH, and the endorphine system. It should be recognized that there are many reserve, redundant or back up systems in the CNS. Even in this small table of selected neurotransmitters there are numerous duplication of functions. Depression can be caused by low levels of DA, NE and 5-HT, while agitation by excess NE or a deficiency of 5-HT, hallucination by excess of DA and deficiency of Ach and euphoria by normal NE function and excess of 5-HT. Thus it appears that following the cocaine induced upset of CNS neurochemical balance, no single substance may be effective to re-establish the neurochemical equilibrium which is necessary for normal processing of information by the

CNS. Thus it may be necessary to dissect at least some of the systems which appear to be "overworked" by cocaine. This analysis is necessary to find the substances which are depleted after heavy chronic cocaine use. Such Precursers or actual substances should be provided during cocaine withdrawal.

It is known that chronic amphetamine abusers develop severe vitamin deficiency, especially the water soluble B complex and C vitamins (Wesson and Smith, 1978). The similar high level sympathetic stimulation by cocaine may also lead to similar vitamin deficiency after chronic cocaine use. Table 6 shows a few examples of vitamins which are known to be involved in both the bio-electricity generating system important for neurotransmission and in the biosynthesis of DA, NE, E and Ach. The substances NAD, NADP, FAD, FMN and TPP are oxidizing agents functioning as hydrogen carriers in the citric acid cycle (Davson, 1964). Each time they transfer hydrogen "high energy" ATP is generated. ATP is the energy source for many biological processes among them the repolarization of neuronal membranes. Thus availability of vitamins which act like coenzymes, namely niacin, riboflavin and thiamin, are necessary for normal neuronal functioning. The tremendous electrical discharge seen during cocaine use makes it necessary that these vitamins are supplied to the CNS in sufficient quantities.

In an effort to learn more about the effects of chronic cocaine abuse on nutrition and vitamin levels, we undertook a pilot study in which we analyzed the vitamin profiles of 26 cocaine abusing individuals on admission to Fair Oaks Hospital (Estroff et al, 1983). These patients met DSM III criteria for cocaine abuse. The diagnosis was confirmed with either a positive blood or urine test for cocaine. The vitamins tested included Vitamins A, B_1 (Thiamine), B_2 (Riboflavin), B_3 (Niacin), B_6 (Pyridoxine), B_{12}, C (Ascorbic Acid), and Folate.

Nineteen of 26 (73%) individuals had at least one vitamin deficiency.

TABLE 6. Vitamins role in brain electrical activity and neurotransmitter synthesis

Substance	Role	Vitamin Source
NAD, NADP	Coenzyme for ATP (Generation of action potentials.)	Niacin, Niacinamide
FAD, FMN	___"___'___"___	Riboflavin (B_2)
TPP	___"___'___"___	Thiamine (B_1)
Zn, Mg, Ca	Cofactors	_____
Tyrosine hydroxylase	Synthesis of E, NE & DA	Folic acid
Dopa-decarboxylase	___"___"___"___"___	Pyridoxine (B_6)
Dopamine-B-hydroxylase	___"___"___"___"___	Ascorbic acid
Acetylcholine	Synthesis	Thiamine (B_1)

Vitamin B_6 (Pyridoxine) was the most commonly seen deficiency with 10 of 25 (40.0%) individuals being affected. The next most common deficiency was Vitamin B_1 (Thiamine) affecting 7 out of 25 individuals (28.0%). Six of 26 (23.1%) were Vitamin C deficient. Only 1 individual was Vitamin A deficient. No individual was B_2 (Riboflavin), B_3 (Niacin), B_{12} or Folate deficient. Five of 25 individuals had higher than normal levels of Vitamin A.

These results suggest that cocaine abuse is associated with multiple vitamin deficiencies principally Vitamin B_6 (Pyridoxine), B_1 (Thiamine) and Vitamin C. These vitamin deficiencies may be specific to the cocaine abuse or may be as a result of malnutrition since cocaine is an anorexic agent and severe cocaine abusers tend to ignore all bodily needs including eating. Metabolic considerations may also be important since Vitamin C is a co-factor of tyrosine hydroxylase, the rate limiting enzyme of norepinephrine synthesis. The high Vitamin A levels may be due to high levels of Vitamin A found in raw cocaine.

Our findings suggest that patients with cocaine abuse should be evaluated for vitamin deficiencies. Treatment of these vitamin deficiencies help stabilize the patient's medical status and makes them more amenable for treatment of their cocaine abuse.

On the lower portion of the table are the names of selected enzymes which are involved in the biosynthesis of DA, NE, E and Ach and have known vitamin cofactors (Kutsky, 1973l; Briggs, 1981). Tyrosine hydroxylase requires folic acid, dopa-decarboxylase, pyridoxine, dopamine B-hydroxylase, ascorbic acid and acetylcholine synthesis, thiamine. It is possible that other vitamins and cofactors are also involved. The question is that the cocaine stimulated severe increase of electrical activity in the CNS use up these enzyme cofactors (vitamins) and neurotransmitter precursors or are they recirculated? More research is needed to specify qualitative and quantitative replacement needs. It is no harm, however, to test all cocaine addicts for vitamin, amino acid and metal deficieny when testing is not available because of laboratory limitations. The physician may wish to replenish water soluble vitamins to withdrawing cocaine addicts of the B complex, C and minerals such as Zn, Mg and Ca. These substances would be excreted rapidly if not needed. Also, supply of neurotransmitter precursors may speed the recovery of the neurochemical equilibrium. In a pilot study L-tyrosine was used in the treatment of cocaine withdrawal symptoms (Gold et al, 1983). Significant decrease in the depression of subjects and their level of anxiety and irritability was observed after treatment with 100 mg/kg daily doses (t.i.d.) of L-tyrosine. Controlled studies to confirm these findings are underway.

Table 7 describes a proposed therapy which may be considered to treat cocaine withdrawal symptoms. Analysis of cocaine effects on es-

TABLE 7. Suggested replacement therapy for chronic cocaine abusers before psychotherapeutic intervention

Reason for use	Substance	Daily dose	Nature of substance
Precursor of DA, NE & E	l-tyrosine	3-5 grams	Amino acid
Precursor of serotonin (5HT)	l-tryptophan	1.5-2 grams	Amino acid
Precursor of acetyl-choline (ACH)	Lecithin	1.5 grams	Phosphotidylcholine
	Choline	.5 gram	Trimethylammo-niumhydroxide
Cofactors and coen-zymes* for synthe-sis and generation of bioelectric energy	Thiamine (B₁)	100 mg	Vitamin
	Riboflavin (B₂)	100 mg	Vitamin
	Pyridoxine (B₃)	100 mg	Vitamin
	Cyanocobalamine (B₁₂)	100 μg	Vitamin
	Niacin	100 mg	Vitamin
	Folic acid	400 μg	Vitamin
	Pantothenic acid	100 mg	Vitamin
	Ascorbic acid	2000 mg	Vitamin

*Available in a single tablet.

sential CNS chemicals maybe analyzed before treatment by drawing blood for comprehensive testing of metals, vitamins and amino acids. It is likely that DA, NE and E depletion after chronic exhaustive cocaine binges cause severe physical fatigue, mental depression and lethargy. These are important symptoms to combat because they may trigger the continuation of cocaine use. As described earlier, a pilot study, using L-tyrosine was successful to reduce depression and irritability during cocaine withdrawal.

In addition based on our analysis of neurotransmitter precursors of 5-HT and acetylcholine are also needed. 5-HT underactivity may manifest in insomnia, depression and agitation these symptoms are often present among the cocaine withdrawal symptoms. Acetylcholine deficiency may result in mental confusion and hallucination which may also add to the psychotic symptomatology seen in some subjects after chronic cocaine use and toxicity. Thus replacement therapy with L-tryptophan and acetylcholine precursers may also be beneficial. Due to the stimulant effects of DA, NE and E, L-tyrosine should be given in the morning while L-tryptophan and lecithin during the evening hours. This is recommended to re-establish normal wake-sleep patterns. The various vitamins are recommended at "semi-mega" doses. These amounts are not considered excessive by current nutritional standards. Many healthy individuals normally supplement their diet with such a daily regimen. The "suggested" replacement therapy is exactly what it's title intends to convey—it is a recommendation. It must be tested to determine its efficacy in subjects withdrawing from cocaine. A pilot study with similar rational reported considerable success using l-tyrosine, l-tryptophan along with Imipramine in cocaine abusers (Rosecan, 1983).

Conclusion

It is established that cocaine has a significant qualitative and quantitative effect on human behavior. In most individuals at small to moderate doses the behavioral effects of cocaine are extremely reinforcing, causing psychological dependence. The most dangerous aspect of cocaine is its delusion producing quality. Subjects dependent on the drug do not see themselves dependent nor do they see any problem in their deteriorating life style, until perhaps the very end often near self destruction. The only safety of cocaine is its high price and low availability which in fact, is changing. Currently cocaine appears to be available in larger quantities and cheaper on the street. This will no doubt increase the cocaine related complications in numbers as well as in severity.

Cocaine was shown to trigger a sympathetic nervous system hyperactivity. The increased release and synthesis of DA and NE elevates the sympathetic tone to very high levels. While the release of 5-HT initially inhibit partly the excitation. Later cocaine related inhibition of serotonin synthesis is the reason for the elimination of the antagonistic and balancing neurotransmitter 5-HT. This further augments the excitatory sympathetic stimulation. This is a possible mechanism for the observed "reverse tolerance."

The biochemical and neurophysiological deficit caused by cocaine related hyperactivity should be treated by replacement therapy using precursors of neurotransmitters and vitamins to reestablish normal neuronal functioning. This should be followed by behavior modification and psychological counseling. Cocaine induced physical dependence makes it necessary to treat the neurochemical imbalance before psychological intervention may be successful.

REFERENCES

Altshuler, H.L. and Burch, N.: Cocaine dependence: psychogenic and physiological substrates. In: Cocaine: Chemical, Biological, Clinical, Social and Treatment Aspects, (S.J. Mule', ed.), CRC Press, Ohio, p. 135, 1976.

Altshuler, H.L., Burch, N.R. and Dossett, R.G.: The electroencephalographic effects of long term cocaine administration to rhesus monkeys, Proc. West Pharmacol. Soc. 19:323, 1976.

Barash, P.G.: Cocaine in clinical medicine. In: Cocaine 1977, (R.C. Petersen,

R.C. Stillman, eds.), N.I.D.A. Research Monograph, U.S. Government Printing Office, Washington, D.C., p. 193, 1977.

Bastos, M.L. and Hoffman, D.B.: Detection and identification of cocaine, its metabolites and its derivatives. In: Cocaine: Chemical, Biological, Clinical, Social and Treatment Aspects, (S.J. Mule', ed), CRC Press, Ohio, p.45, 1976.

Byck, R. and Van Dyke, C.: What are the effects of cocaine in man? In: Cocaine, (R.C. Petersen, R.C. Stillman, eds.), U.S. Government Printing Office, Washington, D.C., 1977.

Caldwell, J.: Physiological aspect of cocaine usage. In: Cocaine: Chemical, Biological, Clinical, Social and Treatment Aspects, (S.J. Mule', ed), CRC Press, Ohio, p. 193, 1976.

Carmichael, F.J. and Israel, Y.: Invitro inhibitory affects of narcotic analgesics and other psychotropic drugs on the active uptake of norepinephrine in mouse brain tissue, *J. Pharmacol. Exp. Ther.* 186:253, 1973.

Davson, H.: Transformation of energy in living systems. In: Textbook of General Physiology, Little, Brown and Co., Boston, p. 181, 1964.

Deneau, G., Yanagita, T. and Seevers, M.H.: Self administration of psychoactive substances by the monkey: a measure of psychological dependence, *Psychopharmacologia* 16:30, 1969.

Dimijian, G.G.: Contemporary drug abuse. In: Medical Pharmacology, Principles and Concepts, (A. Goth, ed.), The C.V. Mosby Co., St. Louis, 7th edition, p. 313, 1974.

Eddy, N.B., Halbach, H., Isbell, H., Seevers, M.H.: Drug dependence, its significance and characteristics, *Bull W.H.O.* 32:721, 1965.

Eidelberg, E., Lesse, H., Gault, F.P.: An experimental model of temporal lobe epilepsy, studies of the convulsant properties of cocaine. In: EEG and Behavior, (G.H. Glasser, ed.), Basic Books, New York, p. 272, 1963.

Estroff, T.W., Dackis, C.A., Sweeney, D.R., Gold, M.S. and Pottash, A.L.C.: The vitamin deficiencies of cocaine abuse, unpublished data, 1983.

Fernstrom, J.D.: Nutrition, brain function and behavior. In: Nutrition and Behavior, (S.A. Miller, ed.), The Franklin Institute Press, Philadelphia, p. 59, 1981.

Gatz, A.J.: Manter's Essentials of Clinical Neuroanatomy and Neurophysiology, F.A. Davis Co., Philadelphia, p. 100, 1966.

Gay, G.R.: Clinical management of acute and chronic cocaine poisoning, *Ann. Emergency Med.* 11:562, 1982.

Gay, G.R. and Inaba, D.S.: Acute and chronic toxicology of cocaine abuse: current sociology, treatment and rehabilitation. In: Cocaine: Chemical, Biological, Social and Treatment Aspects, (S.J. Mule', ed.), CRC Press, Ohio, p. 245, 1976.

Gay, G.R., Newmeyer, J.A., Perry, M., Gregory, J. and Kurland, M.: Love and Haight: the sensuous hippie revisited. Drug/sex practices in San Francisco, 1980-81, *J. Psychoactive Drugs* 14:111, 1982.

Gold, M.S. and Bowers, M.B., Jr.: Neurobiological vulnerability to low-dose amphetamine psychosis, *Am. J. Psychiatry* 135:1546, 1978.

Gold, M.S., Pottash, A.L.C., Annitto, W.J., Verebey, K. and Sweeney, D.R.: Cocaine withdrawal: efficacy of tyrosine, *Society for Neuroscience Abstract*, 9:157, 1983.

Gropetti, A. and DiGuilio, A.M.: Cocaine and its effect on biogenic amines. In: Cocaine: Chemical, Biological, Clinical, Social and Treatment Aspects, (S.J. Mule', ed), CRC Press, Ohio, p. 97, 1976.

Gropetti, A., Zambotti, F., Biazzi, A. and Mantegazza, P.: Amphetamine and cocaine on amine turnover. In: Frontiers in Catecholamine Research, (E. Usdin, S. Snyder, eds.), Pergamon Press, New York, p. 917, 1973.

Gupta, R.C., Montgomery, S.H. and Lundberg, G.D.: Quantitative determination of street drugs in Los Angeles area, *Clin. Toxicol.* 7:241, 1974.

Handbook of Vitamins and Hormones: (R.J. Kutsky, ed.), Van Nostrand Reinhold Co., New York, p. 246, 1973.

Hartman, H.: Schizophrenia: a theory, *Psychopharmacology* 49:1, 1976.

Hatch, R.C. and Fischer, R.: Cocaine-elicited behavior and toxicity in dogs pretreated with synaptic blocking agents, morphine and diphenylhydantoin, *Pharmacol. Res. Commun.* 4:383, 1972.

Innes, I.R. and Nickerson, M.: Drugs inhibiting the action of acetylcholine on structures innervated by postganglionic parasympathetic nerves (antimuscarinic or atropinic drugs). In: The pharmacological Basis of Therapeutics, (L.S. Goodman, A. Gilman eds.), Third edition, Macmillan Co., New York, p. 531, 1965.

Jaffe, J.H.: Drug addiction and drug abuse. In: Pharmacological Basis of Therapeutics, Third edition (L.S. Goodman, A. Gilman eds.), Macmillan Co., New York, p. 298, 1965.

Knapp, S. and Mandell, A.J.: Narcotic drugs: effects on the serotonin biosynthetic-system of the brain, *Science* 177:1209, 1972.

Matsuzaki, M.: Effects of cocaine on the electrical activity of the brain and cardiorespiratory functions and the development of tolerance in the central nervous system. In: Cocaine: Chemical, Biological, Clinical, Social and Treatment Aspects, (S.J. Mule', ed.) CRC Press, Ohio, p. 149, 1976.

Matsuzaki, M.: Comparison of the convulsant effects of cocaine and pseudococaine in the rhesus monkey, *Brain Res. Bull.* 1:417, 1977.

Matsuzaki, M.: Alteration in patter of EEG activities and convulsant effect of cocaine following chronic administration in the rhesus monkey. *Electroencephal. and Clin. Neurophysiol.* 45:1, 1978.

Post, R.M.: Clinical aspects of cocaine: assessment of acute and chronic effects in animals and man. In: Cocaine: Chemical, Biological, Clinical, Social and Treatment Aspects, (S.J. Mule', ed.), CRC Press, Ohio, p. 203, 1976.

Post, R.M. and Rose, M.: Increasing effects of repetitive cocaine administration in the rat, *Nature* (London), 260:731, 1976.

Prioux-Gruyonneau, M., Cohen, Y., Barlet, J., Jacquot, C. and Repin, S.: Effects of cocaine on the release and turnover of noradrenaline, *J. Pharmacol.* (Paris), 6:5, 1975.

Rappolt, R.T., Gay, G.R. and Soman, M.: Treatment plan for acute and chronic adrenergic poisoning crisis utilizing sympatholytic effects of the B1-B2 receptor site blocker propranolol in concert with diazepam and urine acidification, *Clin. Toxicol.* 14:55, 1979.

Resnick, R.B. and Schuyten-Resnick, E.: Clinical aspects of cocaine:assessment of cocaine abuse behavior in man. In: Cocaine: Chemical, Biological, Clinical, Social and Treatment Aspects, (S.J. Mule', ed.), CRC Press, Ohio, p. 217, 1976.

Ritchie, J.M., Cohen, P.J. and Dripps, R.D.: Cocaine, procaine and other local anesthetics. In: The Pharmacological Basis of Therapeutics, (L.S. Goodman, A. Gilman, eds.), Third edition, MacMillan Co., New York, p. 376, 1965.

Rosecan, J.S.: The treatment of cocaine abuse with imipramine, l-tyrosine and l-tryptophan, Abstract VII World Congress of Psychiatry, Vienna, 1982.

Ross, S.B. and Renji, A.L.: Inhibition of the uptake of tritriated catecholamines by antidepressant and related agents, *Eur. J. Pharmacol.* 2:181, 1967.

Rothbeller, A.B.: The effect of phenylephrine, methamphetamine, cocaine and serotonin upon the adrenaline sensitive component of the reticular activating system, *Electroenceph. Clin. Neurophysiol.* 9: 409, 1957.

Rudzik, A.D. and Johnson, G.A.: Effect of amphetamine and amphetamine analogues on convulsive thresholds. In: Amphetamines and Related Compounds, (E. Costa, S. Garattini, eds.), Raven Press, New York, 1970.

Sayers, A.C. and Handley, S.L.: A study of the role of catecholamines in the response to various central stimulants, *Eur. J. Pharmacol.* 23:47, 1973.

Scheel-Kruger, J., Braestrup, C., Nielsen, M., Golembiowska, K. and Mogilricka, E.: Cocaine: discussion on the role of dopamine in the biochemical mechanism of action. In: Cocaine and Other Stimulants, (E.H. Ellingwood, M.M. Kilbey, eds.), Plenum Press, New York, 1976.

Siegel, R.K.: Cocaine and sexual dysfunction: the curse of mama coca, *J. Psychoactive Drugs* 14:71, 1982.

Stripling, J.S. and Ellingwood, E.H., Jr.: Cocaine: physiological and behavioral effects of acute and chronic administration. In: Cocaine: Chemical, Biological, Clinical and Treatment Aspects, (S.J. Mule', ed.), CRC Press, Ohio, p. 167, 1976.

Stripling, J.S. and Ellingwood, E.H., Jr.: Augmentation of the behavioral and electrophysiologic response to cocaine by chronic cocaine administration in the rat, *Exp. Neurol.* 54:546, 1977.

Vander, A.J.: Nutrition, stress and toxic chemicals, The University of Michigan Press, Ann Arbor, p. 198, 1981.

Vitamins in Human Biology and Medicine, (M.H. Briggs, ed.), CRC Press, Boca Raton, p. 121, 1981.

Wallach, M.B. and Gershon, S.: A neuropsychopharmacological comparison of d-amphetamine, l-DOPA and cocaine, *Neuropharmacology* 10:743, 1971.

Wesson, D.R. and Smith, D.E.: CNS stimulants. In: Treatment Aspects of Drug Dependence, (A. Schecter, ed.), CRC Press, West Palm Beach, p. 132, 140, 1978.

CHAPTER 14

Buspirone: A Unique Anxiolytic

Frank J. Ayd, Jr., M.D., F.A.P.A.

Sedative substances have been used throughout history to alleviate the ravages of inordinate pathological anxiety. In the early part of the 20th century, bromides, paraldehyde and chloral hydrate were used extensively, but they fell into disfavor when their cumulative toxic effects became apparent. During the 1930s and 1940s, barbiturates like phenobarbital, secobarbital and pentobarbital became the drugs of choice for relieving anxiety and inducing sleep, yet yet these drugs also developed an unfavorable reputation due to their serious drawbacks: tolerance, physical dependence and withdrawal, and lethality on overdose. Although the introduction of meprobamate, a nonbarbiturate sedative, originally was hailed as a breakthrough in the search for a safe and effective anxiolytic, its dependence/abuse potential and overdose lethality resulted in restrictions of its use as an anxiolytic. An apparent turning point came in the mid 1950s with the confirmation of the anxiolytic properties of the first two benzodiazepines, chlordiazepoxide and diazepam.

That the benzodiazepines are now among the most widely prescribed drugs in the world is attributable to their spectrum of clinical indications (as anxiolytics, hypnotics, anticonvulsants and muscle relaxants), their efficacy, their mild side effect profile, their relative safety when taken in combination with other drugs, and their almost completely suicide-proof qualities when taken alone in overdose. Despite these proven attributes, however, the sedative/hypnotic effects of benzodiazepines prescribed for anxiety may result in unwanted sleepiness, fatigue, lethargy, impaired psychomotor function and possibly serious interactions with alcohol and other CNS depressants. In addition, tolerance, dependency and withdrawal reactions have been reported with nearly every benzodiazepine. As Leo Hollister, an internationally recognized elder statesman in the world of psychopharmacology, has stated: "It would be difficult indeed to persuade most people that the benzodiazepines have not constituted a significant advance over the sedative-hypnotic drugs of the past. Nonetheless, it is becoming increasingly apparent that the advantages are not as great as was originally thought. The nature of progress is such that a clear advantage, albeit a small one, is enough to make older drugs obsolete and newer ones popular. On the whole, it must be concluded that the benzodiazepines have been some of the safest drugs ever introduced into medical practice. Furthermore, they have been among the most widely used. It now remains to be seen which agents (and surely there will be some) will replace the benzodiazepines" (Hollister, 1983). Hence, the search has continued for equally effective antianxiety drugs that may have fewer adverse side effects, less abuse potential and greater specificity.

BUSPIRONE

Buspirone (Buspar*), a lipophilic, dibasic heterocyclic first synthesized as a member of a series of compounds designed as major tranquilizers (Wu, et al., 1972) may prove to be the beginning of the new chapter in the chemotherapy of anxiety. This unique new anxiolytic agent has a pharmacologic profile different from the barbiturates, benzodiazepines, phenothiazines, butyrophenones, tricyclic antidepressants and monoamine oxidase inhibitors. In contrast to the benzodiazepines in particular, buspirone does not have hypnotic, anticonvulsant or muscle-relaxant properties.

MECHANISM OF ACTION

The discovery in 1977 of the brain's so-called benzodiazepine receptor lent credence to the hypothesized existence of specific chemical processes that mediate anxiety. The currently postulated anxiolytic action of benzodiazepines and triazolopyridines is direct occupation of the benzodiazepine receptors, while compounds such as pyrazolopyridines and barbiturates have been shown to alter the apparent affinity and/or number of benzodiazepine and associated gamma-aminobutyric acid (GABA) receptors (Weissman et al., in press). Although buspirone's mechanism of action remains undefined, the drug, its 5-hydroxylated metabolite and its cleavage product 1-(2-pyrimidinyl) piperazine appear to be devoid of direct *in vitro* interactions at this neurochemical locus (Taylor et al., in press).

Buspirone's pharmacological resemblance to dopamine agonists and antagonists, as well as its interaction with dopamine receptors *in vitro* (Riblet et al., 1982; Stanton et al., 1981; Riblet et al., 1981), helped suggest

---

*TM, Mead Johnson Pharmaceutical Division, Evansville, IN

the hypothesis that its dopaminergic action might be the basis for its anticonflict and anxiolytic effects (Riblet et al., 1982). Structurally and pharmacologically, buspirone resembles the atypical neuroleptic clozapine, a dopamine antagonist that inhibits conditioned avoidance response and apomorphine-induced stereotypy in the rat without inducing catalepsy. Buspirone, however, reverses neuroleptic-induced catalepsy while clozapine does not (Riblet et al., 1982). Buspirone also has been shown to produce a dose-related increase in plasma prolactin and a significant increase in growth hormone in humans, suggesting a dopamine antagonist effect at the pituitary gland and a dopamine agonist effect in the hypothalamus (Meltzer et al., 1982). In addition, buspirone is structurally related to the dopamine agonist, piribedil, another compound which reverses neuroleptic-induced catalepsy, although buspirone does not share piribedil's induction of stereotypy, sedation, and potent turning behavior in rats with unilateral lesions of the dopaminergic nigrostriatal pathway (Temple et al., 1982).

Despite these and other data showing that buspirone interacts with the dopaminergic system, other observations suggest that this may not be the primary mechanism of buspirone's antianxiety effect. The buspirone analog MJ 13805 has potent anxiolytic activity but does not bind to [³H]spiperone labeled dopamine sites *in vitro* (Eison et al., 1982), and buspirone's metabolite 1-(2-pyrimidinyl)piperazine also is anxioselective without *in vitro* dopaminergic effects (Garattini et al., 1982). Several investigators have found that buspirone can increase benzodiazepine binding *in vivo*, suggesting that buspirone indirectly affects the GABA-benzodiazepine receptor chloride ionophore complex (Weissman et al., 1984; Garattini et al., 1982; Oakley and Jones, 1983). Indeed, Eison and Eison (1984) state: "Buspirone appears to influence activity in several important midbrain systems, including the prominent mesencephalic dopamine systems (nigrostriatal and mesolimbic), the serotonergic dorsal raphe, and further downstream, the noradrenergic locus coeruleus and cholinergic projections to the cortex and hippocampus." These postulated actions, in addition to buspirone's possible interaction with brain GABA systems, prompted Eison and Eison to conceive of buspirone as a "midbrain modulator." Clearly, elucidation of buspirone's mechanism of action may add substantially to our knowledge of the neural substrates that mediate anxiety.

EFFICACY

Because early animal studies demonstrated that buspirone has psychotropic actions similar to those of antipsychotic agents, the compound was first tested clinically in ten male acute schizophrenic patients. In dosages up to 2400 mg/day, however, it had only a weak and short-duration antipsychotic effect. Two patients had some improvement, two showed minimal improvement and six exhibited a clear deterioration in their clinical status (Santhananthan et al., 1975). Nevertheless, further animal testing suggested that, as a result of its taming effect without ataxia in aggressive rhesus monkeys (diazepam has a similar taming effect but with a consistently higher incidence of ataxia), buspirone would have antianxiety activity in man (Tompkins et al., 1980).

Buspirone's overall efficacy in the treatment of anxiety has been clearly documented in both open and double-blind comparison studies. In general, it has been found to have therapeutic efficacy equal to that of other established anxiolytics: the majority of the studies compare buspirone to diazepam and clorazepate. Buspirone has been given to patients with high scores on a variety of rating instruments, including the Hamilton Rating Scale for Anxiety (HAM-A), Covi Anxiety Scale, Profile of Mood States (POMS), Lipman-Rickels Symptom Checklist (SCL-56), Physician's Questionnaire, Anxiety Entry Checklist, Hopkins Symptom Checklist (HSCL), Raskin Depression Scale and Hamilton Rating Scale for Depression (HAM-D). Analysis of the various comparison studies in which buspirone was administered to hundreds of patients leaves little doubt that it is an effective anxiolytic.

The first double-blind study, conducted by Goldberg and Finnerty (1979), compared buspirone, diazepam and placebo in 56 adult outpatients (aged 20 to 56) with a primary diagnosis of anxiety. Patients had to have a history of anxiety of at least one month's duration, a score of at least 20 on the HAM-A, at least 9 on the Covi Anxiety Scale and a score on the Raskin Depression Scale less than the total score on the Covi scale. Although patients were excluded if they had a history of psychosis, alcoholism or drug addiction, or significant renal, liver or cardiovascular disease, a large number with mixed anxiety and depression were included due to the difficulty in finding patients with only anxiety. During each of the four weeks of the study several rating instruments were used to assess clinical improvement, and patients' vital signs and weight also were monitored weekly. Buspirone patients (N = 18) received an average daily dose of 19.60 mg; diazepam patients (N = 20), 18.66 mg; and placebo patients (N = 18), 21.29 mg. Results, assessed by analysis of covariance, showed buspirone to be as effective on measures of anxiety as diazepam, and significantly more effective than placebo. In addition, buspirone-treated patients had mean depression scale scores 50% lower than those treated with diazepam. Lightheadedness and dizziness were the only side effects reported for buspirone.

In another 4-week double-blind study comparing buspirone and clorazepate in approximately 130 patients, Goldberg and Finnerty (1982) found that buspirone consistently relieved anxiety and depression associated with anxiety. Over 90% of the patients had had symptoms of generalized anxiety for at least 6 months, indicating chronic rather than situational anxiety. The mean daily dosages were 16 mg for buspirone and 20.35 mg for clorazepate. Comparison of the two drugs using several rating scales showed both produced overall equal anxiolytic results, although buspirone tended to be better on specific rating items (depression, inferiority, interpersonal sensitivity, tension, anger/hostility, confusion, dejection and fatigue). Buspirone-treated patients reported fewer side effects, particularly sedative side effects, than patients treated with clorazepate, who needed dose adjustments for sedation more frequently than those taking buspirone.

Rickels, (1982) America's internationally recognized authority on anxiolytics and the benzodiazepines in particular, and his associates at the University of Pennsylvania[18] compared buspirone with diazepam and placebo in a 4-week double-blind study. Among patients screened for the study, 240 met the entrance criteria: a DSM-III diagnosis of generalized anxiety disorder, scores of at least 9 on the Covi Anxiety Scale and 18 on the HAM-A scale, and endorsement of 5 or more items on a 17-item Anxiety Entry Checklist. Initial buspirone or diazepam dosages of 5 mg b.i.d. were increased after four days to 5 mg t.i.d., and after one week most were raised to 5 mg q.i.d. At the end of each treatment week, the physician completed the HAM-A, HAM-D, and a global estimate of anxious psychopathology, while patients completed the HSCL and POMS. Data, analyzed using analysis of covariance, showed significant treatment differences in favor of both drugs over placebo on all rating instruments. Diazepam was slightly more effective in reducing somatic symptom clusters, while buspirone was somewhat better in ameliorating confusion, anger/hostility and fatigue. Although Rickels et al also found that, compared to diazepam, buspirone tended to produce the most improvement in women and patients who had not had previous treatment for their anxiety, other investigators have not reported similar data.

ANXIOSELECTIVITY

Perhaps the most unusual finding in the clinical efficacy studies of buspirone is its anxioselectivity (Taylor et al., 1980). Because all effective antianxiety compounds to date also produce varying degrees of sedation, most clinicians have assumed that sedation is in some way a necessary component of anxiolysis. But, unlike barbiturates, meprobamate, benzodiazepines and other psychoactive drugs in which antianxiety activity and sedative effects go hand-in-hand, buspirone exerts its clinical effect with a relative lack of sedation. As Lader, (1982), England's international authority on anxiety and its pharmacotherapy, has pointed out, "there is no logical reason why calming and sleep-inducing effects should not be dissociable".[20]

In some trials (Goldberg and Finnerty, 1979; Wheatley, 1982; Newton et al., 1982), buspirone has shown an incidence of sedation similar to that of placebo. In others, (Rickels et al., 1982; Lader, 1982), although sedation occurred significantly less often compared to diazepam, some buspirone-treated patients did experience sedation. At the Institute of Psychiatry, University of London, Lader (1982) found that normal volunteers who felt drowsy while taking buspirone described the sedation as largely involving mental state. In contrast, compared to diazepam and placebo, the same subjects rated a feeling of physical tiredness as decreased after buspirone.

Buspirone's low incidence of sedative side effects is important because many effective anxiolytics also are associated with impairment of psychomotor and cognitive skills (Skegg et al., 1979; Kleinknecht and Donaldson, 1975). The most obvious problems with unwanted or unneeded sedation are increased risk of accidents and reduced ability to make critical judgments. The elderly in particular may be more prone to such effects as debilitating falls if their muscular coordination and reaction time are drug-impaired. In addition, those whose livelihood depends on operating machinery may not only suffer economic loss if sedative effects prevent their working, they may be tempted to perform tasks requiring unimpeded motor skills despite their increased risk of accidents.

Most studies designed to test the impairment potential of anxiolytics or sedative/hypnotics use normal volunteers, with the resulting problem that data may not be directly comparable to drug effects in anxious patients. Since anxiety itself may impair psychomotor, cognitive and intellectual performance, anxiolytic drug therapy may in fact produce a paradoxical effect: on the one hand performance may improve as anxiety lessens; on the other, performance may be impaired by the drug. Although further testing in buspirone-treated patients is needed before definitive conclusions about its performance impairment potential can be drawn, results in volunteers are encouraging. Two acute treatment studies disclosed no evidence of skills impairment (Skegg et al., 1979; Mattilla et al., 1982; Seppala et al., 1982). Moskowitz and Smiley (1982) compared the effects of chronically administered buspirone (20 mg/day), diazepam (15 mg/day) and placebo on driving performance in normal volunteers and found buspirone actually tended to improve performance, even after 8 days' ingestion.

THERAPEUTIC INDICATIONS

Since anxiety can be and frequently is secondary to other illnesses, both physical and psychiatric, the physician's first duty is accurate diagnosis. Although anxiety may be the most prominent symptom in many disorders, its etiology should be assessed carefully before any medication is prescribed. Treating only the symptom may in fact result in more suffering on the part of the patient if the true cause of the anxiety is overlooked. For example, anxiety is a common component of depression, schizophrenia and organic brain syndrome, none of which is adequately treated with anxiolytic drugs. Anxiolytics also are not indicated for anxiety associated with physical illnesses such as hypoglycemia or hyperthyroidism unless and until the primary disorder has been treated.

The third edition of the Diagnostic and Statistical Manual (DSM-III) lists the following subclasses of anxiety disorders: phobic (including agoraphobia, social phobia and simple phobia), obsessive compulsive, panic, post-traumatic stress, atypical anxiety, and generalized anxiety. In clinical trials of buspirone, the most commonly reported diagnosis has been generalized anxiety, (Goldberg and Finnerty, 1982; Rickels et al., 1982; Newton et al., 1982; Feighner et al., 1982; Gershon, 1982), the DSM-III criteria for which are listed in Table 1.

Although there are no published data indicating buspirone would be *ineffective* in any particular form of anxiety, benzodiazepine anxiolytics usually have not proven useful for treating phobic and obsessive-compulsive disorders, with the exception of alprazolam which has been shown to be quite efficacious therapy for panic and phobic disorders. It is interesting to speculate whether buspirone may be efficacious for anxious patients who have not responded to benzodiazepines. There is preliminary evidence suggesting that this may be so for a number of benzodiazepine-refractory patients.

DEPRESSION

Anxiety and depression almost always coexist, with one affect primary and the other secondary. Clinical experience has verified that the most effective treatment for either disorder is usually the one directed toward

TABLE 1. DSM-III criteria for generalized anxiety disorder

Nonspecific, persistent anxiety not due to another mental disorder present for at least 1 month in a patient 18 years of age or older who manifests symptoms from 3 of the following 4 categories:

Motor Tension	shakiness, jitteriness, jumpiness, trembling, tension, muscle aches, fatigability, inability to relax, eyelid twitch, furrowed brow, strained face, fidgeting, restlessness, easy startle
Autonomic Hyperactivity	sweating, heart pounding or racing, cold clammy hands, dry mouth, dizziness, light-headedness, paresthesias, upset stomach, hot or cold spells, frequent urination, diarrhea, discomfort in the pit of the stomach, lump in the throat, flushing, pallor, high resting pulse and respiration rate
Apprehensive Expectation	anxiety, worry, fear, rumination, anticipation of misfortune to self or others
Vigilance and Scanning	hyperattentiveness resulting in distractibility, difficulty in concentrating, insomnia, feeling "on edge," irritability, impatience.

alleviating the symptoms of the primary diagnosis. In other words, patients who are primarily anxious and secondarily depressed should be treated with an anxiolytic, while those who are primarily depressed and secondarily anxious should receive an antidepressant. Nevertheless, the differential diagnosis is often far from clearcut and sometimes the patient's response to drug therapy is the only way to confirm an equivocal diagnostic judgment. To alleviate as much suffering as possible in the patient presenting with what is probably anxiety with a high depressive component, the clinician should choose an anxiolytic which also exerts antidepressant effects.

Diazepam has been shown efficacious for both anxiety and depressive symptoms in patients who are primarily anxious (DiMascio and Goldberg, 1978), and several studies have found buspirone as effective as diazepam in this regard. In the first double-blind comparison study of Goldberg and Finnerty (1979), buspirone-treated patients had mean depression scale ratings 50% lower than patients given diazepam. Goldberg and Finnerty (1982) subsequently compared buspirone with clorazepate and found both drugs showed similar antidepressant effects as assessed by endpoint HAM-D results, with a slight trend in favor of buspirone. Because of the high proportion of patients with baseline depressive symptoms in the double-blind comparison study of Feighner et al. (1982), these investigators analyzed the effects of diazepam and buspirone on HAM-D scores. They concluded that buspirone may be particularly efficacious for anxious patients who have a strong depressive component. Thus, buspirone may be like alprazolam in that it has anxiolytic and antidepressant effects in selected patients.

SIDE EFFECTS

In clinical trials, buspirone's overall efficacy has been equal to that of standard benzodiazepines. In terms of side effects, however, it has consistently differed from comparison agents. Since buspirone does not appear to interact with the same neurochemical binding sites as other anxiolytics, in theory its side effects should be different as well. This does seem to be true in practice.

As noted previously, the most conspicuous aspect of buspirone's side effect profile is its relative absence of sedation. Like all active pharmaceutical substances, buspirone does exert some mild to moderate unwanted effects, such as nervousness, headache, dizziness, and nausea. In a number of studies, however, their overall incidence and severity have been significantly lower than those of comparison drugs (Goldberg and Finnerty, 1979; Newton et al., 1982; Feighner et al., 1982). For example, Newton et al. (1982) reported the findings of 10 investigators who treated approximately 700 patients with buspirone in a double-blind fashion, comparing buspirone's side effects with those of diazepam, clorazepate and placebo. In addition to data on incidence and severity of side effects, investigators reported whether they considered a side effect to be related to drug, whether changes in medication were required as a result of the side effect, whether side effects interfered with therapeutic effect, and whether the side effect had been reported by the patient or elicited by the investigator.

Using Fisher's exact test for 2x2 tables to compare overall side effect incidence, Newton et al found that buspirone produced significantly fewer side effects than diazepam, that investigators more frequently considered side effects to be due to diazepam than buspirone, and that more diazepam than buspirone-treated patients required dosage adjustment as a result of side effects. Compared to clorazepate, buspirone produced a comparable incidence and severity of effects, but buspirone was significantly better in terms of side effects interfering with therapeutic effect and investigators believing side effects were related to drug.

When individual side effects were analyzed, buspirone produced significantly less depression, drowsiness, fatigue and weakness than diazepam. Nervousness was the only buspirone effect that occurred significantly more often compared to diazepam (buspirone, 9%; diazepam, 2%; placebo; 1%). In the diazepam/placebo comparison, diazepam also produced significantly more depression, drowsiness, fatigue and weakness; whereas, compared to placebo, buspirone produced a higher incidence of nervousness, headache, and dizziness. Compared to clorazepate, buspirone-treated patients showed a higher incidence of nausea, but a significantly lower incidence of depression and drowsiness.

Although dizziness, headache and nervousness appear to be the most frequently reported side effects in patients (Goldberg and Finnerty, 1979; Rickels et al., 1982; Wheatley, 1982; Newton et al., 1982), dysphoria has been reported in normal volunteers given buspirone in single doses ranging from 20-40 mg (Lader, 1982; Mattilla, 1982; Cole et al., 1982). In a double-blind crossover study designed to assess the acute psychomotor and psychological effects of buspirone with and without alcohol, buspirone 20 mg produced subjective feelings of antagonism, withdrawal, discontent, boredom and sadness 26. Experienced recreational sedative/hypnotics users who volunteered for a study of the abuse potential of buspirone found single doses of buspirone 40 mg equal to placebo in euphoriant effects, but clearly distinguishable in terms of physical unpleasantness and dysphoria 32. In Lader's 20 acute dosage study in normal volunteers, the single buspirone dose of 20 mg produced a feeling of discontent, which he speculates may have been due to the increased incidence of side effects compared to the single 10 mg dosage. Dysphoria was not noted, however, in volunteers given up to 30 mg daily in divided doses.

To date, dysphoric reactions have not been reported in buspirone-treated patients. Two factors, however, could account for this apparent discrepancy between patients and normal volunteers: (a) patients in clinical trials were given buspirone in divided daily dosages; (b) clinical experience usually has verified that the more anxious the patient, the more tolerable is a higher dose of an anxiolytic.

DOSAGE

Most studies have compared buspirone to diazepam on a milligram per milligram basis (5 mg each) and buspirone 5 mg to clorazepate 7.5 mg. Goldberg and Finnerty (1982) originally reported, from data obtained in their unpublished open-dose range study, that buspirone 30 mg (10 mg t.i.d.) appeared to be the effective anxiolytic dose. These investigators subsequently stated, however, that this dose was probably higher than necessary and that when dosages were decreased (mean: 25 mg daily), there was a marked reduction in the anxiety levels of study patients (Goldberg and Finnerty, 1982). Other trials have used comparable dosages, with a mean of about 20 mg/day in divided dosages (Rickels et al., 1982; Newton et al., 1982; Gershon, 1982), although dosages as high as 50 mg/day have been reported (Feighner et al., 1982).

Because high starting doses of any psychopharmaceutical are often associated with adverse reactions and increased toxicity, all patients, and especially the elderly, are best treated with a gentle approach and conservative doses until their therapeutic needs have been adequately determined. To lessen the likelihood that patients will experience unpleasant side effects, buspirone therapy should be initiated with low, divided doses (5-10 mg no more than twice daily). Dosage increases should be gradual.

Since dysphoria has been reported primarily in those given high, single doses, rapid buspirone dosage escalation should be avoided. If a patient does have a dysphoric response to buspirone, this could indicate that the patient is not primarily anxious. In this case, a diagnostic re-evaluation may be warranted.

Even with low starting doses, buspirone usually begins to exert its therapeutic effects within 48 hours. Although there is some indication that the full anxiolytic effects of bupsirone may develop somewhat more slowly than those of comparison benzodiazepines (Lader, 1982; Wheatley, 1982; Newton et al., 1982), these effects also appear to build as therapy continues.

INTERACTION WITH OTHER DRUGS

An important consideration in prescribing any drug is the effect it may have on patients who also are taking other medications. Drug synergism, cumulative effects, altered metabolism and other adverse interactions all may interfere significantly with the therapeutic objectives and make laboratory workups difficult to interpret accurately. Patients often say they take no drugs or only one or two prescribed medications. Closer questioning, however, often reveals use of a variety of over-the-counter preparations (vitamins, laxatives, antacids, analgesics, diet aids, hypnotics, diuretics, "health" foods, topical ointments and salves, cold remedies, and eye, ear and nose drops); social drugs (alcohol, marijuana, cocaine); caffeine-containing foods and beverages; and tobacco products. In addition, although many patients must take medications for various physical ailments, some do not know the names and or/dosages of the drugs prescribed for them. (Asking patients to bring their medications in the original containers can fill in gaps in the medication history). By obtaining as complete a drug history as possible, clinicians can gather not only valuable information about previous response to psychiatric drug treatment, but formulate a rational basis for assessing the possibility of potential drug-drug interactions.

Controlled clinical trials involving approximately 1,000 patients have shown that buspirone's side effect profile generally is unaffected by several medications patients commonly take (Gershon, 1987) Possible interactions were assessed in patients taking buspirone, diazepam, clorazepate or placebo in combination with analgesics, antihistamines/vasoconstrictors, contraceptives, diuretics/antihypertensives, hormones, and sedative/hypnotics. Using Fisher's exact test for 2x2 tables, investigators compared the incidence, severity and duration of side effects; their estimation of the side effects' relationship to the test drug; and the need to reduce dosage. Results showed that like placebo- and clorazepate-treated patients, buspirone-treated patients who also took concomitant medication had side effect profiles no different than patients taking only the test drug. In contrast, patients taking diazepam with other drugs had a significantly higher incidence of side effects than those taking only diazepam, and the presence of concomitant medication adversely affected diazepam's side effect profile.

In general, benzodiazepines are relatively safe when combined with other drugs, yet some potentially serious problems can occur. For example, cimetidine, the most frequently prescribed drug in the world, has been reported to reduce the hepatic metabolism of diazepam and chlordiazepoxide (Klotz and Reimann, 1981). The resulting delayed clearance and increased steady state levels of the benzodiazepine could cause a prolongation of unwanted sedation. Although no studies of the combined effects of buspirone and cimetidine have been reported, buspirone's low incidence of sedation and its relative lack of interaction with other drugs makes it tempting to speculate that it may prove to be a good choice for anxiety in cimetidine-treated patients.

The interaction of benzodiazepines with alcohol also has caused concern because of the increased risk of oversedation with impairment of psychomotor function and cognitive judgment. To ascertain the acute

effects of buspirone and alcohol on psychomotor and psychological parameters, Mattila et al (1982) in a double-blind crossover trial compared
two doses of buspirone (10 mg and 20 mg), lorazepam 2.5 mg, and
placebo taken while study participants drank either an alcoholic or a
nonalcoholic beverage. Both buspirone doses caused negative subjective
effects (participants reported feeling antagonistic, withdrawn, discon-
tented, bored, and sad), but did not significantly modify objectively
assessed performance on psychomotor tests. When buspirone was combined with alcohol, the objective effects were no greater than those of
alcohol alone and the subjective effects were similar to those of buspirone
alone. Alcohol in combination with buspirone 20 mg produced rather
severe drowsiness at 180 minutes and did not alter the negative subjective effects of buspirone. In contrast, alcohol with lorazepam increased
objective skills impairment, was not accompanied by subjective side
effects, and produced positive feelings similar to those of alcohol alone
(social, friendly, content). That buspirone combined with alcohol caused
subjective drowsiness but not objective psychomotor impairment suggests two possibilities. First, buspirone may be safer with alcohol than
other anxiolytics such as lorazepam, which did not give study participants a subjective indication of their decreased performance ability. Second, since alcohol did not alleviate the subjective dysphoria experienced
with buspirone, there may be a reduced likelihood that buspirone would
be ingested to potentiate the effects of alcohol and vice versa.

Moskowitz and Smiley (1982) studied the effects on driving skills of
chronic administration of buspirone and diazepam each alone and in
combination with alcohol. Subjects received divided doses of either buspirone 20 mg (two equal doses q.a.m.), diazepam 15 mg (5 mg q.a.m.
and 10 mg h.s.; reversed on test days) or placebo daily for 9 days.
Simulated driving skills were measured at 4 time intervals on days 1, 8
and 9. On the ninth day, alcohol, in an amount intended to produce a
mean peak blood level of 0.10% was given immediately after the drug
treatment. Subjects receiving diazepam plus alcohol had the largest number of worst skills performances and the smallest number of best performances, whereas the greatest number of best performances occurred
in subjects given buspirone plus alcohol. In addition, buspirone tended
to offset some of the alcohol-induced impairment. Hence, this trial also
suggests that buspirone may be safer than other anxiolytics in combination with alcohol.

CHRONIC ADMINISTRATION

Among the many concerns about benzodiazepines that have surfaced
in recent years is the degree to which these drugs may cause adverse
effects in chronic therapeutic dose users and in abusers. Temporary
withdrawal reactions have been reported following the abrupt discontinuation of nearly all benzodiazepines, particularly if the drug had been

taken for several months. Conclusions, however, often are difficult to draw from these reports because several factors may contribute to the observed effects: (a) patients may have taken more or less of the drug than was prescribed; (b) patients may have taken other drugs (such as alcohol, antihistamines, meprobamate, barbiturates or another benzodiazepine) concomitantly; (c) putative withdrawal reactions may in fact be a resurgence of the symptoms for which the anxiolytic was first prescribed. Nevertheless, the belief that benzodiazepine anxiolytics are overused and abused is becoming widespread, although this belief seems to ignore the fact that the indications for these medications also are widespread. Benzodiazepines are effective not only for anxiety, but for muscle relaxation, convulsions and sleep induction; thus at any given time the percentage of the population requiring drug therapy with a benzodiazepine may be quite large. In addition, a substantial number of anxious patients, such as chronic anxiety neurotics, chronic mixed anxiety-depressives, and borderline personalities, may legitimately require extended periods of anxiolytic/hypnotic drug therapy to alleviate their chronic distress. Despite the many good reasons for prescribing the benzodiazepines, and despite their relative safety, however, growing numbers of physicians as well as the press and other citizens are worried that these drugs may produce a high incidence of tolerance, physical and psychological dependence, and withdrawal reactions of varying degrees of severity. For these reasons, clinical interest in buspirone extends beyond its therapeutic efficacy to its safety in long-term administration and its abuse potential.

At the present time, data are sparse concerning the effects of chronically administered buspirone. Most studies have assessed the drug in relatively short trials (three to four weeks). The length of these is insufficient to compare buspirone's dependency and withdrawal potential with reference drugs such as diazepam, the chronic effects of which are unlikely to surface unless they have been taken for several months. Long-term studies in patients with chronic anxiety are needed to determine if buspirone is superior to benzodiazepines in this regard. Studies in animals and human volunteers, however, suggest that buspirone's potential for dependence and abuse may be negligible.

Chronic administration of substances known to produce physical dependence (such as morphine or barbiturates) have been shown to result in loss of body weight in rats when these compounds are withdrawn (Yanaura et al., 1975). In a study of the potential of buspirone to induce physical dependence, buspirone and diazepam 200 mg/kg were administered daily to rats for 22 days. When the drugs were withdrawn, diazepam-treated animals were observed to have the weight loss typical of dependency-producing drugs, while those given buspirone showed a slight weight gain (Riblet et al., 1982).

Balster and Woolverton (1982) compared the reinforcing properties of buspirone, chlordiazepoxide, clorazepate, and saline in rhesus monkeys trained to self-administer cocaine. Their study, the protocol of which emulates those used to assess the euphoriogenic effects of opioids, sympathomimetic stimulants, barbiturates and phencyclidine, showed that buspirone produced an irregular response pattern similar to that of chlordiazepoxide, clorazepate and saline. That buspirone does not cause physical dependence and is not spontaneously self-administered by primates suggests there is little likelihood that it produces the euphoriant or sedative effects commonly sought by drug abusers.

Cole (1982), one of the most experienced psychoactive drug evaluaters, and his colleagues at McLean Hospital evaluated the abuse potential of buspirone 10 mg and 40 mg compared with methaqualone 300 mg, diazepam 10 mg and 20 mg, and placebo. Most of the 36 subjects in the study were students from upper-middle or upper-class families. All had used casually at least six times sedative-hypnotics such as barbiturates, methaqualone and benzodiazepines in dosages above the usual therapeutic level. Data assessed by analysis of covariance showed participants could distinguish buspirone 40 mg from placebo because at this dose the drug produced physical sedation, discomfort and dysphoria. In addition, buspirone 40 mg was rated as having less desirable subjective effects than methaqualone 300 mg, diazepam 20 mg, buspirone 10 mg, and placebo. The 10 mg dose of buspirone was comparable to diazepam 10 mg and placebo in producing no overt euphoriant or sedative effects. Both buspirone doses evoked less euphoria and stimulation than methaqualone 300 mg and less euphoria than diazepam 20 mg. Subjects identified methaqualone 300 mg as euphoriant, stimulating, and sedative, and rated it and diazepam 20 mg as drugs they would be likely to try again. Cole et al concluded that, because of buspirone's unpleasant effects at the higher dose and its lack of reinforcing effects at the lower dose, the drug is unlikely to be abused by recreational drug users.

CONCLUSION

The theoretical and practical implications of buspirone's therapeutic psychopharmacologic profile are many and varied. Buspirone is clearly as efficacious as comparison benzodiazepines, yet it appears to act independently of benzodiazepine receptors, which heretofore had been postulated as the basis for anxiety mediation. Further investigations into the mode of action of this new compound could result in a better understanding of the pathophysiology of anxiety.

Clinical studies to date consistently have found that buspirone exerts its antianxiety effect without producing the sedative impairment frequently found with benzodiazepines. This not only indicates that buspirone may be a safer choice for patients in whom sedation is unwanted, it implies that anxiolysis is separable from sedation. In addition, buspirone appears to be anxioselective: unlike benzodiazepines it is not a hypnotic, a muscle-relaxant or an anticonvulsant.

Data from some studies suggest that buspirone, besides relieving anxiety, may be useful for patients with a high degree of concomitant depression. In addition, individual investigators have found evidence that buspirone may be helpful for specific anxiety-related symptoms such as aggression and anger/hostility. Clinical trials of buspirone are indicated to determine if its therapeutic indications go beyond those of the benzodiazepines, particularly in patients with anxiety related to agoraphobia and obsessive-compulsive disorder.

Critics of biological psychiatry frequently complain that its practitioners use too many drugs too often, and that what is needed are not more, but fewer psychopharmaceuticals. Those who make this complaint, however, fail to realize that not all patients respond to or can tolerate the side effects of the compounds currently available. Some patients are helped by only one drug, and for these patients that drug can mean the difference between sickness and health. Drugs such as buspirone, which appears to be unique among known psychotropic substances, offer increased hope for our eventual understanding of the chemical events that appear to underly psychopathology. The simple fact is that the more their judicious use can help alleviate the suffering of individual patients. Buspirone may prove to be a welcome addition to our therapeutic options.

REFERENCES

Balster, R.L. and Woolverton, W.L.: Intravenous buspirone self-administration in rhesus monkeys. *J. Clin. Psychiatry* 43:34-37, 1982.

Cole, J.O., Orzack, M.H. and Beake, B., et al.: Assessment of the abuse liability of buspirone in recreational sedative users. *J. Clin. Psychiatry* 43:69-74, 1982.

DiMascio, A. and Goldberg, H.L.: Recognizing and treating anxiety. *Curr. Prescrib.* 4:17-26, 1978.

Eison, M.S. and Eison, A.S.: Buspirone as a midbrain modulator: Anxiolysis unrelated to traditional benzodiazepine mechanisms. In: Drug Development Research, Vol 4. In press, 1984.

Eison, M.S., Taylor, D.P. and Riblet, L.A., et al.: MJ 13805-1: A potential nonbenzodiazepine anxiolytic. *Soc. Neurosci. Abstr.* 8:470, 1982.

Feighner, J.P., Merideth, C.H. and Hendrickson, G.A.: A double-blind comparison of buspirone and diazepam in outpatients with generalized anxiety disorder. *J. Clin. Psychiatry* 43:103-107, 1982.

Garattini, S., Caccia, S. and Mennini, T.: Notes on buspirone's mechanisms of action. *J. Clin. Psychiatry* 43:19-22, 1982.

Goldberg, H.L., Finnerty, R.: Comparison of buspirone in two separate studies. *J. Clin. Psychiatry* 43:87-91, 1982.

Goldberg, H.L. and Finnerty, R.J.: The comparative efficacy of buspirone and diazepam in the treatment of anxiety. *Am. J. Psychiatry* 136:1184-1187, 1979.

Gershon, S.: Drug interactions in controlled clinical trials. *J. Clin. Psychiatry* 43:95-98, 1982.

Hollister, L.E.: The pre-benzodiazepine era. *J. Psychoactive Drugs* 15:9-13, 1983.

Kleinknecht, R.A. and Donaldson, D.: A review of the effects of diazepam on cognitive and psychomotor performance. *J. Nerv. Ment. Dis.* 161:399-411, 1975.

Klotz, U. and Reimann, I.: Elevation of steady-state diazepam levels by cimetidine. *Clin. Pharmacol. Ther.* 30:513-517, 1981.

Lader, M.C.: Psychological effects of buspirone. *J. Clin. Psychiatry* 43:62-67, 1982.

Matilla, M.J., Aranko, K. and Seppala, T.: Acute effects of buspirone and alcohol on psychomotor skills. *J. Clin. Psychiatry* 43:56-60, 1982.

Meltzer, J.Y., Fleming, R. and Robertson, A.: The effect of buspirone on prolactin and growth hormone secretion in man. *Arch. Gen. Psychiatry* 40:1099-1102, 1983.

Moskowitz, H. and Smiley, A.: Effects of chronically administered buspirone and diazepam on driving-related skills performance. *J. Clin. Psychiatry* 43:45-55, 1982.

Moskowitz, H., Smiley, A. and Ziedman. K., et al.: The effects of buspirone and diazepam, alone and in combination with ethanol, upon driving related skills performance. In Abstracts: Eighth International Congress of Pharmacology, Tokyo, 1981. Tokyo, Japanese Pharmacological Society, 1981.

Newton, R.E., Casten, G.P. and Alms, D.R., et al.: The side effect profile of buspirone in comparison to active controls and placebo. *J. Clin. Psychiatry* 43:100-102, 1982.

Oakley, N.R. and Jones, B.J.: Buspirone enhance [^{3}H]flunitrazepam binding in vivo. *Eur. J. Pharmacol.* 87:499-500, 1983.

Riblet, L.A., Taylor, D.P. and Becker, J.A., et al.: Buspirone: An anxioselective drug with similarities to apomorphine. *Soc. Neurosci. Abstr.* 7:865, 1981.

Riblet, L.A., Taylor, D.P. and Eison, M.S., et al.: Pharmacology and neurochemistry of buspirone. *J. Clin. Psychiatry* 43:11-16, 1982.

Rickels, K., Weisman, K. and Norstad, N., et al.: Buspirone and diazepam in anxiety: A controlled study. *J. Clin. Psychiatry* 43:81-86, 1982.

Sathananthan, G.L., Sanghvi, I. and Phillips, N., et al.: MJ 9022: Correlation between neuroleptic potential and stereotypy. *Curr. Ther. Res.* 18:701-705, 1975.

Seppala, T., Aranko, K. and Mattilla, M.J., et al.: Effects of alcohol on buspirone and lorazepam actions. *Clin. Pharmocol. Therap.* 32:201-207, 1982.

Skegg, D.C.G., Richards, S.M. and Doll, R.: Minor tranquillizers and road accidents. *Br. Med. J.* 1:917-919, 1979.

Stanton, H.C., Taylor, D.P. and Riblet, L.A.: Buspirone—an anxioselective drug with dopaminergic action. In: The Neurobiology of the Nucleus Accumbens, (R.B. Chronister, J.F. DeFrance, eds.), Brunswick, ME, Haer Institute, 1981.

Taylor, D.P., Allen, L.E. and Becker, J.A., et al.: Changing concepts of the biochemical action of the anxioselective drug buspirone. In: Drug Development Research, Vol 4. In press, 1984.

Taylor, D.P., Hyslop, D.K., and Riblet, L.A.: Buspirone: A model for anxioselective drug action. *Soc. Neurosci. Abstr.* 6: 791, 1980.

Temple, D.L., Yevich, J.P. and New, J.S.: Buspirone: Chemical profile of a new class of anxioselective agents. *J. Clin. Psychiatry* 43:4-9, 1982.

Tompkins, E.C., Clemento, A.J. and Taylor, D.P., et al.: Inhibition of aggressive behavior in rhesus monkeys by buspirone. *Res. Commun. Psychol. Psychiatry Behav.* 5:337-352, 1980.

Weissman, B.A., Barrett, J.E. and Brady, L.S., et al.: Behavioral and neurochemical studies on the anticonflict actions of buspirone. In: Drug Development Research, Vol 4. In press, 1984.

Wheatley, D.: Buspirone: Multicenter efficacy study. *J. Clin. Psychiatry* 43:92-94, 1982.

Wu, Y.H., Rayburn, J.W. and Allen, L.E., et al.: Psychosedative agents. 2. 8-(4-substituted 1-piperazinylalkyl) -8- azaspiro [4.5[decane-7, 9-diones]. *J. Med. Chem.* 15:477-479, 1972.

Yanaura, S., Tagashira, E. and Suzuki, T.: Physical dependence on morphine, phenobarbital, and diazepam in rats by drug-admixed food ingestion. *Jpn. J. Pharmacol.* 25:453-463, 1975.

CHAPTER 15

A Clinical Psychopharmacologist Remembers and Takes Stock

Heinz E. Lehmann

With the advent of psychopharmacology, a new era for psychiatry opened in the 1950's. Unexpectedly, new scientific, clinical and social—even economic—developments occurred in rapid succession, with important repercussions not only for psychiatry but also for medicine and society in general. In some respects, the situation was comparable to the introduction of antibiotics into the medical world during the preceding decade.

THE STATE-OF-THE-ART OF PSYCHIATRY IN 1950

What was the state of the art of psychiatry at the brink of the new era? Clinicians had psychotherapy to treat the neuroses and other minor functional disorders, at considerable cost in time and money and with often unspectacular results. Our only treatments for major affective disorders and psychoses were unspecific, e.g. electroconvulsive therapy, or shortlived in their effects, e.g. hypoglycemic shock treatment; the latter quite hazardous as well as expensive.

Manic patients and disturbed psychotics had to be deeply sedated or subjected to physical restraints, forced feedings and isolation in seclusion rooms. The fever treatment of general paresis, psychiatry's first major therapeutic success, of which it had been so proud 40 years earlier, had become obsolete when penicillin became available and all but eradicated the disease. Ineffective, and sometimes destructive, lobotomies were inflicted on large numbers of patients.

We had no more than two *theories* to explain mental disorders at midcentury: Freud's psychoanalysis and learning theory, based on Pavlov's classical and Skinner's operant conditioning.

The typical schizophrenic patient of that period could look forward to many years of hospitalization and steady deterioration. Clinicians felt frustrated and powerless, and few competent people were attracted to psychiatry. We had virtually no scientific approach in our attempt to understand the biological substrate of psychopathology, much less treat it. Mental hospitals had become warehouses of apparent incurables, where few psychiatrists could bear to spend more than a few months. The idea of treating an acute psychotic or depressed or manic patient outside a hosptial was unheard of.

When a remitted schizophrenic patient left the hospital and asked us: "Will I stay well?," we told him: "Don't worry." But we knew that 7 out of 10 would be back within a year, suffering a relapse with uncertain response following another course of shock treatments.

ANTIPSYCHOTIC DRUG EFFECTS HARD TO BELIEVE

Then came chlorpromazine and reserpine, the first antipsychotic drugs, in the 1950's. Suddenly, some acute schizophrenic patients became symptom-free within days, and many could be sent home within weeks. It took even those of us who were among the early workers with these drugs more than a year until we really believed that some *pills* could achieve this, that it was not a fluke (Swazey, 1974).

A few years later, antidepressant drugs were introduced and permitted a welcome alternative to ECT. The tricyclics and the MAO inhibitors dealt effectively with depressions, and lithium completed the armamentarium for the affective disorders as a specific remedy for manic episodes. Today it is difficult to grasp that until then we had had, besides ECT, only tincture opii, barbiturates and paraldehyde to fight depression and mania (Lehmann and Klien, 1983).

MAINTENANCE AND SELF-TREATMENT: NEW THERAPEUTIC MODALITIES

It was not known at first, but became clear soon, that the new psychotropic drugs were not only suppressing acute symptoms of psychiatric disorders but could also achieve a kind of prevention, a protection against relapses, by maintaining patients in remission as long as they would comply with the prescribed maintenance pharmacotherapy. Previously, shock treatments had to be administered in hospitals, and their effects were often shortlived. Now, for the first time, psychiatric patients could treat themselves at home and prevent schizophrenic relapses. Others could stop the disruptive cycles of their recurrent affective disorders, and, more recently, it has become possible to prevent the terror of spontaneous panic attacks with self-administered drug treatment. All at once, we were catapulted into the class of physicians able to control serious disorders reliably, like the internist controls diabetes with insulin.

Ironically, in the next few years there was an increase in the diagnosis of manic-depressive disorders, probably in part due to the fact that psychiatrists had been provided with an effective treatment for them.

As a fall-out, the therapeutic breakthroughs solved an old nosological controversy in psychiatry: whether psychotic disorders were on a continuum with neuroses, differing only in severity, or whether there were qualitative differences between the two disorders. The specific action of the new antipsychotic drugs demonstrated clearly that the difference between psychoses and neuroses was, indeed, a qualitative one (Lehmann, 1969).

After the "heroic" era of the forties when empirical, aggressive treatments prevailed, psychiatrists had now come into the golden era of success and optimism. Politicians were dazzled by the prospect of emptying mental hospitals and poured research (NIMH) funds into our coffers—full to overflowing. Now that we had, more or less serendipitously, uncovered the remedies, neuroscientific researchers rushed in to discover why and how the remedies worked. The floodgates were opened to scientific investigation of all aspects of mental illness, using the psychotropic drugs as probes and tools for the study of the disturbed brain's metabolism. The discovery of the causes of schizophrenia, and its cure, seemed to be finally within reach.

We tried not to notice the antipsychiatrists who about this time were coming up with antiscientific ideas about the causes of mental illness and descried the "dehumanization" of psychiatry (Laing, 1968; Szasz, 1970).

Extensive multihospital trials of new drugs gave testimony of innovative, sophisticated methodologies for the design of protocols, the selection of patients and the evaluation of clinical results. New regulations and controls by government agencies monitored the ethical and safety aspects of all new drug trials. The "informed consent" concept acquired wideranging importance.

Psychiatric inpatients poured out of hospitals; the census of public mental hospitals was reduced by 400,000 between 1955 and 1980 (Brill and Patton, 1962). Community mental health centers, outpatient clinics and day hospitals, whose case loads had increased explosively, were expected to take care of them. Moreover, psychiatrists could now treat psychotic patients out of their offices, and primary care physicians learned how to manage mentally ill patients in chronic care, thus multiplying the psychiatric manpower. Even dedicated psychoanalysts recognized the effectiveness of the new drugs (Group for the Advancement of Psychiatry, 1975).

IATROGENIC COMPLICATIONS

Then, in the 1970's, the general euphoria subsided. The new drugs had undesirable side-effects, and now late complications appeared. Tardive dyskinesia, an iatrogenic disorder, never known before, headed the list. Patients who were inadvertently made dependent on benzodiazepines by physicians prescribing them too freely, became other iatrogenic casualties. "Revolving door" patients, most of them noncompliant with prescribed treatment, commuted between hospital and community, sometimes several times a month, and created administrative nightmares of admission and discharge paperwork.

NEW SOCIAL PHENOMENA—NEW PROBLEMS

At the same time, new social phenomena and problems emerged as the result of the psychopharmacological revolution. "Deinstitutionalization" of psychiatric patients—aided and abetted by overly optimistic psychiatrists, zealous civil rights activists and eager politicians—in the first years led to hasty "dumping" of the patients into communities with no provision for them. Many in today's army of the homeless street people are former mental patients, and many are victims of the imprudent policy of poorly prepared, premature deinstitutionalization (Bachrach, 1976).

Another new social problem was the appearance of the "young chronic" patients. There have always been many young, chronic, psychiatric patients, but they were not so visible on our streets. They were quiet and docile when they were cared for in hosptials, but today are streetwise, disturbed, and often still symptomatic, because they do not like to be hospitalized and do not comply with the treatment prescribed for them in the community (Bachrach, 1982).

The public spotlight on mind-altering drugs, including those that produced model psychoses, e.g. LSD—did not go unnoticed by the young people who adopted them, from coast to coast, for their own, non-medical experimentation. The problem of the multi-drug street addicts is still with us, as an evil offshoot of psychopharmacology, and shows few signs of abating (Final report, commission of inquiry, 1973).

THE PUBLIC BACKLASH

All this negative, medical and social fallout now created a backlash in the public media which launched an unrestrained anti-drug campaign that was not only aimed at non-medical drug abuse but also at the legitimate prescription of tranquilizers, mainly benzodiazepines, and then, growing more and more irresponsible and using biased, sensational reporting, began to focus on pharmacotherapy with psychiatric patients in general. Psychopharmacological drugs had grown into a multi-million dollar business and pharmaceutical companies were attacked for their aggressive advertising. Psychiatry's public image being smeared, politicians now became disenchanted and, in the 1970's, cut back severely on research funds. Civil liberties do-gooders, enthusiastic but uninformed, called for controversial court decisions that initiated a creeping loss of psychiatry's autonomy. In the wake of more and more judicial interference, psychiatrists were no longer free to use their best clinical judgement about the indications for hospital admissions and discharges, as well as indications, and even choices, of treatment. A trend toward practicing defensive psychiatry developed that was far from being always to the patient's benefit (Brooks, 1979).

Neuroscientists, on the other hand, remained untouched by these political troubles and forged ahead with their search for biological answers, leaving clinicians who had given them their initial impetus, to grapple with the real-life problems of shortcomings of their clinical tools and the backlash.

PSYCHOPHARMACOLOGY'S LIABILITIES TODAY

Where do we stand today? First, what are the present shortcomings of clinical psychopharmacology?

For years we have been faced with the dilemma of how to manage the schizophrenic patient over time: If, like in the old days of shock therapies, we leave him to his own resources after having successfully treated his acute symptoms, we know, from well established evidence, that he is at 70-80% risk of suffering a relapse within a year. We can reduce that risk to 15 or 20% with maintenance drug therapy, but then incur a 15-20% risk of tardive dyskinesia developing after several years of treatment, with the disorder being irreversible in about a third of the cases. There is at present no effective way of preventing relapses other than maintenance drug therapy, and also no known way of reliably preventing or treating tardive dyskinesia. That leaves the clinician, the patient and his family with a difficult decision to make.

The dramatic success of the antipsychotic drugs in suppressing the florid, positive symptoms of schizophrenia, e.g. hallucinations, delusions, thought disorder and grossly inappropriate behavior, obscured for the first few years the limitations of these drugs in dealing with the chronic negative symptoms, e.g. loss of initiative, emotional blunting and social withdrawal. Pharmacotherapy is relatively ineffective for these residual symptoms which have become the hallmark of today's chronic schizophrenic patients who are pouring from the hospitals into the communities, with few resources to help them. A medical problem has been transformed into a social problem.

For the treatment of depression we have a large array of old and new drugs, but all require from two to three weeks before they become effective, and only about two-thirds of the patients respond to pharmacotherapy. In comparison, electroconvulsive therapy acts faster and in a larger proportion of patients, although it is less convenient to use and often has less acceptable side effects than antidepressant drug treatment. Even when using all our resources, there remain always about

15% of our depressed patients who are treatment resistant and become chronic and frustrating challenges to private physicians and outpatient clinics in the community.

Anxiolytic drugs, too, have their drawbacks. Although effective, relatively safe and causing few immediate side effects, they will produce physical and psychological dependence if prescribed in large doses for more than a few months. They also cause tolerance and, precisely because the drugs are so effective in the short term and relatively free of side effects, patients are often inclined to escalate their doses without authorization (Marks, 1978).

NEW THEORIES—NEW ASSESS

Compensating for all these shortcomings are the many exciting developments in the basic sciences of psychopharmacology, the new discoveries and theories that have opened scientific doors onto vistas psychiatrists could not even dream about thirty years ago.

Within a few years of the discovery of the antidepressant drugs, neuroscientists gave us the first theory of biogenic amines, acting as neurotransmitters, that play a crucial role in the genesis of affective disorders. The theory was suggested by the fact that MAOI type antidepressants, as well as the tricyclics, both increased the availability of noradrenaline and serotonin in the brain. The first did it by blocking their degradation in the nerve cells, the second by blocking the reuptake of these monoamines from the synapse. This led to the hypothesis that a deficiency of one or both of the two monoamines was the biological substrate of a depressive syndrome.

This first, in retrospect somewhat simplistic, hypothesis later gave way to more sophisticated theories based on up and down regulations of noradrenergic and serotoninergic systems, and the scientific focus is now on the cell membrane and the post and presynaptic receptor systems.

It took almost ten years after the discovery of the antipsychotic drugs until the first, and still most unpopular, hypothesis of their mechanism of action was proposed, i.e. the blocking of postsynaptic dopamine receptors. This hypothesis has been extended to the theory which postulates that a hyperactive dopamine system is involved in the etiology of schizophrenia. Again, the theory was the result of deductive, one might say backward, reasoning from the fact that all empirically effective antipsychotic drugs and one pharmacological characteristic in common: they were all blocking dopamine receptors.

The discovery of the encephalins and endorphins in the 1970's opened exciting new avenues in the field of peptides as modulators of transmitter and receptor dynamics. Endorphins even allow us now to explain scientifically some of the strange placebo affects that had always been a theoretical mystery and that our nonpsychiatric colleagues used to scoff at.

OTHER RECENT GAINS

Because of the special contingencies in psychiatry there has always been a need for drugs of low toxicity to prevent accidental or suicidal deaths. With the discovery of the benzodiazepines this need has been filled, at least in the field of anxiolytics.

Psychiatrists have always wished for more objective parameters and criteria, similar to those that are available to physicians in other specialties and permit them a rational and quantitative approach to their treatment methods. Now we do have good insights into the complexities of pharmacokinetics. We can measure plasma levels of psychopharmacological agents down to the nanogram. In addition, a number of promising biological and pharmacological markers are under development for several psychiatric conditions, in particular the affective disorders.

Finally, the development of effective psychopharmacological treatments with powerful drugs created an imperative need for a more reliable diagnostic system, and DSM III, notwithstanding its shortcomings, has provided us, for the first time, with operationally defined psychiatric diagnoses.

The strange paradox is that, as psychiatrists have moved closer to medicine and have become more effective, they also have, perhaps to some dangerous degree, distanced themselves from psychology, the discipline that has traditionally been an integral component of their thinking and practice. The psychiatrist's "art" may thus be in some danger of being crowded out by the fascinating new, and strictly scientific, biological theories and treatments. Our challenge today is to maintain a wise balance between the physical-organic approach to psychiatric disorders and the preservation of our heritage of special insight into the dynamics of the human psyche.

REFERENCES

Bachrach, L.L.: Deinstitutionalization: An analytical review and sociological perspective, Mental Health Statistics Series D, No. 4; DHEW No. (ADM) 79-351, Washington, D.C.: U.S. Government Printing Office., 1976.

Bachrach, L.L.: Young adult chronic patients: An analytical review of the literature, *Hospital and Community Psychiatry* 33:189-197., 1982.

Brill, H. and Patton, R.: Clinical-statistical analysis of population changes in New York State mental hospitals since introduction of psychotropic drugs, *Amer. J. Psychiat.* 119:1., 1962.

Brooks, A.D.: The impact of law on psychiatric hospitalization: onslaught or imperative reform?. In: New Directions for Mental Health Services: Coping with the Legal Onslaught, No. 4 (S. Halleck ed.), Jossey-Bass, San Francisco., 1979.

Final Report of the Commission of Inquiry into the Non-Medical Use of Drugs: Information Canada, Ottawa., 1973.

Group for the Advancement of Psychiatry: Pharmacotherapy and Psychotherapy,

Paradoxes, Problems, and Progress, March, 9(93)., 1975.

Laing, R.: The politics of experience, Penguin, Baltimore, MD., 1968.

Lehmann, H.E.: Problems of Psychosis, International Coloquium on Psychosis, Excerpta Medica International Congress Series No. 194, (November), p. 65-78., 1969.

Lehmann, H.E. and Kline, N.S.: Clinical discoveries with antidepressant drugs. In: Discoveries in Pharmacology, Volume I (M.J. Parnham and J. Bruinvels, eds.), Elsevier Science Publishers B.V., New York., 1983.

Marks, J.: The Benzodiazepines: use, overuse, misuse, abuse. MTP Press Limited, Lancaster, England., 1978.

Swazey, J.P.: Chlorpromazine in Psychiatry—A Study of Therapeutic Innovation. The MIT Press, Cambridge, Massachusetts., 1974.

Szasz, T.: The Manufacture of madness. Dell, New York., 1970.

Index